TRAINING FOR MOUNTAIN BIKING

TRAIN LIKE A PRO

Series Editor: Will Peveler

Rowman & Littlefield's Train Like a Pro series provides nonprofessional athletes, coaches, and trainers with training guides based on scientifically backed information that is both easy to follow and readily implemented. Each book covers the equipment, basic training physiology, specific training techniques, and tips for building a training plan for a specific sport, as well as competition, nutrition, and special considerations. These books are especially beneficial for athletes who have to train while working full-time jobs, as they provide recommendations for how training can be built around a busy schedule.

TRAINING FOR MOUNTAIN BIKING

A Practical Guide for the Busy Athlete

Will Peveler

ROWMAN & LITTLEFIELD
Lanham • Boulder • New York • London

Published by Rowman & Littlefield
An imprint of The Rowman & Littlefield Publishing Group, Inc.
4501 Forbes Boulevard, Suite 200, Lanham, Maryland 20706
www.rowman.com

6 Tinworth Street, London, SE11 5AL, United Kingdom

British Library Cataloguing in Publication Information Available

Library of Congress Cataloging-in-Publication Data

Name: Peveler, Will, author.
Title: Training for mountain biking : a practical guide for the busy athlete / Will
    Peveler.
Description: Lanham, Maryland : Rowman & Littlefield, 2021. | Series: Train like
    a pro | Includes index. | Summary: "A training guide for the nonprofessional
    mountain biker, this book provides elite-level information that is easy to follow and
    readily implemented into a busy life schedule. It covers topics such as equipment
    selection, bike mechanics, developing a training plan that fits your specific needs,
    proper nutrition, and more"—Provided by publisher.
Identifiers: LCCN 2020052941 (print) | LCCN 2020052942 (ebook) | ISBN
    9781538139561 (cloth) | ISBN 9781538139578 (ebook)
Subjects: LCSH: Mountain biking—Training.
Classification: LCC GV1056 .P48 2021 (print) | LCC GV1056 (ebook) | DDC
    796.63071—dc23
LC record available at https://lccn.loc.gov/2020052941
LC ebook record available at https://lccn.loc.gov/2020052942

CONTENTS

ACKNOWLEDGMENTS

I would like to thank my wife, Renee, and our four sons, Grayson, Garrett, Will, and LJ, for supporting me throughout the process of writing this book as well as the other books in the series. My wife was coerced into being in some of the photos as well as taking some of the photos for the book. My son Grayson was also hijacked to take some of the photos as well. Without the support of my family, I would not be able to do much of what I do.

Last but not least, I would like to thank my editors, Christen Karniski and Erinn Slanina, for working with me during this process, putting up with all my questions, and making me sound somewhat intelligent.

INTRODUCTION

The goal of the Train Like a Pro series is to provide elite-level training information that is easily understandable and implemented. Each book in the series will provide you with the following information on the sport: required equipment, a basic understanding of how the body responds and adapts to training, basic training principles, how to develop a training plan, exercise techniques, and basic sport nutrition for performance. Most professional athletes are paid to both train and compete, and therefore their life is built around those work requirements. This series is written for nonprofessional athletes. The majority of individuals reading these books have jobs, families, and other responsibilities that prevent them from working their life around training and competition. Instead, they must find a way to work their training and competition into life. It is important to find a balance that allows you to work, have quality family time, and improve your performance.

The goal of *Training for Mountain Bike Racing* is to provide you with all the basic information to allow you to be successful in the sport of mountain biking. I wrote this book with beginners in mind. It provides information on equipment, training, nutrition, riding for fun, and competition—in short, all the basic information I wish I would have had prior to starting my journey into mountain biking. Whether you are interested in racing or riding for fun, you will gain a lot of useful knowledge from this book.

WHY BECOME INVOLVED IN MOUNTAIN BIKING?

Challenge and Competition

Many people become involved in mountain biking because of the physical and mental challenges the sport provides. It allows you to push your perceived limits to discover what you are made of and what you can accomplish. For many, just completing a mountain bike race is reward enough. For others the drive is competing against fellow athletes to determine who is faster.

One of the unique aspects of mountain biking is that it is an individual sport. This allows people of varying ages and fitness levels to become involved. You can train and race at your own pace and on your own schedule (although it is always fun to train and race with friends!).

Being Outdoors

Mountain biking is appealing to many since it involves exercising outside and enjoying nature. One of the most important aspects about choosing a sport is to find something that you truly enjoy as it will make workouts less grueling and more appealing. While I like road cycling, I truly enjoy riding through the woods on a single track where I get to appreciate the scenery without worrying about being run down by a car.

Health

Improved health is a great motivator for mountain bikers, many of whom become involved in the sport during their pursuit of a healthier lifestyle. Individuals who are physically active are four times less likely to develop cardiovascular disease than those who do not participate in regular physical exercise. This fact is so strongly supported by available research that the American College of Sports Medicine recently implemented the Exercise is Medicine initiative, which is officially supported by the U.S. surgeon general.

Mountain biking provides a challenging but attainable goal for those who wish to get in shape for health or personal reasons. To maximize the health benefits of exercise, 30 minutes of physical activity per day is recommended for most days of the week. During training you will exceed those minimum recommendations and be well on your way to the development of a lifelong healthy lifestyle.

While cardiovascular activity has a strong positive impact on your health, you must first ensure that you are healthy enough to begin an exercise program with no restrictions. Exercise takes your body out of homeostasis (the maintenance of balance within the human body: body temperature, blood glucose levels, etc.) and therefore increases the risk of a cardiovascular incident in those with undiagnosed or unknown heart conditions. You should seek a physician's clearance prior to beginning an exercise program in order to confirm that you are healthy enough to begin. This is especially true for sedentary individuals, older individuals, those who have not had a recent physical, and those with signs of or risk factors for the development of cardiovascular disease.

Racing

Many individuals become involved in mountain biking for the competitive aspect. They enjoy pushing their body, mind, and resolve to the limits. While you will be racing against other individuals, the real race is with yourself. Are you better than you were before? Racing provides an opportunity to push yourself harder than you would in training, and many people thrive on that feeling. There are four main categories for racing mountain bikes: category 3 (beginners), category 2, category 1, and professional. Everyone will start at category 3 and then move up by request after accomplishing a top 5 finish in the current category.

HOW TO GET INVOLVED

While a large number of people would like to compete in mountain biking, many do not get involved simply because the sport can be intimidating and they do not know where to begin. Mountain bikers, as a group, are very accepting and supportive of beginners, and most seasoned racers go out of their way to help those just getting started. Finding a local group of mountain bikers to train with is much easier than you might think.

Local Cycling Clubs

One of the first places to find knowledge and support is your local cycling club. While some areas may have a dedicated mountain bike club, many areas have a cycling club that caters to both road cyclists and mountain bikers. Most clubs get together weekly for training sessions. Local club members can provide some level of coaching, as well as knowledge on local races and shops, and where to bike locally. Most important, they provide a social support group for your involvement in the sport. If you have more than one local club, find the one that best fits your needs. For example, one group may focus more on optimizing performance and racing while another will focus more on enjoying the sport first and look at optimizing performance second. You can usually find information on cycling clubs at your local bike shop or on social media. If your area does not currently have a cycling club, consider starting one yourself.

USA Cycling

USA Cycling is the governing body of cycling in the United States. Mountain biking is one of the many cycling sports that fall under the jurisdiction of USA Cycling. The organization is primarily concerned with sanctioning races, development and enforcement of rules and regulations, development of individual athletes, World Championship and Olympic teams, and overall support for the growth and development of the sport of cycling. Most all mountain bike races are sanctioned by USA Cycling and require a license to participate. Getting involved with USA Cycling is a great way to familiarize yourself with the sport.

Collegiate Mountain Biking

For college students, one of the best ways to get involved with mountain biking is through a collegiate team. Most every collegiate cycling team falls under club sports and does not fall under NCAA jurisdiction, which means that you can earn money and prizes during races, seek direct sponsorship, and work as many hours as you like. As most cycling teams are club sports and have very few, if any, available scholarships, mountain bikers of all levels can join. The downside is that there is very little monetary support from the university and very few programs have scholarships. If your school does not currently have a collegiate cycling team, consider starting one through the university recreation department and USA Cycling. The process is fairly easy and does not require a large amount of work or money.

GEAR FOR MOUNTAIN BIKING

It is very important to have the proper cycling gear for mountain biking. Choosing gear for mountain biking can be a daunting and expensive experience, but with the right information it does not have to be. This book covers the necessary equipment for mountain biking. Some of the equipment mentioned is required, while other pieces of equipment are suggestions for improved performance or comfort. Advice on how and where to purchase equipment will also be covered in this book. Proper maintenance of your cycling gear is extremely important in order to prevent expensive repairs or early replacement of equipment down the road. Keep in mind that the more maintenance you can do for yourself, the less you have to pay to have done. This book will provide information on how to perform basic maintenance that will improve performance and prolong the life of your equipment.

TRAINING AND NUTRITION

To successfully participate in mountain biking, it is vital that you develop and maintain a sound training and nutrition plan. Unfortunately, if you wish to compete, training is not as simple as riding your bike daily. You must develop a plan that incorporates different intensities and distances along with appropriate recovery time in order to optimize performance while preventing overtraining. Most individuals reading this book will have jobs, families, and other responsibilities, and these factors must be taken into account when developing a training program. This book will help you develop a basic training plan that allows you to improve performance without overtraining.

While most cyclists spend a lot of time developing their training plan, they commonly ignore their nutrition plan. To optimize training you must consider type, volume, and timing of nutrition. Your nutritional plan is just as important as your training plan.

1

EQUIPMENT FOR MOUNTAIN BIKING

Due to the equipment required to mountain bike, purchasing gear without proper knowledge or guidance can be very confusing, and it is easy to make a mistake. This chapter will cover the necessary equipment for riding and racing mountain bikes. The beginning of this chapter will provide you with information on the purchase of your first mountain bike and bike fit. The remainder of the chapter will cover related equipment and bike maintenance.

BIKE SHOP

One of the most important decisions to make when looking for a bike is where to buy your bike. Purchasing a bike is a big investment, and you want to work with a shop that will spend the time and effort to make sure you get the correct bike for your needs and budget. While pricing is important, there is much more to a shop than finding the least expensive bike. Most importantly, a good shop is the one that you find yourself in regularly just to hang out and talk with friends. The shop is where you can learn a lot of information on racing, training, equipment, and maintenance. If you have a good relationship with the employees at your local shop, they will bend over backward to help you when you need it. So it is not just about price; it's about the knowledge and atmosphere.

When pricing bikes, it is important to keep in mind that the profit margin on a bike is very small and shops do not have a large amount of room or freedom to drop prices. Many manufacturers will limit how low the bike shop can drop the prices through the dealership agreement. However, I have seen shops that increase the offered price and then drop it down to suggested retail. The one exception to this rule is when the shops purchase deals on close-out models at the end of the year, typically in the fall, which is one of the best times to look for a new bike. As a matter of fact, bike shops make the majority of their money through maintenance and the sale of accessories.

A good shop will spend time to ensure that you are getting the bike and accessories you need. The staff should ask about your short-term and long-term goals, riding experience, and budget. These questions will allow you and the expert to work together to come up with the best bike that fits your current needs and budget. Regardless of whether you are purchasing an entry-level or high-end bike, the staff should spend time to help you find the bike you need and ensure that it fits properly. While rare, I have seen staff brush off customers when they found out they were interested in buying an entry-level bike as opposed to a high-end bike. Luckily this is not the norm; most all staff are very enthusiastic when it comes to helping newcomers to the sport, regardless of their budget. If the staff does not seem eager to help you, then it is time to visit another shop.

CHOOSING A MOUNTAIN BIKE

The bike itself (see fig. 1.1) is going to be the single most expensive piece of required equipment you will purchase, and therefore budget is going to be a major factor for most individuals. An entry-level mountain bike will cost between $300 and $600; a good beginning race bike will cost between $700 and $1,100. There are significant differences in performance between an entry-level bike and a race-level bike. There is an inverse relationship between cost and weight; as cost increases, weight decreases. Highly skilled labor and better materials are required to make a bike lighter while still maintaining structural integrity, which in turn increases manufacturing costs. In addition, as price increases performance, reliability and durability also increase. It is important to note that it does not require an expensive bike to mountain bike. It just requires a bike. Keep in mind that when you are losing a race by minutes, spending extra money for a lighter bike to shave seconds off your time is not overly cost effective. Work on the engine first, and then worry about the bike.

Due to the cost of new bikes, many people purchase a used bike for their first bike, and this approach is a perfectly good one. Buying used allows the individual to get more bike for their money. Bikes are similar to cars in that the

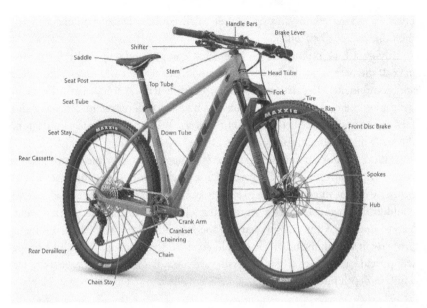

Figure 1.1. **Mountain bike anatomy.** *Fuji.*

value drops immediately after purchase. You can typically find a used entry-level race bike that is a few years old for the same price as an entry-level mountain bike. As long as the bike has been well maintained, then it will be a good first purchase. I advise having a bike mechanic look over the bike prior to purchase to ensure that the bike is in working order. Mountain bikes take a lot of punishment and I have had more than one used bike come into the shop where the cost of repairs was more than the bike was worth. Do not be afraid to work with your local shop when purchasing a used bike. Most shops understand why you are looking for a used bike and will help you in the process. Shop staff know that you will be coming in to buy accessories and for maintenance of your used bike and will want to treat you right. For more information, you can look up the original specifications and price of the used bike on the manufacturer's website in their archives. If the price is not listed, you can search online for the original price.

There are specific benefits to buying new as opposed to used. Typically, the warranty on a used bike does not transfer to the new owner. Frame warranties range from five years to lifetime depending on the company. Components, forks, and wheel sets typically have only a one-year warranty from defects starting on the day of purchase. There are also other perks to consider when purchasing new. Some shops offer free or discounted basic maintenance with the purchase of a new bike.

Buying a bike online can be somewhat complicated, especially for beginners. If the bike is used, you cannot be confident in the condition of the frame and components. Regardless of new or used, it will be somewhat difficult to determine the correct size to purchase. There are differences in geometry and measurement methods between manufacturers. When buying from a local shop, the staff will take the time to properly fit you to the bike.

While it is understandable that budget is going to be one of the main deciding factors when purchasing a bike, proper fit is paramount. A bike that does not fit properly will be uncomfortable to ride, may be difficult to handle properly, and could lead to overuse injuries. Purchasing a bike that does not fit properly may lead to greater cost in the long run. If the bike shop does not take the time to properly fit you on the bike, you should go to a different shop. Some bike shops will provide a standard fit for free with purchase of a bike, but charge extra for a full, in-depth micro fit.

Frames

While there are different categories of mountain bikes, this book focuses on training for cross-country riding and racing. There are two main categories of mountain bikes that I will cover. The first is a hardtail mountain bike, which has a front suspension fork but no rear suspension. The second is a full-suspension bike that has both front and rear suspension.

Hardtail

Hardtail mountain bikes, as implied by the name, do not have rear suspension systems. This category of bike consists of a traditional bike frame with a suspension fork for dampening vibrations when riding rough terrain. With less technical requirements, in relation to a full-suspension bike, these bikes are less expensive and require less maintenance. Hardtail bikes are also going to be lighter at any level in relation to full-suspension bikes. A hardtail bike allows you to gain a better feel of the terrain as you ride over it, resulting in a more technically proficient ride. Hardtail bikes excel on fast, nontechnical trails.

Full Suspension

A full-suspension bike (see fig. 1.2) has a rear triangle that is separate from the main frame triangle and is attached through pivot points and suspension. This allows the rear triangle to move separate from the main frame triangle, resulting in a smoother ride. A full-suspension bike provides a much more comfortable ride in relation to a hardtail as more of the bumps and vibrations of the terrain are absorbed by the suspension system. As full-suspension bikes have greater mechanical requirements, they are typically more expensive in relation to similar-level hardtail bikes and have greater maintenance requirements. There is a justifiable debate on loss of power from the pedal to the drive train due to the movement of the rear triangle on a full-suspension bike. However, with advancements in suspension systems, this is less of a concern in relation to older model full-suspension bikes. Full-suspension bikes are great for those who ride very bumpy technical trails, older riders, or anyone looking for a more comfortable ride.

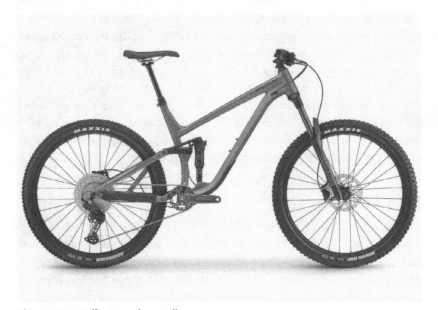

Figure 1.2. Full suspension. *Fuji.*

Frame Material

Another concern when purchasing a mountain bike is frame material. The most common materials used for mountain bike frame production are carbon fiber, aluminum, and titanium. However, as the vast majority of mountain bikes are constructed from either carbon fiber or aluminum, the following discussion will focus on these two materials only.

The most popular frame material used today is carbon fiber. Carbon fiber can be manipulated to produce an extremely light frame that is stiff yet comfortable. The carbon fibers can be arranged in a manner that limits horizontal movement while allowing small vertical displacement to occur. The carbon fiber arrangement allows the frame to be stiff during a sprint and provides vibration dampening so that trail vibrations are lessened, making for a more comfortable ride. These properties produce a frame that has little flex when power is applied to the pedals and is very comfortable to ride. Carbon fiber also allows manufacturers to produce tube shapes that could not be achieved with any other frame material. Carbon fiber also has a longer fatigue life in relation to any other frame material. The downside to carbon fiber is the high cost of manufacturing the frames, which in turn increases the cost of purchase. Also keep in mind that you will crash when mountain biking, which could damage the bike frame.

Of the two discussed materials, aluminum is the most affordable. Aluminum bikes are a great choice for those on a budget. If worked correctly, aluminum is light and provides a fast and stiff ride. The stiffness of the aluminum frame, though, will easily transfer trail vibrations and can make for a bone-jarring ride. However, with the addition of front and rear suspension systems, an aluminum frame can provide a smooth ride. Do not overlook an aluminum-framed bike just because it is not carbon fiber. A well-made aluminum frame can outperform a cheaply made carbon frame and may be a better choice.

Wheels

For a long time, mountain bikes only came in one wheel size: 26 inches. Next came the 29-inch wheel that allowed for greater rollover and more efficient riding. However, the 26-inch wheel accelerated much faster. This led to the development of the 27.5-inch (650b) wheel that split the differences between the 26-inch wheel and the 29-inch wheel, allowing for quick acceleration, good rollover, and efficiency. Another factor that would affect the choice of wheel size is height. Smaller riders may prefer a 27.5-inch wheel over a 29-inch wheel. At the time of this writing, both 27.5- and 29-inch wheels were equally common.

Component Groups

Another consideration when purchasing a bike is the component group. The component group consists of the shifters, the front and rear derailleurs, the crankset, the rear cassette, and sometimes the brake set. As component groups increase in quality, they decrease in weight and increase in durability and function. Unfortunately, the cost of component groups also increases with quality. While there are other companies that make component groups, the two primary companies are Shimano and SRAM.

Within each companies' lineup, they have different levels of component groups, which start with entry level and end with professional level. As the level names can change with new lineups each year, I encourage you to visit the websites of each company to get a rundown on the current component lineup. This will give you an idea of what you are dealing with when you purchase a bike.

When choosing your component group, you must consider the front crankset and rear cassette. One of the main considerations is gear development, which is the distance the wheel travels in one pedal stroke. A unique aspect of cycling is that it combines man and machine in order to produce movement. Because the bike is a simple machine, you can use math to determine gear development and ultimately speed. The formulas for determining gear development and speed are:

Gear development (GD) = (# of chainring teeth ÷ # of cog teeth) × diameter of wheel in inches × 3.14 mph = GD (in feet) × rpm × 0.0114

Sample Problem

Chainring teeth = 36
Cog teeth = 19
Wheel size = 29 inch
Revolutions per minute (rpm) = 90
GD = (36÷19) × 29 × 3.14
GD = 172.53 inches
172.53 ÷ 12 = 14.38 feet
mph = 14.38 feet × 90 rpm × .0114
mph = 14.75 mph

This formula will allow you to calculate cycling speed in mph with any given ratio at a specific cadence. However, this may be harder to translate into mountain biking as the ability to climb within your comfort zone and to accelerate on flat and downhill sections are more of a concern. It's important to choose a crankset with the appropriate chainrings and a rear cassette with a suitable range of cogs that allows you to both climb and descend within your current limits.

When choosing a crankset, first determine if you want a triple, double, or single front chainring. I will discuss the two ends of the spectrum first; a triple and a single chainring. A triple front chainring offers a much wider spread of gears in relation to a double or single chainring. While there is a lot of crossover (repeated gear ratios) with a triple chainring, the GD range for gear ratios outweighs a double or single. A triple is heavier and requires greater shifting in relation to a double or single. The triple chainring is good for beginners, because it offers much easier gears for climbing. The downside is that it also requires more shifting and can lead to shifting issues if the drive train is not set up correctly or is of low quality. A single chainring reduces weight, virtually eliminates a dropped chain (due to deeper teeth), and eliminates front shifting. However, the gear development range is greatly decreased and requires a high level of physical fitness. A single is good for flat, fast courses and cyclists with a higher fitness level. A double chainring decreases the overall range in relation to a triple but requires less shifting, and there is less crossover. A double is a good halfway point between the triple and single. I suggest test-riding a triple, double, and single prior to buying. Make sure that there is at least one descent hill on your route in order to get a good feel of the range of gears available. Keep in mind that the larger the chainring, the harder it will be to pedal and the faster you will go.

A rear cassette consists of a number of cogs, typically 7 to 12, that you will shift between to alter gear ratios. The larger the rear cog, the easier it will be to pedal and the slower you will go. The more cogs you have on a cassette, the wider the gear range you will have, providing greater options when riding. Entry-level bikes will typically come with a 7-speed cassette, and as the level of bike increases, so too does the number of cogs. A 12-speed cassette is currently the largest you can get and will be found on most high-end bikes.

FIT

Once you have purchased a bike, it will need to be fit to your specific anthropometrics, or body measurements. Proper bike fit is vital for injury prevention, performance, and comfort. Overuse injuries are not uncommon in mountain bikers. If you ride for one hour at 80 rpm, you would pedal 4,960 revolutions during that time period. If you are in an improper cycling position that applies undue torque on the joints of the lower extremities (primarily the knee), it can lead to the development of an overuse injury. In this section I will discuss basic bike fit for mountain biking. However, there are a couple points to keep in mind. The first is that it is extremely difficult to fit yourself on a bike; you will need assistance in your fit. The second is that a bike fit is similar to computer programming in the concept of "junk in, junk out," meaning that an improper fitting session will result in an improper fit. For this reason, it is important to know how to fit or seek out an expert in the area of bike fit. However, if you follow the guidelines provided in this section, you will be able to produce a good basic fit.

Most good shops will provide a bike fit at no charge when you purchase your bike. Some shops will do a basic fit at no cost in order to make sure that the bike is the correct size, but will charge for a more detailed fit. However, there should never be a charge for a basic fit. If the shop will not take the time or make the effort to fit you on your bike, then consider visiting another shop.

Through this process, the fit expert may need to swap out parts, typically the stem or seat post, in order to optimize fit. Most shops will keep extra stems and seat posts on hand for the bikes they carry in stock so that alterations can be made during the fitting process. If they do not have the correct size available at the shop, they can order it from the manufacturer. They should change the parts out at no cost to you, unless you request an upgrade. If you choose to upgrade parts during this process, then you should expect to pay. There are two common ways it typically plays out when you choose to upgrade parts. The first is that you pay full price for the part and keep the old part as a spare. The second is that you pay the difference in cost between the two parts and the shop will keep the part removed from your bike. These are both common and accepted practices.

Performance vs. Comfort

In an attempt to improve performance, mountain bikers can adjust their bike fit to assume an aggressive ride position. However, it is important to consider comfort as well. An ideal position will be one that optimizes performance, decreases the risk of injury, and is comfortable to ride. Bike fit for a mountain bike varies from a road bike to allow you to maneuver over rough terrain.

Frame Size

One of the most important aspects of bike fit is to ensure that you purchase the correct frame size. The anthropometrics of the mountain biker cannot be altered to fit the bike, so the bike must be altered to fit the cyclist. However, the bike can only be altered within a limited rage, which is predetermined by frame size and geometry. If the frame is too small or too large, you will be unable to achieve a proper fit.

There are various generic formulas that estimate frame size for each individual. Most of these formulas will get you in the ballpark but are not overly accurate. The best way to determine correct frame size is to have the bike properly fit to you. The exception to this rule would be if you ordered a bike from a manufacturer who takes very detailed measurements for their specific formula in order to customize a frame specifically for you. However, even if you order a customized frame, it's still necessary to go through a detailed bike fit.

Crank Arm Length

Crank arm length is measured in millimeters and is engraved on the back of most crank arms. If the crank arm is not marked, simply measure from the center of the bottom bracket to the center of the pedal axle to determine length. Crank arms come in 165, 170, 175, and 180mm lengths. The crank arm length is dependent on bike frame size: smaller frame sizes come with shorter crank arm lengths, and larger sizes come with longer crank arm lengths. Though most bikes will come with 170 or 175mm crank arm lengths, extra-small bikes will come with 165mm and extra-large bikes may come with 180mm lengths.

Because crank arm lengths on stock bikes are proportional to frame size, there is typically no need to alter the crank arm length for the majority of individuals. Consult with a professional bike fitter prior to altering crank arm length.

Cleat Position

When using clipless pedal systems, it is important to properly position the cleat in order to prevent injury and optimize performance. The first step is to determine the fore and aft alignment of the cleat. For the vast majority of cyclists, the cleats should be positioned so that the metatarsophalangel joint (MTP), commonly referred to as the ball of the foot, is centered over the pedal axle when the clip is engaged with the shoe (see fig. 1.3). Individuals with larger than average feet may want to consider moving the cleat back slightly, placing the MTP joint

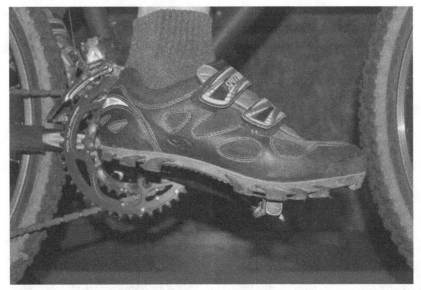

Figure 1.3. Cleat position over pedal. *Grayson Peveler.*

just in front of the pedal axle. This will relieve stress on the Achilles tendon and the ligaments on the bottom of the foot.

The next step is to adjust the medial and lateral alignment of the cleat. For most individuals the cleat should be centered on the shoe. Clipless pedal systems have enough float (amount of rotation allowed by the pedal without the cleat disengaging from the pedal) that there is typically no need to alter medial and lateral alignment away from the centered position for most individuals. However, in extreme cases of internal or external rotation, alteration to cleat alignment should be considered.

Saddle Adjustment

Now that the foot is properly positioned on the pedal, it is time to adjust the saddle. Adjustment of the saddle should focus on saddle tilt, saddle height, and saddle fore and aft positions. Keep in mind that you will frequently move positions while mountain biking. Therefore, there is more leeway when it comes to fitting a mountain bike as opposed to a road bike. The first step in this process is to adjust saddle tilt. It is recommended to keep the saddle tilt level on a mountain bike. If the saddle is tilted too far down, the cyclist will continually slide down to the nose of the saddle and then push back along the seat. This back and forth motion across the seat can lead to chaffing and saddle sores. If the saddle is tilted too far up, then the nose of the saddle can apply unnecessary pressure to the groin area. You can use a bubble level in order to determine if the saddle is level.

After determining that the saddle position is correct, set the saddle height. While there are various methods suggested for determining saddle height in lay literature, use of a 25–35-degree knee angle has been supported in scientific literature. I typically recommend a 25–30-degree knee angle (or more correctly, knee flexion) for road bikes and a 30–35-degree knee angle for mountain bikes. If using a 30–35-degree knee angle on a mountain bike, it will slightly lower the saddle height, in relation to a 25–30-degree angle, allowing for more freedom of movement across rough terrain. Depending on where and how you ride, you may need to lower the saddle to achieve more than a 35-degree knee angle. While a 30–35-degree knee angle may provide the most economical height for pedaling, it is not optimal in all situations for mountain biking. The more technical the terrain, the more you will need to lower your saddle for optimal control of the bike, more vertical movement for your bottom, and a lower center of gravity. All these factors affect your ability to traverse obstacles. Those interested in riding trials or traversing difficult obstacles and large drops will want a very low saddle. This lower saddle setup does make it more difficult to pedal efficiently while seated and can result in overuse injuries. You will have to find that happy medium between optimal cross-country performance and the ability to effectively traverse obstacles. A 30–35-degree knee angle is a good place to start and then lower as needed.

To measure knee angle, you need a goniometer (device used to measure joint angles in degrees). A goniometer can be purchased from a medical supply store for approximately $15. Begin by placing the bike in a stationary trainer. Mount the bike and pedal until you are comfortable on the saddle. Once you are comfortable, stop pedaling with the crank arm perpendicular to the floor in the six o'clock position. Ensure that the pedal is parallel to the ground. Center the goniometer over the lateral femoral condyle (located at the knee) with the stationary end of the goniometer pointing down and centered on the lateral malleolus (ankle bone). Rotate the other end of the goniometer until it is pointing up and centered on the greater trochanter of the femur (at the hip joint). See fig. 1.4.

It is important to correctly locate these bony landmarks in order to properly measure joint angle. After measuring joint angle with the goniometer, adjust the seat height up or down until the appropriate knee angle is obtained. Take two to three measurements to ensure the accurate seat position.

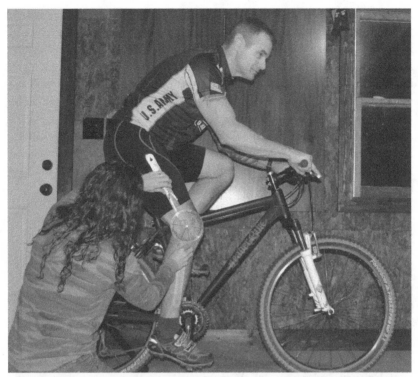

Figure 1.4.   Knee angle. *Grayson Peveler.*

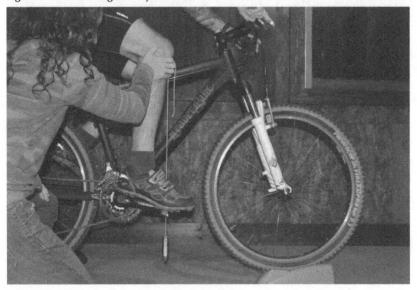

Figure 1.5.   Knee over pedal. *Grayson Peveler.*

After saddle height has been determined, the saddle should next be adjusted fore and aft. For this step you will need a plumb line, which can be purchased from your local hardware store for about $2. Pedal until you feel comfortable, and then stop with the crank arms parallel to the ground, with the right leg in the three o'clock position. From the right leg, drop the plumb line from the tibial tuberosity. The typical recommendation is that the plumb line should be centered over the pedal axle, as shown in fig. 1.5.

Keep in mind that moving the seat forward will effectively lower the saddle, and moving the seat back effectively raises the saddle. If the saddle was adjusted significantly during this step, go back and measure saddle height and adjust accordingly.

Handlebars

Do not adjust your handlebars until your lower body is dialed in correctly. Adjusting the handlebar is much more subjective in relation to setting up the bike for the lower body. When adjusting the handlebar, look at reach (stem length) and drop (handlebar height). While lower handlebars (the drop) result in a more aggressive riding position, they put a lot of weight on your hands. Find the height that allows for optimal handling while not causing your hands to go numb from the excessive front-leaning weight. The reach is affected by top tube length and stem length. You cannot change the length of the top tube, but you can alter the length of the stem. Stem lengths typically range from 30 to 120mm. Choose a stem length that comfortably fits your reach. You do not want to be too crunched up with a short stem or too stretched out with a long stem. The shorter the stem, the more responsive the bike will be to movements of the handlebars. A stem that is too long will make it harder to optimally distribute your weight on a downhill section. A shorter stem allows you to get behind your seat, resulting in less weight on the handlebars during downhill riding. Conversely, a long stem allows you to keep weight on the front wheel when climbing. This prevents the front tire from lifting off the ground on steep climbs. As you will be doing a lot of both climbing and descending on a trail, it's important to find a stem length that allows you to optimally handle both.

Record Your Fit

Once you have your bike appropriately adjusted to your body and riding style, record your fit. This will allow you to keep track of your bike measurements so that you will have them for future reference. This also allows you to make adjustments to your bike if the saddle slips down or you purchase a new bike.

To start with, it is good to keep a copy of the geometry chart for your specific bike. This enables you to compare the geometry of your current bike and a new bike. Next, record the key measurements of your bike fit:

Saddle height. Most commonly measured from the center of the pedal axle to the top of the saddle with the crank arm in the six o'clock position. However, it can also be measured from the center of the bottom bracket to the top of the saddle.

Saddle fore and aft. Distance measured by dropping a plumb line from the nose of the saddle and measuring the distance from the string to the center of the bottom bracket.

Cockpit length. Measured from the front of the saddle to the center of the handlebars.

Drop. Measure the drop in height from the top of the saddle to the top of the handlebars using a level and a tape measure.

OTHER GEAR

Helmet

One of the most important pieces of equipment you can purchase is your helmet. Though bike crashes are not a frequent occurrence (hopefully), it is inevitable that you will eventually experience one. I cannot emphasize enough the importance of always wearing a helmet. Helmets are required at all mountain bike races.

There are a few things to consider when purchasing a helmet. Since you will at some point crash while mountain biking, a good helmet is necessary. All helmets sold in the United States are required to meet minimum standards. Some companies work to exceed the required minimum standards.

A helmet should not only provide protection but also dissipate heat well. You want a helmet that provides optimal ventilation to reduce heat buildup when riding on hot days. Air vents in the helmet allow air to pass through the openings, dispersing heat through convection and evaporation.

When purchasing a helmet, it is important to choose one that fits your head securely. A helmet that moves around loosely will not provide adequate protection. The helmet should fit snugly and not move around on your head.

However, it should not be so tight that it is uncomfortable. If the helmet is not comfortable, you will be less likely to wear it when riding.

Shoes and Pedals

Clipless pedals are used to lock the cyclist's shoe in place while pedaling. A cleat, which is specific to the model of cycling pedal, is attached to the bottom of a rigid cycling shoe using screws. This cleat will lock into place when force is applied downward into the pedal. The system locks the shoe to the pedal, preventing the cyclist from pulling the foot straight up and out during the pedal cycle. To disengage from the pedal, cyclists merely twist their heels away from the bike.

The shoe and pedal combination provides an interlocking platform that will increase overall performance. Economy increases due to the ability of the leg to unweight during the upstroke of the pedal cycle and improved overall pedal kinematics. The increased interaction of the cycling shoe and pedal provides a more stable platform for power production and transfer to the pedal. Lastly the solid connection to the bike increases bike-handling skills.

When you purchase your new bike, do not be surprised if it does not come with clipless pedals as most new bikes do not. The reason for this is that there is such a large selection in pedals, and pedal style is somewhat of a personal choice. There are a few things to consider when purchasing pedals.

The style of pedal will determine engagement, disengagement, float, and weight. While some will argue that engagement and disengagement with the shoe is better with one style as opposed to another, ease of engagement and disengagement is more a function of practice. You will become accustomed to the style you choose, and it will become second nature after a while. As previously mentioned, to engage (clip into) the pedal, place the front of the cleat into the front of the pedal and push your heal down. To disengage (unclip), twist your heel away from the bike. Prior to riding in clipless pedals for the first time, practice clipping in and out of the pedals by placing your bike in a trainer.

Float refers to the distance traveled prior to the cleat disengaging from the pedal, measured in degrees. This allows your foot to naturally rotate during the pedal cycle. Too much or too little float can lead to the development of overuse injuries. Float varies by brand and model. Choose a model that provides the right amount of float based on your individual biomechanics. Most pedals allow for adjustment to float.

Cost is another consideration when purchasing pedals. The price of pedals ranges from $40 to $400 and varies by brand and model. You will need to purchase clipless pedals that best fit your budget, needs, and comfort.

Also look for a pedal system that sheds mud easily. It is inevitable that you will ride muddy trails during your time mountain biking. When the cleat on your shoe or the pedal becomes caked in mud, it can be difficult to lock back into the pedal. Some pedal systems retain mud more than others. Do some research and find a set of pedals that do not clog up under muddy conditions. The Crank Brothers Egg Beater pedals are good for muddy conditions.

The second part of the equation is the cycling shoe itself. Once you have determined the pedal and cleat system you would like to use, then you will need to choose a pair of cycling shoes that are specific to mountain biking. Mountain bike shoes will have a stiff sole for the transfer of power and possess deep treads for traction when you have to dismount. The shoe will close with either Velcro or ratchet straps. Avoid shoes that close with laces. Cycling shoes range from about $70 to over $400.

Clothing

When planning for mountain biking, invest in a good pair of cycling shorts. A pair of cycling shorts can make the difference between a nice enjoyable ride and a pain-filled torture test. The chamois in a cycling short will provide protection between your bottom and groin area and the saddle. It is designed to reduce contact stress and reduce friction. Keep in mind that thicker does not always mean better, and chamois that is too thick will feel uncomfortable. A good chamois is designed so that it is thicker in parts that contact the saddle and thinner in other areas so that it does not bunch up between your legs. Because you will be moving in and out of the saddle, moving behind the saddle for descending, etc., you do not want to wear baggy cycling shorts as they will get caught on the saddle.

A cycling jersey is also beneficial when riding trails. Jerseys will typically have three large pockets in the back used for carrying food and extra supplies. This is ideal especially for longer rides. In the unfortunate event of a crash, the material of the cycling jersey will offer some form of protection against rash. Lastly, cycling jerseys are breathable and provide greater cooling potential during a ride on a hot day, as compared to a cotton shirt.

Outerwear and Foul Weather Gear

You can mountain bike year-round and therefore have to take changes in weather into account. You cannot take a prolonged break from training just because it is cold and wet outside. So, unless you live in an area with optimal weather year-round, you will eventually need to invest in foul-weather gear that allows you to train outside in relative comfort. Some items to consider purchasing are: rain jacket, wind vest, cold weather jacket, winter cycling tights, arm and leg warmers, cap, gloves, and shoe covers. There is nothing worse than being miserably cold and wet on a ride.

Hydration Pack

It is important to stay hydrated when riding. Not only does a hydration pack hold a lot of water, but you will drink more frequently because the drinking tube is hanging by your chest and you can easily drink while riding. Water bottles require a lot more movement and effort and therefore you will drink less. Hydration packs are also great for carrying your repair kit, food, and any other gear you may need.

Cycle Computers

If you are going to train on a bike, it is vital that you use a cycle computer to assist in your training. Cycle computers range from $20 to over $500 depending on the functions of the system. The basic $20 systems provide current/average/ maximum speed, odometer, and trip distance, whereas the top-end systems provide the basic functions plus many of the following additional functions: power, heart rate, training zones, cadence, and GPS data, and can be later downloaded to a computer for evaluation. I recommend purchasing a cycle computer with the minimum of the basic functions plus cadence ($30–$40). If you are also going to purchase a heart rate monitor, then look at the overall cost of purchasing a cycle computer, a GPS, and a heart rate monitor separately, and compare that to the cost of purchasing one system that will do everything. Some companies produce a GPS and heart rate system to use while cycling, and then the cyclist can later download the data for training evaluation. If you are riding in areas where it is easy to become lost, a dedicated GPS system is ideal to help you find your way back to your vehicle.

Heart Rate Monitor

It is vitally important to monitor and control workout intensity during training, and heart rate is an excellent indicator for levels of intensity. While you can measure pulse rate with your fingers and a watch, it is not as accurate and convenient as using a heart rate monitor.

A heart rate monitor consists of a transmitter and a receiver. The transmitter fits around the thoracic region just below the pectoralis major. When placing the transmitter below the chest, it is important to center the transmitter midline. The transmitter should be tight enough not to move around, but not so tight as to be uncomfortable. The transmitter should be wet and placed against the skin in order to pick up the electrical impulse of the heart contractions. The receiver acquires the signal from the transmitter and displays heart rate. The receiver can be a dedicated watch, your cycle computer, or your cell phone.

A dedicated heart rate monitor system will possess various functions that are useful for maintaining intensity and evaluating performance. Heart rate monitors vary in price based on function (from $40 to over $300). An entry-level heart rate monitor that provides heart rate and time only will start at around $40. I recommend purchasing a heart rate monitor that at least has zone alarms. This will allow you to set alarms that sound when you go below (typically not a problem) or above (usually the problem) your training zone for the day. If you are going to train in a group, use a heart rate monitor that is coded so that you do not pick up another cyclist's heart rate as you train.

You can also purchase a heart rate monitor strap with Bluetooth capabilities and pair it with your smart phone in order to get GPS data as well as heart rate. For many people this will be the most affordable and viable option as most people already own a phone. There are very good applications that are free or minimum cost that you can download on your phone. These applications will not only provide heart rate but also distance traveled, speed, and grade. Once your workout is complete, you can then analyze the data. As a coach, I find this feature invaluable. I can examine an athlete's heart rate in relation to alterations in grade, speed, and distance. One downside to using your phone for training is during the winter months. The cold can drain your battery quickly, and I have had my phone shut down 2 miles into a run when I started with almost 100 percent battery life.

When choosing a heart rate monitoring tool, there are other options to consider as well, but these are the basics. A word of caution here: I have seen many athletes spend a lot of money on cycle computers and heart rate monitors, but then never really use them. At that point, the heart rate monitor or cycle computer just becomes an expensive toy as opposed to a powerful training tool. Before purchasing an expensive heart rate monitor, seriously consider how you will integrate the system into your training program.

Power Meters

Power meters are often used to measure training intensity in cycling. However, use of power meters when mountain biking is not as straightforward as during road cycling. Mountain bike terrain changes continually, and power output is mandated by the terrain more so than in relation to road cycling. There are four basic methods of measuring power: at the bottom bracket, at the crank set, at the rear hub, and at the pedals. Pedal power systems for mountain bikes were released in 2019. Each one of these systems has benefits and drawbacks. Using a pedal system to measure power output allows the users to more easily change measurement systems from one bike to the next.

While power meters are an excellent tool for determining training intensity, they are expensive, costing more than most people spend on their first bike (from $700 to over $3,000). Keep in mind that mountain biking is very tough on equipment. Power meters also require more understanding and effort to properly incorporate them into training. I have met more than one person who rides with power but never really uses it to optimize their training. Prior to purchasing a power meter, look into what is required to incorporate the tool into your training program and how to use the system. While it does take a little effort to properly use, it can pay off tremendously for those who want to be competitive.

BIKE MAINTENANCE

It is extremely important to keep your bike well maintained in order to increase its longevity, ensure optimal performance, and save money on repairs. Of all the equipment that you purchase, the bike is the most expensive and often the most neglected. Something as simple as cleaning the bike will add years to the components.

This section is not designed to offer in-depth bike maintenance. Instead, it is designed to cover cleaning and basic maintenance of the bike. If you come from a cycling background, much of what is covered you probably already know. For both beginners and those with experience, I recommend purchasing an in-depth bike maintenance book. Learning to conduct all your own repairs will allow you to save time and money.

Cleaning

Cleaning is one of the most overlooked bike maintenance procedures. Mountain biking will always leave your bike dirty, and muddy days are the worst. While it is not necessary to completely break down and wash your bike after every ride, it is important to at least wipe it down after every ride. When you ride, you sweat, and sweat is very corrosive to metal. Wiping the bike with a wet cloth will remove the sweat and protect your bike. Periodically, and after any muddy ride, the bike should be completely washed. The "periodically" recommendation will vary from individual to individual. Those that ride many hours per week will need to wash more often than those who ride fewer hours per week. Also, wet and muddy conditions will require more frequent washing.

To conduct a complete wash, you will need the following: bucket of soapy water, soft sponge, soft bristle brush, water hose, and chain-cleaning brush. Do not use a high-powered setting on the hose to wash your bike. This could lead to water being forced into areas that are greased to reduce friction. If water is forced into these areas, grease will be displaced, friction will increase, and parts will wear prematurely. Even with a gentle water flow, avoid spraying directly into the bottom bracket area, headset area, and wheel hubs.

The first step in the procedure is to clean the drive train as this will be the dirtiest area. Start by cleaning the chain. You can use an old toothbrush or a tool specifically designed for chain cleaning. While soapy water will work, consider using a degreaser for this portion of the cleaning. Next use a soft-bristled brush to clean the front chainrings and rear derailleur pulleys. Use a long-bristled brush to clean the rear cassette. After washing the rest of the bike, remember to dry the chain by running it through a dry cloth, and then lubricate it with an appropriate bicycle chain lube. Cleaning and lubing the chain will greatly prolong the life of your drive train. A dirty drive train prematurely wears down the rear cassette teeth, the front chainring teeth, and the chain itself.

Once the drive train has been cleaned, wash and rinse the rest of the bike. Upon completion, dry the bike thoroughly. While tedious, try to remove any water standing inside the bolt heads as they tend to rust over time.

Maintenance Procedures

Listed below are simple maintenance procedures designed to help you complete basic maintenance on your bike. For those interested in more detailed information, I recommend picking up a good bike maintenance book or finding good videos that step you through the process.

Removing and Replacing Wheels

When removing the front wheel, first identify what type of axle you have. Most all new mountain bikes will have a thru axle that will come with a quick-release lever or a hex head that will require a wrench. Thru axles will pass through the hub and screw into the opposite side of the fork. Both axles are removed from the bike in the same manner. For the hex head thru axle, use a hex wrench to loosen the axle until it slides free. With the quick-release system, pull the lever back and use the lever to unscrew the axle until it is free. Once the thru axle is removed, the wheel will drop out. If you have disc brakes, it is important that you do not engage the brake lever when the wheel is removed. It is advised to place a brake-pad spreader between the brake pads when the wheel is removed. This will prevent the brake pads from becoming stuck together if the brake is initiated without the wheel connected. In a pinch you can use a piece of cardboard folded over. To replace the wheel, just reverse this process.

On older bikes you will have what is called a skewer with a quick-release lever. On these, there are either V-brakes or disc brakes. To remove the front wheel, first open the V-brakes, if you have them, in order to allow the tire to slip between the brake pads. If you have disc brakes, there is nothing you need to do with the brakes. Next, push down on the skewer to release the tension on the wheel axle. On the opposite side of the skewer, loosen the tension-adjusting nut. You do not have to remove the nut. Only loosen the nut until there is enough space for the skewer to clear the tabs located on the fork. To replace the wheel, reverse this process.

To remove the rear wheel, begin by shifting the chain to the smallest cog on the rear cassette. This lines the rear derailleur up with the smallest cog and aids in removing the wheel by providing more slack to the chain. Some rear derailleurs will have locking mechanisms that will allow you to lock the rear derailleur out of the way as you remove the wheel. Rear derailleurs with a clutch will require that you disengage the clutch prior to removing the wheel. Once the derailleur is out of the way, remove the thru axle as described above with the front wheel. Manually move the derailleur down and back so that the wheel can be removed easily. As with the front wheel, do not engage the brakes with the wheel off. If the rear wheel is going to be off for travel or for a prolonged period of time, install a brake-pad spreader between the brake pads. Reverse this process to reinstall the back wheel.

For older bikes with skewer systems, open and loosen the skewer as described with the front wheel. Remove the chain from around the cassette and the wheel is free. If the bike has V-brakes, open the brakes as mentioned above prior to attempting to remove the wheel.

Brakes

Brakes are typically low maintenance and require only slight adjustments from time to time. All new mountain bikes come with disc brakes. Disk brakes consist of a disk brake caliper that contains two brake pads and a disk brake rotor that is attached to the wheel hub. The brakes function by pinching the rotor between the two disk pads when the brake lever is engaged. Disk brakes can either be cable or hydraulic activated.

One of the most common problems with disc brakes is when the rotor rubs against the pads while riding. When the disk brakes are out of alignment, there are two primary causes: the disc brake caliper is out of alignment or there is a bent rotor. There are other causes (loose hub, loose rotor bolts or lock ring, or brake pads not resetting correctly), but those are beyond the scope of this book. The first thing to do is to make sure that your wheel is correctly installed and tight. Once it is established that the wheel is on correctly, you can then begin to align the calipers. To align the calipers, loosen the caliper bolts so that the caliper can move. Next, pull the brake lever, which allows the caliper to move and center on the rotor. Hold the brake lever down and retighten the caliper bolts. Once the caliper bolts are tightened, test the brakes to determine if the problem has been resolved.

If the rotor is still rubbing, the next step is to check the rotor to ensure it is straight. Using a wheel-truing stand and a rotor-alignment gauge is the most accurate way to true a rotor. However, few people own those tools and will instead use the brake calipers. This is also the method to use when out on the trail. Look down through the caliper, spin the wheel, and see if the rotor is bent and touching to one side or another. If you are having trouble seeing the rotor, place a white sheet of paper on the opposite side. The contrasting color will make the rotor more visible during this process. If the rotor is bent, use a rotor-truing tool to straighten the rotor by bending it back to true. Make small adjustments each time. The rotor does not have to be perfectly straight as long as it is not touching the brake pads.

Derailleurs

One of the more common issues you will run across is misaligned derailleurs leading to poor shifting. There is nothing more annoying than being unable to smoothly shift from one gear to another, especially during a race. Most people are intimidated when it comes to derailleur adjustments. However, if you know the basics, adjustment is easy.

If you have a two- or three-chainring crankset, you will have a front derailleur. Once the front derailleur is properly set, it is rare that you will have any problems with it. The first step is to ensure that the height and angle of your derailleur is correct. To check height, move the derailleur out to the point where the outer portion of the derailleur is over the top of the outermost chainring. You should have about a 2mm gap between the derailleur and the chainring. To check rotation, look down from the top of the derailleur and ensure that it is parallel (in line) with the chainring.

Next, ensure that your low- and high-gear limit screws are correctly set. The low- and high-gear limit screws are not used to adjust shifting. Instead they are used to set the inner and outer limits of derailleur movement. If the low-gear limit screw is not set correctly, then you will drop the chain toward the frame when shifting to the small ring from the large. If the high-gear limit screw is not set correctly, then the chain can move past the large ring and off when shifting from the small to the large ring.

Start by placing the bike in a stand so that you can turn the crank arms and shift gears as you work. First shift the chain to the small chainring on the front and the largest cog on the rear cassette. Release the shift cable by loosening the cable-retention bolt so that there will be no tension on the front derailleur during this process. In this position there should be about a 1mm gap between the inner derailleur plate and the chain. If there is too much or too little a gap, adjust the low-gear limit screw. Locate the low-gear limit screw (typically marked with an "L") on the front derailleur. Using a screwdriver, loosen or tighten the low-gear limit screw until a gap of 1mm is obtained. Only use small turns of the screwdriver as it does not take much to move the derailleur. Attach the derailleur cable to the derailleur by sliding the cable behind the cable-retention bolt, pulling out the slack, and tightening the bolt.

Next, set the outer limit with the high-gear limit screw. Shift the chain to the largest gear on the front and the smallest gear in the back. Again, you should have about a 1mm gap between the outer derailleur plate and the chain. Locate the high-gear limit screw (typically labeled with an "H") and adjust until a 1mm gap is obtained. Now shift back and forth between the chainrings on the crankset. The chain should move quickly and smoothly.

Problems more frequently occur with the rear derailleur adjustment and shifting. The first thing to set with the rear derailleur is the limit screws. First shift the chain onto the large chainring in the front and the smallest cog on the rear cassette. Loosen the cable-retention bolt and remove the cable. The guide pulley of the rear derailleur should line up perfectly with the rear cog. The high-gear limit screw on the rear derailleur prevents the chain from being thrown off the smallest cog and into the frame. Adjust the high-gear limit screw until the guide pulley is correctly aligned. Pull the slack out of the rear derailleur cable, place it behind the retaining bolt, and tighten. Next, shift the chain to the small ring on the front and the large on the back. With your hand, push the derailleur toward the spokes of the wheel to ensure that it is up against the limit screw. The guide pulley should now line up perfectly with the largest cog. If it does not, adjust the low-gear limit screw until it does. The low-gear limit screw is used to prevent the chain and derailleur from going into the spokes.

After the limit screws are set, shift up and down the cogs on the rear cassette to ensure that the chain transfers smoothly from one cog to the next. If the chain does not shift smoothly, then adjust cable tension by turning the barrel adjuster located on the rear derailleur until the chain moves smoothly up and down the cogs. If you are still having problems shifting, check to make sure that the rear derailleur bolt, which holds the derailleur to the frame, is tight and that your derailleur hanger is not bent.

Chain

Over time, chains wear and need to be replaced. Depending on the quality of the chain, how well the chain is cared for, and riding conditions, a typical chain will need to be replaced every 1,000-2,000 miles. Regularly cleaning and lubing will increase the longevity of the chain and the rest of the drive train. Use a chain gauge to determine wear on your chain, and replace the chain once it has lengthened due to wear.

To remove a worn chain from your bike, remove a link pin using a chain tool. Center the chain tool over a link pin, and then tighten the handle until the pin is pushed out the other side of the link. Next, back off the chain tool, separate the link, and remove the old chain. If the chain has a removable master link, then just remove this link. When purchasing a new chain, ensure that you purchase the correct size chain. There is a difference in thickness between a 9-, 10-, 11-, and 12-speed chain.

The new chain will have to be sized for your specific bike. There are various methods for determining chain length; I will mention two. The first method is to line up the old and new chains side by side and count links. This will ensure that you are replacing the old chain with a correctly sized chain. Keep in mind that the old chain has elongated and you cannot just line them up side by side and cut the chain based on length alone. This is why you need to count links or line the chains up link by link.

The second method does not rely on the old chain to determine length. Run the chain over the big ring in the front and the small ring in the back and through both derailleurs. Pull the chain together, applying tension to the rear derailleur until the two pulleys are aligned in a vertical line underneath the small cog. Align the chain, and mark the chain in order to remove the excess links. If the new chain is connected with a pin and chain tool, make sure that you have a roller end and a plate end. If the new chain uses a master link, then ensure that you have two roller ends and a gap for the master link. Use the chain tool to break the chain where it was marked, and then connect the two ends of the chain. The new chain will have come with either a new pin or master link to connect the chain. If you are using a pin, place the pin into the pin hole and use the chain tool to push the pin all the way through. Once you feel the pin seat into position, carefully break off the excess pin sticking out. The pin is scored and designed to be broken off. If your chain has a master link, then connect the two roller ends using that link.

Tires and Tubes

One of the unfortunate facts about cycling is that tubes puncture and tires become worn and need to be replaced. Tires should be replaced when they become worn and lose traction, when any type of bulge or deformation appears, and when gashes occur. You should conduct a quick inspection of your tires prior to any ride. The tube should be replaced any time it does not properly hold air. Do not keep riding on a tube that has a slow leak, because at some point it will become a large leak. Keep in mind that it is normal for tubes to lose some pressure overnight, and this is why it is important to check tire pressure and pump up the tires prior to every ride. An improperly inflated tire can lead to a pinch flat.

The steps to replacing a tube or tire are virtually the same. The first step is to deflate the tire if it is not already. Next use tire levers to separate one side of the tire from the rim. Place the tire lever between the tire and wheel rim and pry the tire bead up and over the rim. Place the hook on the end of the tire lever around a spoke. Move around the rim about two inches and use another tire lever in the same manner. From this point, the tire should easily roll up and over the rim. If not, then use a third tire lever. Next remove the tube from the tire. If you are replacing the tube due to a flat, then discard it. If you are not replacing the tube, set it to the side. At this point you will have the tube out and the tire half on and half off the rim. If you are replacing a punctured tube, carefully run your fingers along the inside of the tire looking for any sharp protruding objects and removing any that you find. It would do you no good to replace the tube if the object that caused the puncture is still imbedded in the tire. If you are replacing the tire, remove the tire completely by pulling the remaining tire bead up and over the rim. Next, place one bead of the new tire over the rim. At this point you will have a tire that is half on and half off the wheel regardless of whether you replaced the tire or not.

The next step in this process is to place a small amount of air in the tube, giving it shape. Insert the valve stem through the hole located on the rim of the wheel and place the tube inside the tire. Once the tube has been fully placed inside the tire, begin pushing the tire bead back over the wheel rim. Start at the valve and work your way around the tire in both directions at the same time. Throughout this process you should ensure that the tube does not get caught between the tire bead and the rim. Once your hands meet on the opposite side, push the last section up and over the rim. At times pushing the last section of tire bead over the rim can be somewhat difficult. Resist the urge to use the tire levers to force the bead over the rim as this could damage the tube and you will have to start all over with a new tube. Instead, just keep working the bead up and over and it will eventually go. Once the tire is fully on the rim, go around the wheel and ensure that the tube is placed up inside the tire. If any of the tube is caught between the tire and the rim, it will rupture when you add air. The last step is to inflate to the desired PSI. The recommended PSI varies from tire to tire but is typically around 35 PSI. The maximal pressure will be stamped on the sidewall of the tire.

Using tubeless tires for mountain biking completely eliminates pinch flats, and punctures will seal quickly with the liquid tubeless sealant that is placed within the tire when it was positioned on the rim. Remove the tire using the same process as mentioned above. If you are replacing the tire with a new one, just dispose of the old one. If you plan to reinstall the old tire, make sure to wipe out all the old sealant. Next, wipe the old sealant off the rim and clean it.

To install a tubeless tire, make sure that the valve stem is tight before beginning. Check the tire for directional arrows, and then place one side of the tire onto the wheel. Next, push the second side of the tire onto the rim beginning at the valve and working your way around both sides, stopping so that there is about 8 inches of the tire bead still outside the rim. Measure out the recommended amount of tire sealant and pour it into the opening. Rotate the tire so that the liquid sealant stays at the bottom as you bring the open section to the top. Finish putting the tire onto the wheel. If the bead is too tight, you can use a tire lever or soapy water to help get the last bit of the tire seated on the rim.

Inflate the tire using a compressor or a floor pump. If you are having trouble inflating the tire with the floor pump, you may need to use a compressor instead. After the tire is inflated to max pressure, circle the liquid sealant around the tire to ensure that it covers the beads on both sides. This will help prevent leaks at the bead. Every few hours reinflate to max pressure as needed and circle the sealant around the tire again. Repeat this process until the tire holds air, and then inflate to the desired riding pressure.

Wheels

From time to time wheels will move out of true. This can be due to spokes loosening over many miles of riding or due to the direct impact that naturally occurs when mountain biking. When a wheel comes out of true it will wobble from side to side as it spins. Learning to true your wheels will save you time and money in the long run. While truing a wheel may seem intimidating, it is relatively easy, though it does require a truing stand and spoke wrench.

Remove the wheel from the bike and place it in a truing stand. Spin the wheel and slowly tighten the calipers of the truing stand until you hear the caliper scrape. At this point there should be sections of the wheel that move freely past the calipers and others that touch as it passes. It is also possible that one section of the wheel will make contact with the caliper on one side and another section of the wheel will make contact with the opposite caliper as it comes around. Stop the wheel at the point the caliper touches, loosen the spoke on the side of the wheel that touches, and then tighten the spoke opposite the side of the rim that touches. Only turn the spoke wrench ¼ to ½ turn each time. Spin the wheel to see if it clears. If it does not clear, repeat the first step. Once the rim clears, tighten the caliper again until it touches and repeat the process. In most all cases, it will not be possible to perfectly true a wheel and a 1–2mm gap between the rim and the caliper is normal.

Seat Post

While seat posts do not require a lot of maintenance, there are a few key points to remember. Over time the seat post will slide down. For this reason, it is important to either mark your seat post or take a measurement from the center of the bottom bracket to the top of the saddle. After adjusting the seat post, always remember to tighten the seat collar bolt to the manufacturer's suggested torque. This will ensure that you do not damage the seat post or frame while also minimizing the chances of the seat post slipping.

Always lubricate the seat post prior to placing it in the frame. For a metal seat post that will be inserted into a metal frame, use normal bike grease. The lubrication will help prevent the seat post from seizing and help keep water from entering the frame. If either the frame or the seat post is composed of carbon fiber, then a special carbon fiber grease is used. Never use normal bike grease on carbon. The specialized carbon fiber grease is designed to prevent the seat post from slipping as well as prevent water from entering the bike frame.

When adjusting the seat post, make sure that the minimum insertion limit mark is never showing. If it is showing, then purchase a longer seat post and replace the old one. Periodically check the seat post for cracks or damage.

Changing Pedals

From time to time you will need to remove your pedals. You will need either a pedal wrench, a thin wrench designed to fit between the crank arm and pedal, or a hex wrench depending on the model of pedal on your bike. The drive side pedal is threaded normally, but the non-drive side, left side, is reverse threaded. Always remember that turning the wrench toward the back of the bike will loosen the pedal and turning the wrench to the front of the bike will tighten the pedal regardless of the side you are on. While it might require some torque to break a pedal free, the pedals should go on and off smoothly.

Repairs on the Trail

It is inevitable that you will run into mechanical issues while on the trail, and it is unlikely that they will occur in the parking lot as you start or finish a ride. In most cases you will be far enough from the trail head that walking back in cycling shoes will be undesirable. There are three keys to ensuring that you ride back in and not walk: that you carry the proper tools, that you have knowledge on bike repairs, and that the malfunction is within the scope of your knowledge, tools, and ingenuity.

The first thing you need is an adequate repair kit to cover all the basic repairs you may encounter on the trail. While there are other options, most people choose to carry their repair kit in their hydration pack or in a saddle bag that attaches under the seat. The repair kit should contain the following:

- Spare tube and patch kit. The patch kit is for those occasions when you flat more than once.

- Small tire pump of CO_2 inflator. I prefer a mini-pump over a CO_2 inflator. While the pump takes longer and requires work, it is reliable and can be used more than once.
- One to three tire levers to assist in removing the tire to change a flat.
- Small multi-tool. Choose a lightweight multi-tool that contains a wide assortment of tools you will need on the road. An ideal multi-tool will have the hex wrenches you will need, chain tool, rotor truing tool, and spoke wrench.
- Master link for the chain.
- Zip ties for makeshift emergency repairs.
- Cash for emergencies.

You should also consider carrying your cell phone with you in case of an emergency. Keep your cell phone in a waterproof container to keep it dry. Keep the mind-set that the phone is for emergency purposes only and not to socialize. When riding, pay attention to your surroundings and avoid using the phone for social reasons.

When conducting a repair on the trail, it is important to move as far off the trail as possible. This may require you to move up or down the trail from where you stopped originally. This frees up the trail for other riders.

2

BASIC TRAINING PRINCIPLES, PHYSIOLOGY, AND PSYCHOLOGY

This chapter provides the necessary training background required for you to better determine how you will plan and implement your training program for mountain biking. In order to create and adhere to a quality training program, it is important to understand how your body will respond to the stress applied during training and competition. The body responds to stress in very predictable ways, which has allowed for the development of principles that can be predictably and directly applied to your training and competition. Gaining an understanding of these basic principles will help you to make better training choices.

BASIC TRAINING PRINCIPLES

Training Adaptations

Training adaptations are how the body responds to the applied training stimulus over time. These adaptations can either be positive or negative depending on the type, volume, and intensity of the training stimulus. The goal of proper training is to manipulate these three factors in order to elicit a physiological response that will lead to positive training adaptations and increased mountain bike performance. Incorrectly manipulating these factors can lead to improper physiological adaptations and, therefore, no alterations to performance. Additionally, improper training can lead to negative adaptations and subsequent decreases in performance.

Individual Differences

The principle of individual differences states that not every individual responds to the same training stimulus in the same manner. For example, some individuals recover quicker and can handle a higher training volume or intensity. Others may require longer recovery periods and therefore cannot handle higher volumes or frequent high-intensity bouts of training. You will need to individualize your training program so that you optimize training volume and recovery time.

While most individuals are born with approximately 50 percent slow twitch muscle fibers (good for endurance) and 50 percent fast twitch (good for anaerobic exercise), some individuals are born with a greater percent of slow twitch or fast twitch fibers. Therefore, some individuals will be predisposed to greater improvements in endurance or anaerobic activity. Mountain biking is an endurance event, and therefore an individual possessing a higher percentage of slow twitch fibers has the potential to improve to a higher level in relation to an individual who does not. Current training status is also an obvious factor. Those that have been training longer will be able to handle greater volume and intensity than beginners.

Athletes and coaches will often overlook individual differences and use a generic boxed training program that does not vary based on individual progression and can often hinder progress by delaying it. Conversely, if the training program is too strenuous, it can lead to overtraining and burnout. That said, it is okay to use a boxed training program to begin with, but adjustments to volume and intensity need to be made based on your response to that program.

Progressive Overload

The progressive overload principle states that the training stimulus needs to be continuously increased, allowing for adequate recovery between bouts, so that performance will improve. You can increase stimulus by either increasing volume or intensity. For mountain bike training, volume is increased by either increasing duration (distance or time) of training sessions or frequency (number of sessions). Intensity is altered by changing how hard the workout session is conducted. Volume should always be increased prior to increasing intensity. Make sure you can complete the distance before focusing on how fast you can complete it. Increasing intensity prior to increasing volume also increases the risk of injury.

Principle of Hard and Easy

The hard–easy principle states that you cannot train hard every day and instead must alternate hard and easy days to optimize training adaptations. While this principle does oversimplify the problem, it does work, especially in the development of a training program for the beginning mountain biker. When designing a workout program, it is important to alternate your hard and easy days so that you will have ample time for recovery. Too many hard days in a row will result in overtraining due to lack of recovery between bouts. Examining intensity is one way to determine your hard and easy days. Interval sessions are examples of hard days. Whereas rides below the anaerobic threshold would be considered easy days. Keep in mind that your long ride of the week is also considered a hard day, even though it is below threshold.

Recovery

Too often cyclists focus so much on training that they forget one of the most important components of increasing performance: recovery. Training is catabolic (molecules are broken down into smaller constituents) in nature, ultimately resulting in protein synthesis after the training bout. To optimize the body's response to the training stimuli, it is vital that adequate recovery occurs between bouts.

Alternate hard and easy days to optimize recovery. It is important to monitor intensity so that you do not ride too hard too often. This is a common mistake made by most beginning mountain bikers. During recovery it is also important to focus on recovery nutrition in order to refuel and optimize protein synthesis. Also important is to maintain a minimum of eight hours of good sleep every night.

Overtraining

One of the most common threats to mountain bike performance is overtraining. In most all cases, a cyclist will compete better 10 percent undertrained as opposed to 1 percent overtrained. To optimize performance, cyclists continually walk the line of optimal performance and overtraining. Overtraining occurs when adequate recovery is not allowed between bouts and is often the result of a sudden increase in volume and/or intensity, or an accumulation of a small imbalance of recovery and training.

As a mountain biker, be aware of how your body responds to training, and know the signs and symptoms of overtraining. Common signs for overtraining include:

- Multiple sessions of decreased performance. One bad day does not necessarily indicate overtraining. However, multiple days of decreased performance do indicate overtraining.
- Feeling of constant fatigue.
- Poor attitude.
- A feeling of dread about training.
- Abnormal sleeping patterns.
- An increase in resting heart rate measured on multiple days. An increase on one day may indicate that you have not recovered from the previous day's workout or that you may be dehydrated. However, if the increase in resting heart rate persists over multiple days, it is a strong indicator of overtraining.
- Consistent overuse injuries.
- Chronic illness due to a lowered immune response.
- Abrupt changes in body composition.

Specificity of Training

Training adaptations are specific to the training stimulus applied. In simpler terms, train the body in the manner in which you would like for it to adapt. For example, as a mountain biker it would not make sense for you to run and spend very little time on the bike. Mountain biking is an aerobic sport; therefore, the majority of training will be designed to enhance your aerobic capacity. At this level, specificity of training seems fairly obvious. However, specificity of training can also apply to the not so obvious.

Specificity of training can even apply to your cycling position. You should conduct your training on the bike that you plan to race on, and if you have two bikes, make sure that the setup is exactly the same for both.

Detraining

Detraining occurs when you decrease or remove the training stimulus, which leads to a decrease in performance and loss of training adaptations. Put quite simply, if you do not use it, you lose it. Common reasons for detraining include injury, illness, and improper off-season training. Typically detraining begins after two weeks of inactivity. This does not mean that you lose all adaptations after two weeks of no training. It just means that there is a measurable difference after that amount of time.

Detraining is one of the biggest fears of most mountain bikers, which often leads to overtraining. Many cyclists believe that taking a few days off from training will negatively impact performance. However, taking a couple days off on occasion will not hurt your performance and could, in fact, be beneficial if you are overtrained. However, do not use the fear of overtraining as an excuse to take multiple days off on a regular basis.

If you must scale down or completely stop training due to illness or injury, it will not take too long to get back to where you left off. When returning to mountain biking, do not try to start at the same volume and intensity where you left off. Instead, start back up slowly and work your way back to where you were before you stopped. Start by increasing volume first, and then increase intensity. Coming back too quickly can lead to injury and further delays in training. This is especially true if the time off from training occurred due to injury.

Consistency

Your training plan should be well laid out and consistent in terms of frequency of training. One of the common mistakes that beginners make is to train haphazardly; they might train four days a week for a couple weeks, then two days the following week, and then one day a week for the next couple weeks. In this scenario, increases in performance would be unlikely or minimal at best.

Inconsistent riding may also lead to injury. Trying to automatically pick up where you left off in training places too much stress on the body. For the best gains and to reduce the risk of injury, follow your training program. If life gets in the way, which it does, then alter your training program to minimize the impact.

Frequency

Frequency is defined as how often you train. This can be measured in days or the number of training sessions. Beginning mountain bikers should train a minimum of three days per week, with a day off between workouts. This method allows you to train harder on workout days and then recover prior to your next workout. Training only three days per week will be just enough to get you across the finish line; however, it will not get you to the finish line quickly.

To determine frequency of your workouts, first consider your current fitness level. As a beginner, you should start on the lower end and work your way up.

Also consider time management. Family, work, school, and other commitments have to be considered when developing a training schedule. Find a way to balance all aspects of your life so that you are ultimately happy. For me, family will always come first, then work, then training.

Duration

Duration is the length of your training session, which will be determined by the goal of that session. Most often, training duration will be determined by the desired intensity for that session. Duration and intensity are inversely related, meaning as one goes up, the other must go down. You cannot race a 20-mile trail at the same pace you would race a 10-mile trail. As the distance increases, the intensity will decrease.

You can determine the length of your training sessions by specifying a time limit or a specific distance. For mountain biking, I usually prefer distance over time because it allows for a more precise measure. If the goal for the day is a mid-distance ride at an easy pace, it makes more sense to state that you will ride for 6 miles at a heart rate that is equal to your easy training zone and then mark the time when you are finished. This will give you more precise measures as opposed to riding at an easy pace for 1 hour and 30 minutes. However, you must keep in mind that due to the varying nature of mountain bike trails, a relatively flat 6-mile trail will take much less time in relation to a 6-mile trail with a lot of climbing. With the exception of ultra-endurance events, you should be able to complete the distance of the race prior to race day to ensure that you have an enjoyable competition.

Intensity

Intensity is the "how hard" of training, and it is extremely important to properly manipulate in order for appropriate training adaptations to occur. The hard–easy principle, mentioned previously, is one method of manipulating training intensity. There will be weeks when you will have more than one hard day in a row, but they must be purposeful and planned carefully.

Intensity levels can be categorized into three basic stages: below anaerobic threshold, at anaerobic threshold, and above anaerobic threshold. When training or racing, you will be at one of these three physiological intensities. Intensities below threshold involve workouts that are below race pace—active recovery training, easy mid-distance training, and long slow distance. At threshold training consists of race pace and tempo work (short tempo work may actually be above threshold). Above threshold training is interval and overreaching training. Knowing and understanding intensity levels allows you to better plan a training regimen to ensure that you do not overtrain. How to properly determine intensity levels will be discussed in the following chapter.

Warm-Up

It is important to warm up prior to exercise in order to optimize performance and decrease the risk of injury. While a direct link between a warm-up and a decreased risk of injury has yet to be determined, there is a strong correlation between injury rates and lack of a warm-up. When examining sport performance, warming up facilitates three important aspects. First, the warm-up will redirect blood flow to working muscles. Second, there will be an increase in cardiac output due to an increase in both heart rate and stroke volume. And third, muscle temperature will increase, which improves muscular performance. It typically takes about two minutes to sufficiently increase cardiac output, increase muscle temperature, and redirect blood flow to the point that oxygen supply is equivalent to demand in the working muscles. All these factors will result in increased performance.

A warm-up for mountain biking should consist of about five minutes of easy riding, followed by about 5 to 10 minutes of stretching, and then finished off with another bout of riding. If it is a low-intensity training ride, then you can go right into the ride after the brief stretching. If it is a hard training day (tempo work or intervals) or a race, you will need to adjust the second warm-up ride accordingly. When warming up for a race, the second warm-up ride should consist of short intervals that take you to the race pace of the distance you are racing for that particular event.

Your warm-up should end about 5 to 10 minutes prior to the start of the race. You do not want to miss the start of the race. One method that many cyclists use is a stationary trainer. It is not as ecologically valid as warming up on the trails, but it is more practical as it allows you to warm up right by the start line.

Cool-Down

Conducting a cool-down after a workout is an important part of your training program. An active cool-down will slowly bring your heart rate down and prevent blood from pooling in your legs. If you suddenly stop after a hard bout of exercise and blood pools in your legs, it could result in dizziness. While dizziness under these conditions is not overly common, it is not uncommon.

As you pedal during active recovery, the muscle pump in the legs will assist with blood return to the heart and prevent blood from pooling in the legs. An active cool-down will also help clear blood lactate after high-intensity bouts. A cool-down will not prevent the development of delayed onset of muscle soreness, however.

A cool-down should consist of 5 to 15 minutes of easy pedaling followed by 10 to 15 minutes of stretching. The harder the workout, the longer the cool-down should be. Cool-down after a recovery ride should take much less time than cool-down after an interval session.

Delayed Onset of Muscle Soreness

If you work out, it is inevitable that you will experience delayed onset of muscle soreness (DOMS). This is the pain you feel the day after a workout. It will typically last one to three days, depending on the extent of the muscular damage. In severe cases, DOMS can last much longer. There is a common misconception that DOMS occurs due to a buildup of lactic acid. However, this is not the case. DOMS occurs due to tiny tears in muscle tissue during eccentric contractions (when muscle lengthens during the contraction). Edema then develops, and as the swelling continues, it begins to push on nerve endings, resulting in pain. As cycling has no eccentric load, DOMS will typically not occur from riding. Your legs may be fatigued the next day, but not sore from DOMS. There are a few exceptions to this general rule. The first exception is if you ride a fixed-gear bike. Slowing down or stopping with the pedals produces an eccentric load. Another exception is pushing your legs beyond their limits to the point of cramping. And the last main exception deals with trails that are extremely bumpy or have big jumps, as every time you absorb the impact with your legs, it is an eccentric load.

BASIC PHYSIOLOGY

Physiology Overview

In order to correctly apply training principles for optimal performance, it is important to have a basic understanding of physiology as it applies to sport. This understanding will help you to determine the type of training stimulus that will best lead to adaptations for increased performance in mountain biking. There are many "experts" that claim to have the best method for increased performance. Some of these methods work well, but many times these methods are unsubstantiated fads that will not lead to increased performance and in some cases lead to a decrease in performance. The more informed you are on the subject, the better you will be able to make an educated decision.

Knowledge of physiology as it is applied to sport performance will also help you determine if your body is correctly adapting to the applied training stimulus. If you understand the physiological adaptations that should occur, then you can better gauge the degree to which your training program elicits these changes.

The key to understanding physiology comes from two terms driven into my head through eight years of school (undergrad through Ph.D., not eight years of undergrad!): form and function. Every element of the body is formed for a specific function. Adaptations, occurring due to training, may even slightly alter form in order to improve function. Understanding the function of a system, organ, hormone, substrate, or enzyme will allow you to determine the effect of each on human performance. The first part of this section will cover basic physiology in order to provide a foundation that will help you to grasp the physiological adaptations that occur due to endurance training.

Cardiorespiratory Endurance

The cardiorespiratory system is comprised of the cardiovascular system and the respiratory system. The cardiovascular system is comprised of the heart and blood vessels and is responsible for the movement of blood through the body. Movement of blood through the body is vital as it is responsible for transporting oxygen, glucose, free fatty acids, hormones, and other key substrates to the working muscle. Equally important are the byproducts that blood carries away from the working tissue (carbon dioxide and lactate).

The respiratory system is comprised of air passages and lungs and is responsible for the transport and diffusion of gasses. Air moves through the air passageways, bringing in vital oxygen to the lungs where it is diffused across the respiratory membrane and into the lungs. Carbon dioxide crosses the respiratory membrane into the lungs and then is exhaled into the atmosphere.

The cardiorespiratory system is key during endurance performance and many times will limit performance based on the individual's current fitness level. There are adaptations that occur due to endurance training that greatly improve the body's ability to transport blood and oxygen. These adaptations will be discussed later in this chapter.

Heart

The heart is a specialized muscle (myocardium) designed to pump blood through the body. The heart differs from other muscles in that it is the most oxidative muscle in the body; it is designed to conduct the electrical impulse rapidly, and the signal for contraction originates in the muscle (sinoatrial node). The heart consists of four chambers (left and right atria and left and right ventricles). Pulmonary circulation (right atrium and ventricle) is designed to pump oxygen-poor blood returning from the body into the lungs. Systemic circulation (left atrium and ventricle) is designed to pump oxygen-rich blood to the body.

I will make a long, complicated story short. Oxygen-poor blood returns to the right side of the heart and then is pumped to the lungs where CO_2 is released from the blood and O_2 is picked up. The oxygen-rich blood then travels to the left side of the heart where it is pumped out to the body. The blood then travels through smaller and smaller arteries until it reaches arterioles and then capillaries at the tissue. This is where oxygen, nutrients, water, carbon dioxide, and other byproducts are transported to and from the tissue. As the capillaries leave the tissue, they connect to venules and then veins before returning to the heart.

The heart is not strong enough to pump blood down through the body and then back up toward the heart against gravity from the lower extremities. There are mechanisms in place that assist with blood return to the heart. The first is called the muscle pump. Muscles in the leg contract rhythmically, causing blood to be pushed upward during the contraction phase. When the muscles relax, one-way valves in the veins prevent the blood from flowing back down. The second method is the respiratory pump. Changes in thoracic pressure due to breathing aid in blood return to the heart.

Cardiac Output

Cardiac output is the volume of blood pumped per minute and is a product of stroke volume and heart rate ($Q = SV \times HR$). Stroke volume is the volume of blood pumped from the left ventricle in each beat, and heart rate is defined as the number of times the heart beats each minute. Cardiac output responds to exercise by increasing linearly with increases in intensity until max intensity is reached. Heart rate also increases linearly with an increase in intensity. Stroke volume can nearly double from resting but will only increase to about 50 percent of maximal intensity, and then it levels off. So after about 50 percent of max intensity, all increases in cardiac output will come primarily from heart rate only.

Autoregulation of Blood Flow

Autoregulation of blood flow concerns the redirection of blood flow based on tissue need. Blood flow is redirected by altering blood vessel diameter through vasoconstriction and vasodilatation. As we move from a resting state to an exercising state, metabolism substantially increases. Going for an easy ride can increase metabolism six to nine times above resting levels. Because the metabolic demand of the working muscles increases substantially during exercise, a greater amount of blood flow must be sent to the working muscle to increase the delivery of oxygen and nutrients. During exercise, blood flow is redirected to the working muscles, skin (for cooling), heart, and brain and reduced in areas where it is less needed, such as the digestive system and kidneys. During rest, approximately 20 percent of blood flow travels to the muscles. During exercise, as much as 80 percent of blood flow can be redirected to muscles.

Understanding this concept is vital for a complete understanding of the body's response to exercise. For example, autoregulation of blood flow explains the body's response to exercise after eating. You have probably eaten a meal and then exercised at some point in your life. Even if you are not completely miserable exercising right after a meal, the experience is never as comfortable as you would like it to be and your performance is subpar. The reason behind this is that your digestive system is in direct competition with the working muscles for blood flow. Due to fight or flight, the sympathetic response will win out over the parasympathetic response and greater blood flow will go to the muscles. However, a greater amount of blood will be redirected to the digestive system compared to exercising without prior food consumption. Because of the redirection of blood flow to the digestive system, your performance will decrease and your stomach may become upset.

When exercising in the heat, a greater amount of blood flow will be redirected to the skin for cooling than if you were training in a thermo-neutral environment. Dissipating heat is vital for survival and will take priority over blood flow to muscles. Due to this, performance decreases in a hot environment.

Blood

Blood is made up of around 55 percent plasma, 45 percent red blood cells (erythrocytes), and less than 1 percent white blood cells (leukocytes) and platelets. Hematocrit, the ratio of red blood cells in relation to whole blood, is used to measure the particular makeup of an individual's blood. The average hematocrit for a male is around 45, and for a female it is around 42.

Blood plays five major roles: transportation, heat transfer, acid base balance, coagulation, and immune response. While all five are important, we typically concentrate on the first three in exercise physiology as they have the greatest impact on performance. Each red blood cell contains a large volume of hemoglobin molecules, which are responsible for the transportation of oxygen. Hemoglobin is comprised of a globin protein and a heme ring. The heme ring contains four iron molecules, and each of these iron molecules can bind one oxygen. This is why those who suffer from iron deficiency feel fatigued and have difficulty exercising.

Blood is extremely important when it comes to heat dissipation. Water makes up about 90 percent of plasma, which is why plasma is an excellent mechanism for heat transfer. Heat is transferred from the core and the working muscles to the blood where it is dissipated at the skin's surface. Plasma is also important for cooling as it provides sweat for evaporation through the skin; this statement is oversimplified as plasma moving from the blood vessels to the interstitial space to the skin is a complicated process.

It is vital that the acid base balance (pH) is maintained in order for the body to correctly function. Keep in mind that pH levels differ depending on the location in the body. The average muscle pH is about 7.1 whereas the average blood pH is around 7.4. It does not take a large drop in pH before physiological systems are affected. A drop in muscle pH from 7.1 to 6.9 will begin to negatively impact energy systems, leading to a decrease in performance. Blood helps maintain pH through the use of chemical buffers.

Gas Exchange

Cyclists need to be concerned with gas exchange in the lungs and tissue (primarily muscle). Henry's law states that gas dissolves in liquids because of three factors: partial pressure of the individual gas, solubility of a specific gas in a specific fluid, and temperature. While all three affect how gases dissolve in liquid, partial pressure is the main driving force behind gas exchange in the body. The types of fluids and gases do not alter in the human body. However, temperatures do, and this change affects the oxyhemaglobin disassociation curve, but the main driving force is the partial pressure of each gas.

To understand the importance of partial pressure, it is important to know Dalton's law: the sum of each individual pressure of each individual gas is equivalent to the total pressure of the mixture of gases. At sea level the atmospheric pressure is equivalent to 760 mmHg, which gives you the total pressure of the mixture of gases (air). What becomes important for understanding gas exchange is the partial pressure of each individual gas in the mixture. Oxygen makes up 20.93 percent of the total mixture, resulting in a partial pressure of oxygen (PO_2) equal to 159 mmHg. Carbon dioxide makes up .03 percent of the total mixture, resulting in a partial pressure of carbon dioxide (PCO_2) of .2 mmHg. Lastly, nitrogen accounts for 79.04 percent of the total mixture, resulting in a partial pressure of nitrogen (PN_2) of 600.7 mmHg. One thing to keep in mind is that atmospheric pressure alters as you leave sea level. If you were to leave sea level and travel to the top of Mt. Evans in Colorado, the atmospheric pressure would decrease to around 460 mmHg. Because the atmospheric pressure decreases and there are no alterations to the percent of each individual gas, the partial pressure of each gas will decrease.

The alveoli are air sacs at the end of air tubes located in the lungs, which are responsible for oxygen and carbon dioxide exchange. Gas exchange occurs across the respiratory membrane, which lies between the alveoli and the capillaries. While the PO_2 in the atmosphere at sea level is equivalent to 159 mmHg, the PO_2 will decrease to around 105 mmHg in the alveoli. At rest, oxygen-poor blood will return to the lungs at a PO_2 of around 40 mmHg. The pressure differential of 60 mmHg will cause oxygen to move from the alveoli to the capillaries. Because alveolar PO_2 is maintained at 105 mmHg (it is not a closed system), oxygenated blood will leave the heart at a PO_2 of around 100 mmHg.

The alveoli PCO_2 remains at a constant 40 mmHg. The PCO_2 of blood returning to the heart will be approximately 46 mmHg. While the pressure differential is not as large compared to oxygen, carbon dioxide diffuses at a much greater rate across the respiratory membrane than oxygen. Therefore, the gradient does not have to be as large.

Muscle

Skeletal muscle originates and inserts on bone and crosses at least one joint. Therefore, the primary purpose of skeletal muscle is human movement. There are over 600 muscles in the human body, and it is important that you be able to name and identify all of them (just kidding). But it is important that you learn the primary muscles used in mountain biking in order to ensure proper strengthening and flexibility of those muscles.

Each skeletal muscle is composed of numerous muscle fibers. These muscle fibers are classified by characteristics and divided into slow twitch (type I) and fast twitch (type II with subcategories of IIa, IIx, and recently discovered IIb) muscle fibers. Slow twitch fibers are highly oxidative, fatigue resistant, and optimal for endurance performance. Type II, fast twitch, fibers are larger compared to intermediate and slow twitch fibers, and are more glycolytic, produce more force, and are good for events that require anaerobic energetics, strength, and power. These fibers contract and relax very quickly, but fatigue easily, which means they are great for initiating a sprint for the finish line.

Intermediate fibers are technically classified as a fast twitch fiber but fall between fast twitch and slow twitch. The reason IIa is classified as fast twitch is that it is slightly more glycolytic as opposed to oxidative. While you cannot alter fiber type through training, you can increase metabolic capabilities with intense training. If you were to train seriously for power, strength, or anaerobic performance, then intermediate fibers would shift toward greater glycolytic characteristics. If you were to train seriously for endurance performance, then oxidative processes would increase. Intermediate fibers will never be as oxidative as slow twitch fibers or as glycolytic as other fast twitch fibers; the properties will shift toward type of training. Intermediate fibers recruitment will increase as intensity increases.

Slow twitch fibers are of the utmost importance for cyclists as they are primarily oxidative muscle fibers. Slow twitch fibers do not activate as quickly as fast twitch and do not produce as much force. However, they are slow to fatigue and ideal for endurance activities.

Distribution of muscle fiber type is genetic, and most people are born with 50 percent slow twitch and 50 percent fast twitch (including intermediate). Some individuals are born with a greater amount of one type of fiber or another. Elite-level endurance athletes will typically possess up to around 80 percent slow twitch fibers. Whereas an elite-level Olympic lifter can have around 65 percent fast twitch fibers. The predominate theory is that muscle fiber types cannot change from one type to another through training. Muscle fiber distribution can be determined through a muscle biopsy, which is expensive and painful, and therefore typically not recommended.

Muscle fibers are arranged in functional groups called motor units. Each motor unit consists of only one type of muscle fiber and is innervated by a motor neuron. A slow twitch motor unit will have a small amount of muscle fibers, 10–180, and a fast twitch motor unit will contain anywhere from 300 to 800 muscle fibers. The number of motor units in a muscle is highly dependent on the size of the muscle. The numbers range from around 100 in a small muscle to over 1,500 in a larger muscle.

It is important to understand how motor units function as well as how they are recruited to contract. When the signal to contract travels down the motor neuron to the muscle fibers of the motor unit, all muscle fibers in that unit will contract. This is known as the all-or-none response. It is like a light switch; it is either on or off. However, not all the motor units in a muscle will contract during a task. We recruit only those motor units necessary to accomplish the task at hand.

Motor units are recruited in a specific pattern based on the size of the motor unit. Due to this, slow twitch motor units are recruited first, followed by intermediate fibers and then fast twitch fibers. Recruitment is designed for optimal economy. When cycling, you will recruit only the minimum amount of motor units to accomplish the task; primarily slow twitch fibers. The higher the intensity, the more intermediate and fast twitch fibers will be recruited. As these fibers are not very oxidative, you will fatigue sooner at higher intensities. Through training, neuromuscular recruitment patterns alter, allowing you to become more proficient at the skill. This adaptation improves economy and ultimately performance.

Energy Systems

Energy is required in order for human movement to occur. Competing in mountain biking requires repetitive muscle contractions and significant increases in metabolism. As you move from resting to exercise, metabolism increases exponentially. Going from resting metabolism to an easy ride increases energy requirements six to nine times those of resting requirements.

Humans derive energy from the ingestion of food. There are three primary sources for energy: lipids, carbohydrates, and proteins. The two main sources used for energy in the human body are lipids and carbohydrates. With the exception of extreme situations (starvation), protein will never provide a substantial source of energy. The main job of protein involves anabolic processes in the body. Carbohydrates are stored as glycogen in the muscles and liver and transported in the blood as glucose. Glycogen stores are limited to around 2,000 kCals. Lipids are stored as triacylglycerol (commonly referred to as triglycerides) in muscle and adipose tissue (under the skin and around organs). Storage of lipids varies greatly among individuals, with the average being 60,000–80,000 kCals. Naturally the volume of stored lipids can vary greatly as well. Excess protein is not stored in the body. Regardless of the source, all ingested food must be converted to adenosine triphosphate (ATP) in order for it to be utilized as fuel in the human body.

Energy systems are frequently categorized into aerobic and anaerobic systems. Aerobic systems are those systems that require oxygen for the metabolic processes to occur, and anaerobic systems are those that do not require oxygen for metabolic processes to occur. Under each of those broad categories are specific energy systems. There are four basic energy systems that provide ATP for human movement. It is important to understand each of these energy systems because it will affect training and your choice of nutrition.

Stored ATP

The first system is stored ATP in the muscles. While commonly classified as a system, stored ATP is more of a source than an actual system. Stores are limited, and therefore reliance on this system as a major energy source is also limited. Stored ATP will only provide energy for about two to three seconds before stores are depleted. Energy for the muscle contraction is provided when a phosphate is cleaved from ATP, leaving adenosine diphosphate (ADP) and a phosphate. This process does not require oxygen and provides energy quickly for immediate contraction. The remaining three energy systems are methods of producing ATP for energy. Once ATP is generated through these systems, a phosphate must be cleaved off to release the energy for muscle contraction.

ATP-PC$_r$ System

The second system is the ATP-PC$_r$ system. Phosphocreatine (PC$_r$) is stored in the muscle and is key in producing ATP. During this process, a phosphate is cleaved from PC$_r$ and donated to an ADP in order to form ATP. The ATP-PC$_r$ system is limited by PC$_r$ stores in the muscle and can only function as a major energy system for about 10 to 15 seconds. This system is anaerobic in nature and does not require oxygen to function. It takes about two minutes of recovery for PC$_r$ stores to replenish. This is a key consideration when planning rest intervals during resistance training.

Anaerobic Glycolysis

The next energy system is anaerobic glycolysis, which provides ATP through the catabolism of glucose and glycogen. This process does not require oxygen and can provide energy for up to 1.5 to 2 minutes. Anaerobic glycolysis produces two to three ATP per glucose or glycogen molecule. A decrease in pH is the limiting factor for energy production during anaerobic glycolysis. Muscle pH will decrease due to the hydrogen buildup that occurs during glycolysis. Glycolysis is a complex chemical process that stops at the creation of pyruvate. During anaerobic glycolysis two hydrogen bind with pyruvate to form lactic acid, which in turn will lose one hydrogen, becoming lactate. Lactic acid production is based on intensity level, which determines the speed of glycolysis and oxygen availability for metabolism.

Lactic acid is often considered as bad. However, this assumption is not correct as lactic acid is formed in order to decrease acidity. As mentioned previously, pyruvate picks up the excess hydrogen to decrease acidity. This binding is only temporary, and lactic acid releases the hydrogen ions and is converted into lactate (a salt molecule). Lactic acid itself is not the problem; instead it is the buildup of hydrogen. Hydrogen ions greatly increase acidity and will interfere with muscle contraction. The pain felt during high-intensity exercise, such as intervals, is the body's mechanism to signal you to slow down or come to a stop. Upon completion of exercise, lactic acid will be converted back into fuel through specific pathways and therefore should not be considered a waste product. Lastly, lactic acid is not responsible for delayed onset of muscle soreness.

Oxidative Phosphorylation

The first three systems provide energy quickly and without oxygen. As even the shortest mountain bike race will last longer than two minutes, the first three energy systems will not be used as the primary energy source through the race. Instead, oxidative phosphorylation will be used as the primary energy system for activity lasting longer than two minutes. Oxidative phosphorylation, as the name suggests, relies on oxygen for ATP production. There are two major pathways for energy production that fall under oxidative phosphorylation: the oxidation of carbohydrates and the oxidation of lipids. Duration and intensity will determine reliance on carbohydrates and lipids. Longer duration and lower intensity training will rely heavily on the oxidation of lipids, and higher intensity, shorter duration training will rely more heavily on the oxidation of carbohydrates. Typically, you will be using 80–100 percent carbohydrates at race pace during competition. During a recovery ride, you will be utilizing 60–80 percent lipids.

The first pathway under oxidative phosphorylation is the oxidation of carbohydrates, which produces ATP through the catabolism of glucose and glycogen. This process is often termed "aerobic glycolysis." The steps in aerobic glycolysis are the same as those used in anaerobic glycolysis. The main difference is that instead of pyruvate being converted to lactic acid, it is converted to acetyl-CoA, which moves on to the Krebs cycle (citric acid cycle) for ATP production. Aerobic glycolysis produces 36 to 39 ATP from one molecule of glucose or glycogen. The limiting factor for oxidation of carbohydrates is the amount of stored glycogen. As mentioned previously, the average stores of glycogen are equivalent to about 2,000 kCals. A runner will use approximately 100 kCals of glycogen per mile during a marathon. By mile 20 the runner would have utilized the 2,000 kCals of stored glycogen. Once glycogen stores are depleted, fatigue sets in.

The second pathway involves the oxidation of lipids. This process requires more oxygen, more chemical processes, and more time. However, ATP production is much greater with the oxidation of lipids. One triacylglycerol will produce approximately 460 ATP. With 60,000–80,000 kCals of lipids stored in the body, it would be impossible to completely deplete them during exercise. When fatigue occurs due to limitations of oxidative phosphorylation, it occurs due to depletion of glycogen stores.

VO_2 Max

Mountain biking is an endurance sport, and an individual's ability to perform is highly dependent on the athlete's ability to transport and utilize oxygen. There is a very strong correlation between an athlete's oxidative capacity and their performance during endurance events. Due to this, it has become common practice to test an endurance athlete's $VO_{2\,max}$ in order to determine current fitness level. $VO_{2\,max}$ is the body's maximal ability to deliver oxygen to the working muscles and the muscles' ability to use that oxygen to produce energy for movement. As $VO_{2\,max}$ increases with training, so too will endurance performance.

$VO_{2\,max}$ can be increased through proper training. The adaptations that occur due to endurance training are designed to increase oxygen transport and utilization. So as training increases, $VO_{2\,max}$ increases, and so too does performance. The extent to which $VO_{2\,max}$ can be increased through training is highly dependent on genetics; while everyone can increase $VO_{2\,max}$, improvements are limited by a predetermined genetic ceiling.

$VO_{2\,max}$ can be expressed in absolute (l/m) or relative (ml/kg/min) terms. Expressing $VO_{2\,max}$ through relative terms is the preferred method as it more accurately represents endurance performance relative to body mass: milliliters of oxygen consumed per kilogram of body mass each minute. As there is a strong linear relationship between $VO_{2\,max}$ measures and endurance performance, it is often used to predict performance. Certain measures are expected by gender and training status. $VO_{2\,max}$ increases with training, and there are gender differences in measures. The gender differences are due to the physiological differences between males and females. The expected ranges of $VO_{2\,max}$ for males are 45–50 ml/kg/min for sedentary, 55–65 ml/kg/min for trained, and ≥ 70 ml/kg/min for elite. The expected ranges of $VO_{2\,max}$ for females are 35–40 ml/kg/min for sedentary, 45–55 ml/kg/min for trained, and ≥ 60 ml/kg/min for elite.

$VO_{2\,max}$ is measured during a graded exercise protocol conducted in a laboratory setting. Testing is typically conducted on either a treadmill or cycle ergometer (stationary bike). As mountain biking involves cycling, you will receive more accurate numbers if you complete the protocol on a cycle ergometer. The graded exercise protocol starts easily, and intensity increases at regular time intervals until complete exhaustion. Most protocols consist of two- or three-minute stages. Intensity increases during the treadmill protocol by increasing both speed and grade. Intensity increases during the cycle protocol by increasing resistance on the cycle ergometer. During the graded exercise protocol, gas exchange of O_2 and CO_2 is measured using an automated metabolic cart. This requires the participant to wear an airtight mask that allows them to breathe in room air and breathe out into a gas-mixing chamber. From the gas-mixing chamber the air is analyzed for O_2 and CO_2.

Measurement of $VO_{2\,max}$ requires expensive specialized equipment and trained personnel to run the test and evaluate the data. Due to these facts, testing is expensive. Testing will typically run between $100 to $300 depending on the facilities, testing personnel, and other services offered. However, testing can sometimes be conducted at local performance centers and universities. The best option would be to contact the exercise physiology (kinesiology, physical education, and exercise science) department at your local university. Most researchers there are always looking for subjects and will offer low cost or free testing.

Before spending your money on $VO_{2\,max}$ testing, do your homework. I have seen a disturbing trend toward performance centers purchasing cheap metabolic carts that do not accurately measure VO_2. An accurate metabolic cart costs around $23,000, making the purchase and upkeep of the system somewhat prohibitive for many centers. Metabolic carts can be purchased for much less, but do nothing more than estimate VO_2. If the metabolic cart does not have an O_2 and CO_2 analyzer, do not waste your time, effort, or money. Prior to scheduling an appointment, ask what make and model metabolic cart will be used for testing, and do your homework. You can estimate $VO_{2\,max}$ using simple performance measures that are free and easy to accomplish. So it does not make sense to pay money to have an inaccurate machine estimate $VO_{2\,max}$.

ANAEROBIC AND LACTATE THRESHOLDS

Threshold terminology is used a lot in sports performance, but few actually understand or know how to correctly apply the concept. The two most common terms used are "anaerobic threshold" and "lactate threshold." Anaerobic threshold is defined as the point at which metabolic processes begin to switch from aerobic energetics to anaerobic energetics. Lactate threshold is defined as the point at which lactate production exceeds the body's ability to remove it. Human bodies are always producing lactate, even at rest, but it is removed from the system before it builds up. As intensity increases, lactate production increases, and there will come a point when production will exceed removal. As intensity increases, reliance on glycogen as a fuel source increases to the point that hydrogen is being produced at such a rate that it begins to build up, leading to a decrease in pH. To offset this decrease, two hydrogen will bind with pyruvate to form lactic acid. This is unstable and a hydrogen is released, forming lactate.

There are two common methods for measuring lactate threshold. The first involves plotting blood lactate as intensity increases in order to determine the inflection point. The second method is referred to as onset of blood lactate accumulation and is marked at 4 millimoles per liter of blood. Using 4 millimoles per liter of blood is somewhat arbitrary and not overly accurate, however. Therefore, it is typically not used to determine threshold. To obtain lactate threshold using either method, a graded exercise protocol would be conducted where resistance is systematically increased every three minutes until exhaustion. Blood would be taken at the end of every workload and analyzed for blood lactate.

A third and less common method for determining anaerobic threshold is termed "ventilatory threshold" (VT). This is the point at which ventilation increases exponentially and is easily calculated from data collected during a $VO_{2\,max}$ test. Ventilation increases as a direct response to the increased CO_2 production that occurs due to buffering excessive hydrogen. While I have a blood lactate analyzer in my lab, I generally prefer using VT because it is accurate, easy, and I do not have to draw blood.

Regardless of the method used to determine anaerobic threshold, it will be expressed as either a percentage of max or relative to heart rate. An untrained individual can have an anaerobic threshold of about 70 percent of max, whereas an elite cyclist will have a threshold of around 90 percent of max. In order to use anaerobic threshold to monitor training intensity, you will need to know heart rate at threshold.

Knowing your anaerobic threshold is just as important as knowing your $VO_{2\,max}$. It can even be argued that it is more important. The higher your anaerobic threshold, the faster your race pace will be. Not only do you want to focus your training on increasing your $VO_{2\,max}$ but also on increasing your anaerobic threshold. Changes in anaerobic threshold occur quicker and have a greater impact on performance in relation to changes in $VO_{2\,max}$. Do not get me wrong, increases in both are important and should be a focus of your training plan.

TRAINING ADAPTATIONS

Adaptations to Endurance Training

Almost every adaptation that occurs due to endurance training is designed to increase the delivery of oxygen to the working muscles and increase the oxidative processes that occur within them. The entire point of your training program is to elicit these adaptations in order to improve performance. The purpose of this section is to identify the primary adaptations and explain the importance of each.

With endurance training there will be an increase in overall blood volume. Red blood cells will increase in order to boost the oxygen-carrying capacity of the blood. Plasma volume will also increase but to a greater extent. Plasma increases due to two primary reasons. The first is in response to the increased red blood cell volume. Plasma is the fluid portion of the blood responsible for the smooth transfer of the more viscous red blood cells. So if there is an increase in red blood cells, there will be a corresponding increase in plasma. Plasma volume also increases in response to the heavy sweating and plasma loss that occurs during exercise. The increased plasma volume will assist in heat dissipation and thermoregulation because there is a large increase in plasma volume in relation to the red blood cell increase; hematocrit will decrease in trained individuals.

Increased blood volume would do no good if delivery at the muscles was not also increased. In response to the greater demand, capillary density will increase at the tissue, primarily the working muscles. The increased capillary density will supply more blood to the working muscles, allowing greater gas, nutrient, and metabolic byproduct exchange.

Improved cardiac function also occurs as an adaptation to endurance training. As mentioned previously, cardiac output equals stroke volume multiplied by heart rate ($Q = SV \times HR$). With endurance training, there will be an increase in stroke volume, which affects both cardiac output and heart rate. Stroke volume increases due to three primary reasons. The first is that there will be a healthy enlargement of the left ventricle, allowing a greater volume of blood to enter. Second, the increased blood volume will result in a larger volume of blood returning to the heart and therefore greater filling. Third, the cardiac muscle will produce a more forceful contraction. Because SV has increased, there will be a corresponding decrease in HR at any submaximal intensity, because cardiac output for that given submaximal intensity has not greatly altered. This is why endurance athletes have low resting heart rates. Max heart rate does not alter with training and remains relatively constant. Due to the increase in stroke volume and no alteration in max HR, there will be an increase in cardiac output with endurance training.

Alterations to muscle fiber will also occur with endurance training. Type I muscle hypertrophy develops, leading to improved performance. Slow twitch muscle hypertrophy is often overlooked because it is not as visibly noticed in relation to the type II muscle hypertrophy that occurs due to strength and power training. Type one muscle fibers will greatly increase their oxidative capacity. Type IIa (intermediate fibers) will shift toward oxidative properties. There will also be an increase in myoglobin to increase oxygen-carrying capacity within the muscle. Mitochondria (the oxidative powerhouse of the cell) will increase, leading to an increase in oxidative processes. There will be an overall increase in all oxidative enzymes as well.

Changes to energy sources will also occur due to endurance training. There will be an increase in glycogen stores. Glycogen stores for the average individual will be around 2,000 kCals. An elite endurance athlete will store around 2,500 kCals. Lipid stores will decrease in adipose tissue and increase in muscle. This will provide greater stores in the muscles readily available for production of ATP. Lastly, you will begin to utilize fat at a higher percentage earlier during prolonged exercise in order to spare glycogen.

The last adaptation is an increase in lactate threshold, due to a decrease in lactic acid production and an increase in lactate clearance. While endurance training, especially tempo work, will increase lactate threshold, anaerobic training is key to increasing lactate threshold.

Adaptations to Anaerobic Training

Anaerobic training will result in various adaptations that will increase your anaerobic capacity, allowing you to maintain high-energy outputs for a little longer period of time. One of the main adaptations that occurs due to anaerobic training involves an increase in anaerobic threshold due to an increased buffering capacity. As mentioned previously, during high-intensity exercise, which relies on anaerobic glycolysis, hydrogen builds up in the system. This buildup of hydrogen results in a decrease in pH (increased acidity). There are two primary methods used to buffer this decrease in pH. The first is that two hydrogen will bind with pyruvate to form lactic acid, and the second is when sodium bicarbonate binds with hydrogen to form carbonic acid. When you increase your buffering capacity, you greatly increase the intensity you can compete at as well as the duration you can hold the intensity. The increase in anaerobic threshold also occurs because of an increase in glycolytic enzymes that enhances energy production through glycolysis. There is also an increase in pain tolerance in individuals who train anaerobically. With just eight weeks of high-intensity training, you can significantly increase your anaerobic threshold.

Another adaptation to anaerobic training is an increase in muscular strength. This adaptation correlates with the strongest increases in anaerobic performance. This concept has been reverse engineered by strength-and-conditioning coaches for years, with great effect. While these increases in strength from anaerobic training are great for improved performance alone, coaches have realized that implementing strength-and-power-training programs will in turn improve the athlete's anaerobic performance.

Anaerobic training will also improve motor unit recruitment and the stretch-shortening cycle, both of which will increase the muscles' ability to contract forcefully and quickly. This improvement occurs due to an increase in motor unit recruitment, an increase in the firing rate of the recruited motor units, and an improved stretch-reflex response.

Adaptations to Resistance Training

Off-season resistance training is a vital part of a yearly training plan and will be discussed later in this book. When you begin an off-season resistance training program, you will see a large increase in the first eight weeks of training. Keep in mind that eight weeks is an average number that assumes you have not been active in resistance training. When someone new to resistance training begins a program, they will see somewhat steady gains for about the first eight weeks and then level off. This is because the first eight weeks of training result in neuro-muscular adaptations that improve performance without a correlating increase in muscle fiber size (hypertrophy). These neuromuscular adaptations consist of increased motor unit recruitment, increased synchronization of motor unit and muscle activation, and a reduction in the golgi tendon organ (the sensory organ that limits force development as a protective mechanism) threshold.

After the first eight weeks of resistance training, you will begin to see increases in muscle fiber diameter (hypertrophy). To understand hypertrophy, it is important to first have an understanding of basic muscle structure. A muscle is made up of fasciculi bound together by connective tissue. Each individual fasciculus is made up of a bundle of muscle fiber, and each muscle fiber is made up of a bundle of myofibril. Within the myofibril you have actin and myosin, which work together to cause a contraction of the muscle. Hypertrophy occurs due to an increase in the number of actin and myosin within each myofibril and an increase in the number of myofibril within each muscle fiber. To date, there is no strong evidence to support an increase in the number of muscle fibers within a muscle (hyperplasia) in humans.

PSYCHOLOGICAL TRAINING

We focus so much on the physiological and biomechanical principles of sport and often overlook the psychological factors of sport performance. Your psychological state can directly impact your physiological performance on many levels. For example, your heart rate will increase in anticipation of a workout or competition without any increase in physical demand. The greater the anxiety, the higher your heart rate will be prior to participation. There is nothing wrong with an anticipatory increase in heart rate, and as a matter of fact, starting your warm-up with a higher heart rate is beneficial. This section is not designed to give you an in-depth knowledge of sport psychology, but instead will hit on some key factors that will help with your performance.

Anxiety

Anxiety is a feeling of apprehension, nervousness, or fear that is in response to an event. While anxiety is a psychological construct, there is a corresponding physiological response. Anxiety results in an increased activity of the sympathetic nervous system leading to an increase in cardiac output, redirection of blood flow, tightening of muscles, and gastrointestinal distress. It is quite common to feel anxious about an upcoming competition or event, and everyone experiences anxiety prior to a race.

Being anxious is not entirely a bad thing as it triggers your fight or flight response and prepares your body for the competition. However, it is not good to be overly anxious. Focusing on your anxiety prevents you from focusing on the competition at hand and can lead to negative physiological responses (tight muscles, gastrointestinal distress, etc.).

Attention and Focus

When both in training for races and when racing mountain bikes, it is important to focus on the trail so that you can pick the ideal path along the trail and respond to any obstacles. Your bike will go in the direction of your focus. If you are riding at the edge of a ditch and your focus is on the ditch and not the trail, you will start moving toward the ditch. Instead, focus your attention on where you want to go and not where you do not wish to go. "Selective attention" is the term used to describe an athlete's focus on performance-relative cues while ignoring all nonessential cues. It is important to block out all the commotion going on around you and focus on the trail and your bike-handling skills.

Visualization

If you can visualize a movement or a sequence of movements, it will greatly increase your ability to perform those movements. This theory holds true for anything from jumping a fallen log to leaning through a curve at high speed. Visualizing the movement in your head as you produce the movement allows you to better conduct the movement. In order to effectively use visualization, it is important to know and understand the appropriate sequencing of the techniques.

The ability to correctly use visualization is a learned process and takes time to master. Video recordings of performance can help the athlete with visualization. Often, with beginners, it is hard to visualize proper technique. For example, a coach will explain to an athlete that he or she is conducting the technique incorrectly and the athlete does not understand because he or she feels it in fact is being done correctly. When the coach shows the athlete the video and details what is being done incorrectly, the athlete can now better visualize what to change as well as the correct technique.

Desensitization

Desensitization is the process by which you work to reduce the impact of a stimulus. It is a normal human reaction to feel fear when making a big jump or flying through a corner turn. Although that is a normal reaction, it is counterproductive to becoming a competent mountain biker. With time and training you will become desensitized to these factors and respond more appropriately. However, this does not mean that you should be fearless. A little fear is a good thing.

To work on the desensitization process, simply get accustomed to those factors of mountain biking that scare you. For example, if you are afraid of jumps, start off small and increase the size of the jumps as you become accustomed to the current height. Soon the jumps you were afraid of will come easy and you will wonder what you were ever worried about.

Motivation

Motivation is the force that drives the way you respond to situations. Motivation is not always simple and straightforward. Often motivation is multifaceted, complicated, and not always clear. Everyone reading this book will have different motivations for getting involved in mountain biking: for the competition, to get in shape, or simply the love of being outdoors. Most often, though, there is more than one factor that motivates someone to get involved. Taking the time to sit down and understand your motivation to train will allow you to better focus on your training plan and long-term goals.

Motivation can either be intrinsic (from within) or extrinsic (from outside sources). Intrinsic motivation will have the largest impact on your performance in the long run as the focus comes from your own desires. Intrinsic motivation is driven by your desire to excel, curiosity, love of the sport, desire to learn, desire to be challenged, etc. As your desires are self-motivated, it is less likely that you will experience burnout or frequent changes in attitude toward training and competing. Intrinsic motivation leads to greater learning, greater focus, greater self-confidence, and greater satisfaction.

Extrinsic motivation can be either beneficial or harmful to performance. Examples of extrinsic motivation are monetary reward, trophies, external praise or lack thereof (from a coach, parents, friends, etc.), contract or scholarship, etc. The problem with extrinsic motivation is that it is completely out of the athlete's control, and there is a danger that the athlete will focus their self-worth on these extrinsic factors. Extrinsic motivators can also lead to anxiety. Extrinsic motivators work best when the athlete has strong intrinsic motivation and the extrinsic motivation is not overemphasized. Also, those who focus solely on extrinsic motivators will burn out easier and will not develop as quickly.

Setting Goals

When developing a program, it is important to establish long- and short-term goals in order to develop a long-range training plan. When working with a new athlete, I first want to know their long-term goals. This allows me to determine their overall motivation for training and to build a successful program for them to reach those goals. It is difficult to develop a plan without knowing where you want to go.

Goals should be challenging, while remaining realistic and attainable. It is okay to set a high goal, such as becoming a professional mountain biker. However, it is not realistic to set the goal for your first year of training. It is always a good idea to talk over your goals with your coach so that you can get them set and develop a plan. In order to set your goals, ask yourself the following questions:

- Overall, what do I want to accomplish? (fitness, competition, being outdoors, or any combination of the three)
- What is my current fitness level?
- What is my current skill level?
- How much time can I dedicate to training?
- What are my logistical challenges?

These are some of the basic questions you can use to help determine your goals. It is important to think about each question and answer each as honestly as possible.

As mentioned, when setting goals, it is important to set both short- and long-term goals. Look at it like a ladder. If you only had the bottom and top rungs of the ladder it would be virtually useless, and you would be unable to climb to the top (your ultimate goal). Adding rungs (short-term goals) to the ladder between the bottom and the top will allow you to climb easily and ultimately reach your goal. The journey to reach your ultimate goal can be difficult, long, and at times discouraging. Short-term goals give you something to strive for along the way.

After determining your long-term and short-term goals, write them down so that you will have them for future reference. The act of writing down your goals makes it much more likely that you will stick to those goals. Place your goals where you can see them daily so that they will provide motivation along your journey.

Do Not Make Comparisons

One of the worst mistakes a mountain biker can make is to compare their progression with the performance level of other mountain bikers. This is doubly true when a beginner attempts to compare their current level to an elite-level cyclist. It is important to remember that the elite mountain biker started where you currently stand and progressed to an elite level through hard training and dedication. Do not focus on whether you are better than someone else. Instead, focus on whether you are better today than you were yesterday. If the answer is yes, then you are going in the right direction. If the answer is no, then you need to evaluate your motivation, consistency, and training plan to determine why and make appropriate changes.

This concept does not mean that you should not realistically determine where your performance level is in relation to others if you plan to compete. Never compete before you are ready as it may lead to disappointment if your performance level is not where it needs to be.

3

AREAS OF TRAINING

This chapter will cover the various areas of training that you should focus on in order to improve your mountain biking. While mountain biking is an aerobic sport, there are other areas you should focus on in order to optimize your performance, including anaerobic training, flexibility training, and off-season resistance training.

AEROBIC TRAINING

Aerobic training is designed to improve your cardiorespiratory endurance. As aerobic capacity is the primary component of mountain biking, the greatest volume of your training will be in this area. As mentioned previously, determining training intensity is important if you want to improve your mountain biking performance. The majority of your training will be conducted below anaerobic threshold, with a small portion at or above threshold. The following methods can be used to control training intensity.

Determining Intensity

Determining Intensity Using Speed

Speed is often used to control intensity in mountain biking. However, it is a poor overall measure. There are factors that greatly impact speed when mountain biking. The first and most obvious is terrain. You will be able to maintain an overall faster speed on a flat, rolling course as opposed to a course that requires a lot of climbing. This factor makes it impossible to compare intensities between two different trails. However, you can compare speeds between different rides on the same trail. While many courses are blocked from wind, it is still possible for wind to play a factor when using speed as a measure of intensity. Headwinds will make you ride slower and tailwinds will increase your speed.

While using speed has its drawbacks, it is still an easy and practical tool. But do not fall into the trap of trying to obtain a personal best every time you train. You should stick with the specific goal of that training session and make adjustments only based on the environmental conditions (wind, hills, etc.). Keep in mind that you should not compare average speeds from one course with another.

Time can be used as a marker set for improved performance. To do this, ride at race pace on the same trail in similar environmental conditions more than once to determine if your training is working and whether or not positive adaptations are occurring. If times are faster, then you know the program is working. However, if times have declined or have not improved, look at your training and recovery program to determine if changes need to be made. Marker sets should be performed periodically and not every time you are on the trail. Treat a marker set as a race. Make sure that you are well recovered, well hydrated, well fueled, and well rested prior to any marker set. Your goal is to measure improvements in performance and not how tired you are from your interval training the previous day or the fact that you only got three hours of sleep the night prior.

Determining Intensity Using Heart Rate

Using heart rate to determine intensity may seem a little daunting. However, it is a very easy method to implement into your training and is a good tool for setting levels of riding intensity. Heart rate shares a linear relationship with intensity from rest to maximal effort, meaning that as intensity increases, so too does heart rate in equal measure.

Recently, though, there has been a trend toward not relying on heart rate for determining intensity levels, due to the day-to-day variability in heart rate. While it is true that heart rate varies from day to day, it does not invalidate heart rate as a useful tool. Being aware of normal heart rate variability allows you to better understand heart rate and better implement heart rate monitoring into your training program.

Hydration levels and recovery have a strong impact on heart rate. As you become dehydrated, blood plasma volumes decrease, which in turn leads to a decrease in stroke volume (volume of blood ejected from the heart with each beat). A decrease in stroke volume results in an increase in heart rate at any resting or submaximal (also known as submax) intensity level. Mountain bikers who are training in the summer have a tendency to stay chronically dehydrated. On long hot rides, heart rate can gradually increase due to dehydration.

Heart rate will also remain elevated during recovery from training due to replenishing energy systems, cooling the body, and anabolic (tissue-building) processes. During easy days, heart rate returns to resting levels fairly quickly. However, after a hard day of training, resting and submax heart rates can remain elevated for a period of time.

One last factor to keep in mind is cardiovascular drift, which is an increase in heart rate without an increase in intensity during prolonged steady exercise, particularly in a hot environment. Cardiovascular drift is typically a result of dehydration. During prolonged exercise, plasma volume decreases due to sweating, which leads to a decrease in blood volume, resulting in a decrease in blood return to the heart and a subsequent decrease in stroke volume. In order to dissipate heat from the body's core, more blood will be sent to the skin for cooling, which also decreases venous return and stroke volume. Cardiac output (volume of blood ejected from the heart each minute) is the product of heart rate and stroke volume. Because cardiac output must be maintained in order to sustain a specific intensity, heart rate must increase to compensate for the decrease in stroke volume. Do not be surprised if your heart rate begins to creep up on a long ride, especially if it is hot outside.

A heart rate monitor is the best method for measuring heart rate, because it detects the electrical impulse of the heart contractions. You can also count pulse rate at either the carotid artery (located at the neck) or the radial artery (located at the wrist). However, this method is not as accurate when compared to using a heart rate monitor. When purchasing a monitor, look for one with a chest transmitter as they are the most accurate.

To use heart rate as a training tool, you need an anchor point. The most common anchor point used is heart rate max. Heart rate max is the highest heart rate measured at maximal intensity. In order to determine your max heart rate, either conduct a $VO_{2\,max}$ test or perform hill repeats at maximal effort. $VO_{2\,max}$ testing requires specialized equipment and provides a greater amount of information than performing hill repeats. $VO_{2\,max}$ testing is discussed in detail in chapter 2.

But you do not need a laboratory or sophisticated equipment to determine max heart rate. You can simply perform hill repeats at maximal intensity. Find a hill that is about half a mile to a mile long. Warm up for about 15 minutes, and then climb the hill as fast as possible. If you are not completely exhausted at the top of the climb, you did not climb hard enough. The idea here is to achieve your max heart rate. Repeat the climb two to four times and record the highest heart rate achieved. Upon completion, cool down by riding 10 to 15 minutes.

The problem with using intervals to determine max heart rate is that it requires you to repeatedly engage in maximal effort bouts. This is not typically recommended for beginners; you may want to consider estimating max heart rate instead. There are various formulas that will help you make a close estimate. These formulas are not overly accurate but will provide a ballpark anchor point that will be relatively accurate for most individuals. Once you establish a good training plan and fitness level, I recommend ditching the estimated max HR and conducting hill repeats or a $VO_{2\,max}$ test to determine your true max heart rate.

Example Formula

$220 - age = HR_{max}$

Example: $220 - 41$ years of age = 179 beats per minute (bpm)

$210 - (age \times .5) - (body\ weight\ in\ pounds \times .05) + correction\ factor = HR_{max}$

Correction factor = + 4 for males and + 0 for females

$210 - (41 \times .5) - (180 \times .05) + 4 = 184.5$ bpm

Now that you have established max heart rate, you will next need to determine intensity based on heart rate. Training zone heart rates will set the parameters of your training session for that day by providing an upper and lower heart rate limit. This is where the training zone alarm on your heart rate monitor comes into play. It allows you to train without constantly checking your heart rate monitor to determine if you are in or out of your training zone. Here are four basic heart rate training zones:

Zone 1—Active Recovery

- 50 to 65 percent of max heart rate.
- Beginners will typically stay closer to 50 percent.
- Training below 70 percent ensures that it is an active recovery day.

Zone 2—Aerobic

- 70 to 80 percent of max heart rate.
- For beginners, 80 percent may be too high and you may want to consider staying closer to 70 percent.
- This is where the majority of your training will occur.

Zone 3—Threshold

- 80 to 90 percent of max heart rate.
- This will be your race pace or tempo training.

Zone 4—Interval

- 90 to 100 percent of max heart rate.
- This will be your high-intensity training above threshold.

You can also set heart rate training zones using heart rate at anaerobic threshold. If you know the heart rate that corresponds to your current anaerobic threshold, you can set training zones based on that anchor point. Anaerobic threshold will change with training, and the better race shape you are in, the higher your anaerobic threshold will be. The common four zones when using threshold heart rate are:

Zone 1—Active Recovery	25 percent or more below threshold heart rate
Zone 2—Aerobic	25 to 10 percent below threshold heart rate
Zone 3—Threshold	± 10 percent of threshold heart rate
Zone 4—Interval	> 110 percent of heart rate threshold

The reason that an upper and lower heart rate is given with each training zone is due to day-to-day heart rate variability, which makes it somewhat impossible to stay at a single fixed heart rate for each given zone. The majority of your mountain bike training will focus on heart rate training zones one and two. Naturally, if you are climbing a steep hill on those days you may have to go out of your zone in order to climb the hill. However, it's best if you can slow down and take the hill easier to stay within your zone.

Heart rate training in zone three occurs at race pace and is used for threshold training. However, do not use heart rate to limit yourself during a race. As a mountain biker it is important to learn to pace yourself on feel and known distance in a race situation. Mountain biking is a self-paced event, and you will develop pacing strategies. Use of a heart rate monitor to control intensity during a race may limit your race performance. Instead, learn to pace based on how you feel at race pace. You may still want to wear a heart rate monitor during the race in order to evaluate performance afterward.

When coaching, I was not concerned about heart rate during interval training and typically used time or power measurements for them. Intervals are conducted at high intensities, and heart rate can even continue to climb briefly after a high-intensity interval.

Determining Intensity Using Power

Cycling power meters are considered the optimal method for determining intensity during cycling. However, due to the expense and knowledge level required to correctly integrate a power meter into your training, the use of power meters is beyond the scope of this book. Prior to purchasing a power meter, do some in-depth reading so that you can make an educated decision based on your ability and willingness to apply power to training.

Determining Intensity by Feel

Determining intensity based on feel is a valuable tool that is often applied incorrectly or overlooked altogether. Mountain bikers who have been racing for a while are able to pace correctly for different training zones based on known distance and how they feel (peripheral feedback). Beginners typically have a difficult time correctly gauging intensity, especially during a race. They may go out too fast, experience fatigue, and then slow down, leading to a poor performance time. Instead of going out too fast, focus on maintaining a pace that you can hold throughout the entire race. Research has shown that using an even-paced race strategy is ideal for optimal performance during endurance sports. With mountain biking, speed and effort will alter greatly with terrain. However, you can keep an even pacing strategy by basing it on how you feel. Through experience you will learn to correctly pace during a race.

There are a couple simple methods that help you to control intensity through feel, the first of which is the talk test, which is extremely simple to use and, yet, very effective. The talk test allows you to determine if you are below, at, or above threshold. If you are training below threshold, you should be able to hold a decent conversation. The closer you get to threshold, the harder it will be to hold a conversation. At threshold you should only be able to get out a short sentence at most. Above threshold you may get out one or two words at most.

The next method, a bit more complicated, uses a rating of perceived exertion (RPE) scale to determine intensity (numbered scale indicating level of fatigue). You can use the Borg scale, one of the most common RPE scales used in exercise science, which runs from a rating of 6 (no exertion) to 20 (maximal exertion), to correlate to an average resting heart rate of 60 bpm and max heart rate of 200 bpm. Or, use the OMNI scale (rating of 0 [extremely easy] to 10 [extremely hard]), which has become the preferred RPE scale because it is more logical in nature.

Prior to using an RPE scale to determine training intensity, and accurately correlate an RPE number to how you feel, it is important to first anchor it during a graded exercise protocol. A graded exercise protocol starts off at an easy level and increases intensity every two to three minutes (depending on the protocol). During the graded exercise protocol, you will establish an RPE every minute by determining how you feel at that point. This allows you to anchor all numbers from first to last.

ANAEROBIC TRAINING

Anaerobic training is the high-intensity training that will be conducted above threshold in order to improve your anaerobic capacity. As mountain biking requires frequent significant increase in power to climb steep hills, you will encounter many anaerobic bouts within a race. Interval training is the best method for increasing your anaerobic abilities.

There are multiple ways to conduct interval training, and I will discuss a few of those methods. To begin, most cyclists conduct interval training incorrectly. They go out as hard as they can each interval with their power output decreasing with every subsequent interval. This is called overreaching interval training, and it has a place within a well-designed program. However, the mistake many cyclists make is that they conduct overreaching intervals every time they conduct intervals. The majority of your interval training should be conducted so that the last interval is at the same power output as the first interval, but you can barely hold the output during the last interval. If you can barely hold the power output during the first interval, then your power output will continuously drop throughout the remaining intervals. The first through last intervals should be conducted at a level that is challenging yet allows you to maintain the assigned power output for every interval.

Interval training can be conducted either seated or standing. I recommend doing the majority seated, and then add in some standing intervals as you will be out of the saddle from time to time when climbing. It is true that pedaling seated at a higher cadence is more efficient in relation to pedaling at a lower cadence while standing. However, the reality of mountain biking is that, due to the terrain, you will be out of your saddle climbing multiple times during a race.

Intervals can also be conducted in either long-time intervals or short-time intervals. You can conduct short-time intervals from 60 to 120 seconds each.

If you pick 90 seconds for your intervals, then each individual interval for that session will be conducted at 90 seconds. This type of interval really pushes your anaerobic abilities. You can also do longer interval sessions (5- to 10-minute intervals) that really work on pushing up your threshold for race pace.

A rest period between intervals is another key concept to consider when conducting interval training. You must make sure that energy systems and neuromuscular fatigue are addressed between bouts. However, currently there is no concrete evidence to state what the exact work-to-rest ratio should be at different interval time lengths. The typical recommendation is that the work-to-rest ratio for intervals that last 60 to 120 seconds should be approximately 1:3, and for intervals that last about 3 to 5 minutes, the work-to-rest ratio should be 1:1. So, if you are conducting a 60-second training interval (work), then your recovery period should be 180 seconds (rest). If you are conducting 5-minute intervals (work), then your recovery period should be 5 minutes (rest). The rest interval can either be conducted actively (very easy cycling) or passively (no cycling). Either will work, but I tend to recommend active recovery during long sessions. Keep in mind that active here actually means that you are pedaling very easily and slowly.

You can also conduct fartlek sessions where the intervals are not timed specifically and instead you pick up the pace at random intervals and recover in between. Typically, I recommend that you feel well recovered, but not necessarily completely recovered, between intervals. This can be something fun that you do with your friends. Assign everyone a number, one through however many are riding with you, and the intervals start in number order. Line up by number and start down the trail. When the first cyclist decides to start the interval, they quickly pick up speed without a word, and everyone else attempts to keep up. During the recovery phase, the first rider goes to the back of the line and then rider two will decide when to pick up the pace again. Keep repeating this process throughout the ride.

Overreaching intervals can be used periodically to maximize stress on the physiological systems of your body. Unlike normal interval training, overreaching intervals will have continuously slower intervals as the training session progresses. Each interval is conducted as fast as you can ride, which will result in slower intervals as you fatigue with each subsequent interval. Overreaching intervals should be used sparingly as they place high stress on the body.

FLEXIBILITY

Flexibility is your ability to move each joint through the complete range of motion for that particular joint. Maintaining a dynamic range of motion and proper flexibility is very important for the sport of mountain biking. However, flexibility is often overlooked by many athletes, resulting in decreased performance and overuse injuries.

There are different methods used to increase flexibility. However, this book will only focus on the two primary methods and when to use them. The first method used to increase flexibility is called static stretching. When conducting a static stretch, slowly move into the proper position for that specific stretch and hold it for 10–30 seconds. When you move into the stretch, only go to the point of slight discomfort. Never go until you feel pain as it is counterproductive, causing the muscle to tighten during the stretch.

The second method of stretching I recommend is dynamic stretching. This method requires that you move through the full range of motion for a particular joint in a dynamic manner without holding a stretch. Dynamic stretching is used during warm-ups for competition in order to increase range of motion and optimize performance.

Both static and dynamic stretching have a place in your training and competition. There is currently debate on whether static stretching is harmful prior to competition. Some research states that power and speed are reduced when static stretching is used, as opposed to dynamic stretching. However, the current pool of research is not conclusive. I would recommend dynamic stretching going into your competition and training, and static for after. Static stretching is key when it comes to increasing range of motion and should remain an integral part of your training program.

As mountain bikes are pedaled with legs and not arms, it is easy to understand why many cyclists will ignore the upper body. However, because mountain biking is conducted on rough trails, the upper body and core do a lot of work to maintain the dynamic stability of the bike. Therefore, it is important to conduct stretching on all parts of the body.

Static Stretches

Neck

When stretching the muscles of your neck it is important to include rotation, flexion, extension, and lateral flexion.

- Begin by rotating your head to the left as far as it will turn and hold, then repeat this process to the right.

- Take your neck into flexion by trying to touch your chin to your chest and hold the stretch. Next move your head into extension by rotating your chin toward the ceiling and hold.
- Take your head into lateral flexion to the right by taking your right ear toward your shoulder. Hold that position, and then repeat this process to the left.

When stretching the neck, it is very important to not apply a large force or to conduct these movements in a fast or bouncing manner.

Anterior Shoulder Stretch

This stretch is designed to stretch the anterior deltoid and pectoralis major. Raise your arm until it is parallel to the floor and place your hand on any object that will not move (such as a wall, door frame, etc.). Next rotate your upper body away from the arm that is being held in place, stretching the anterior muscles of the shoulder.

Posterior Shoulder Stretch

The posterior shoulder stretch focuses on the posterior deltoid and muscles of the back. Horizontally draw your right arm across the chest, then place your left hand on the elbow and apply pressure to stretch.

Behind the Head Stretch

This stretch focuses on the triceps and latisimus dorsi. Raise your right arm above your head, and then flex at the elbow until your hand is behind your head. Reach up with your left hand to grab your elbow and apply pressure to the left. Repeat this process with the left arm.

Abdominal Stretch

As the name indicates, this stretch will focus on the abdominal muscles. Lie prone and place your hands palm down on the floor. Push upward with your arms, leaving your lower body flat on the floor.

Calf Stretch

The calf muscle (triceps surae) is made up of the gastrocnemius and soleus muscles. To stretch the calf muscle, stand on a raised surface with the fore part

of your foot on the surface and the heel hanging off the surface. Allov
to go down by placing the foot in dorsiflexion. To concentrate on tl
nemius, keep the leg straight during this process. To focus more on
slightly flex at the knee and repeat the process. Placing the knee iı
places slack on the gastrocnemius and allows a greater focus on the sc
is important because even at the bottom of your pedal stroke your kne

Hamstring Stretch

The basic hamstring stretch does much more than just stretch the ł
This stretch is also great for the muscles of the lower back. If you can
toes and pull the foot into dorsiflexion, it will also stretch the calf.
stretch can be conducted standing, I advise conducting the stretch seate
your legs together and straight out in front of you. Bend forward at the v
as far forward and down as possible. Grab your toes and pull the foot
flexion. If you cannot reach your toes, grab as far down the leg as you cı
this process, keep your legs straight and do not allow a lot of bend at tl

Modified Hurdle Stretch

The modified hurdle stretch (see fig. 3.1) primarily concentrates oı
strings and muscles of the lower back. Sit on your bottom with yo

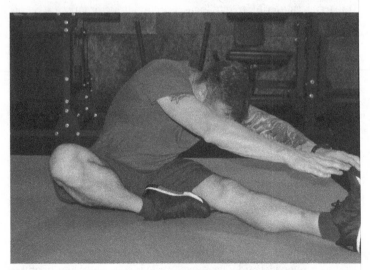

Figure 3.1. Modified hurdle stretch. *Will and Renee Peveler.*

straight out in front of you and your right leg flexed at the knee with the bottom of your foot in contact with your left leg. Bend forward and attempt to place both hands on your left foot. Repeat this stretch with the right side.

Straddle Stretch

This stretch primarily focuses on the hamstrings, adductor muscles, and muscles of the lower back. Sit on your bottom with your legs spread wide (horizontal split). Lean your body over your left leg attempting to touch your foot with your right hand, and then repeat the movement on your right leg. Once you have completed those movements, bend toward the floor in the middle.

Quadriceps Stretch

The quadriceps stretch is typically conducted incorrectly by trying to push the heel into the gluteus maximus while in flexion. Instead, reach behind your body and grab your right leg with your left hand, then place the knee into flexion and pull rearward. Repeat this process with the other leg. If you have trouble balancing on one leg during this process, move to a wall and place your free hand on the wall for balance.

Adductor Stretch

The adductor stretch (butterfly stretch) focuses on the adductor muscles. Sit on the floor and place your knees into flexion with the soles of your feet touching. Grab your feet and place your elbows on your legs. Push down on your legs with your elbows and bend forward at the waist.

Hip Stretch

This stretch concentrates on the gluteus maximus and hamstrings. Lie supine with both legs straight out. Bring your right leg up by flexing at the hip. As you bring the leg up, allow the knee to go into flexion. Place your hands behind the knee and pull. Repeat this process with the left leg.

Supine Twist

This stretch focuses on muscles around the spine, the external oblique and gluteus muscles. Lay on your left side, keeping your left leg straight and bending

your right knee. Your left arm should be perpendicular to your body and lying on the ground with your right arm on top of the left. Keeping your right leg in place, rotate your upper body toward the right, placing your shoulders flat on the ground; your right arm should now be on the ground and perpendicular to your body. Repeat this process on your right side.

Dynamic Stretches

Wrist Rotations

Wrist rotations are conducted by rotating both wrists clockwise for about 15 seconds and then reversing to counterclockwise for another 15 seconds.

Cross-Body Arm Swings

To conduct the cross-body arm swings, horizontally abduct your arms and then adduct them across your chest with one arm slightly above the other as they cross. Alternate which arm is above and below with each swing.

Elbow Circles

With arms slightly raised from your sides, make circles from the elbow. You will not actually have rotation at the elbow, it will be more like circumduction with slight shoulder movement. Start by going counterclockwise for 15 seconds and then clockwise for another 15 seconds.

Arm Circles

Rotate your arms from the shoulders in a 360-degree circle (circumduction). Conduct arm rotations to the front for 15 seconds, and then rotate them to the back for 15 seconds.

Trunk Rotation

Place your feet a little wider than shoulder-width apart and abduct your arms until they are approximately parallel to the floor, then rotate as far as you can go to the left and then back as far as you can go to the right.

Butt Kicks

Butt kicks can be conducted in place, or while walking or jogging. As your foot comes off the ground, drive the heel to your butt with each step. Alternate legs as you perform the dynamic stretch. When you first start this movement, your heel may not reach your butt. This is okay, just get your heel as high as you can.

High Knees

High knees can be done in place, or while walking or jogging. When the foot leaves the ground, bring your knee as high as possible toward your chest. Alternate legs as you do this dynamic stretch.

High-Knee Hip Circles

Conduct this movement in place. Bring your knee up high toward your chest and then rotate the leg away from your body and then back to the ground landing in your starting position. Alternate legs as you conduct this movement. After 15 seconds reverse this movement (rotate from the outside in).

Leg Swings

You can conduct leg swings with or without support. If you need support for balance, place your hand on a wall or non-moveable object. Without bending your knee, kick your leg forward as high as possible and then allow it to swing down and behind you as far as possible. After 15 seconds switch to the other leg and conduct leg swings for another 15 seconds.

Lateral Leg Swings

Lateral leg swings are similar to leg swings, but instead of front to back you will swing your leg from side to side (abduct and adduct). Kick your leg to the side, and then allow it to come down and cross in front of your stationary leg. After 15 seconds switch to the other leg and conduct leg swings for another 15 seconds.

Supine Leg Circles

To conduct supine leg circles, lay on your back and bend at the hips until your thighs are perpendicular to the floor and then move your feet in circles. Move your left foot clockwise and your right foot counterclockwise. After 15 seconds reverse each foot for another 15 seconds.

OFF-SEASON RESISTANCE TRAINING

Off-season resistance training has been shown to greatly improve endurance performance in the upcoming race season. Other than keeping your off-season endurance base, resistance training is the most valuable tool you have in the off-season. You will not see improvements in your oxygen-carrying capacity, as the adaptations to the resistance training are not designed to increase cardio-respiratory endurance. Instead you will see improvement on a neuromuscular level; primarily improvements in the stretch-shortening cycle and motor unit recruitment and synchronization.

When adding a resistance program to your off-season training plan, remember that it is only a small portion of your plan and not the main part of your program. You will need to slightly reduce your normal off-season volume and replace it with your resistance training. Do not try and put your resistance training on top of your normal off-season volume. You do not need a high-volume resistance routine as you are not trying to become a body builder. Your resistance workout should take about 40 minutes for your total time lifting.

It is important that you learn the proper technique for every lift you plan on using in your program. The use of improper technique is one of the most common causes of injury in the weight room. Lift in a controlled manner that follows the correct technique precisely. If you cannot maintain the proper lifting form, then reduce the weight until you can.

As a mountain biker you will not have a lot of eccentric loading during your normal training routine (unless you ride a fixed-gear bike). However, all the resistance training techniques that you will use will have an eccentric load. Therefore, it is important that you work into your off-season resistance training slowly. Your legs will be strong enough to lift heavier than you should starting out. It is important to be aware of this in order to avoid the common error of lifting too much and then being so sore that you cannot walk for a week.

While each lift requires specific techniques, there are general guidelines that go with all lifts:

- Maintain proper technique throughout the movements. Don't try to use momentum to get through a lift where the resistance is too heavy. If the resistance is heavy enough to require you to alter proper form, you should decrease the weight to maintain form.

- Movements should be conducted in a controlled manner and at a constant speed. The speed should not be explosive and fast, nor should it be super slow.
- Correctly grip the bar at all times in order to prevent the bar from rolling out of your hands.
- Do not attempt to lift weights that are too heavy for your current fitness level. This is a common source of injury. Remember to let your ego go. It does not matter how much you are lifting as you are not training to be a power lifter. You are training to be the best fighter you can become.
- Work large muscle groups before working small muscle groups. If you work the small muscle groups first, they will become too fatigued to allow you to adequately work the large muscle groups. For example, if you work the triceps brachii first and then work the pectoralis major, your triceps will be too fatigued and give out prior to the pectoralis major fatiguing. Instead, work the pectoralis major first and then the triceps.
- Never hold your breath. Inhale during the eccentric load and exhale during the concentric load. Holding your breath during a lift will result in a larger spike in blood pressure than normal (blood pressure always spikes during lifting), which will cause a large decrease in blood pressure when the lift stops, resulting in dizziness.
- For safety, always use a spotter with free weights.
- Use collars on the barbells in order to keep the weight from shifting on the bar. It only takes a slight shift in the bar to cause a weight to slide, which results in a catastrophic event as the plates start sliding off the bar.

One of your first steps is to determine frequency by determining the length of the program and how many days per week you use resistance training. The typical off-season resistance program should last 6 to 12 weeks. The first 1 to 2 weeks of training will be used to slowly work your way into the program, and the last week will be used to taper off into the preseason. It is possible to conduct a maintenance phase through the first portion of the preseason. Once you determine the length of your off-season resistance training program, you need to determine how many days per week you will conduct the program. Do not continue resistance training into your season.

Resistance training should be conducted two to three days per week—typically Monday, Wednesday, and Friday. Not all three of those days have to be in the weight room lifting weights. You can work on plyometrics or sports-specific resistance training (over-geared hill repeats) during one of those sessions.

The next step is to determine your sets and repetitions. Sets are the number of times you perform the exercise, and repetition is the number of times you lift or perform the movement per set. Research has shown improvements occur with one to three sets. Since you want to get in and out, I typically recommend two sets for the majority of exercises in the program.

Improvements in endurance performance after off-season resistance training have been demonstrated with high weight at low repetitions (4–6 repetitions), moderate weight at moderate repetitions (8–12), and low weight at higher repetitions (up to 30 repetitions). While they all have resulted in improved performance, I typically stay away from high weight and low repetitions due to the increased risk of injury associated with heavy lifting. I recommend 8 to 15 repetitions when lifting weights. When conducting body management exercises (muscular endurance: push-ups, crunches, etc.), the goal is muscular endurance, and therefore do not limit yourself to 8 to 15 repetitions. Instead, do as many as you can with the goal of conducting at least one more repetition each training session. For example, if you conducted 16 pull-ups on your first set on Monday, then your goal should be at least 17 reps on the first set during your workout on Wednesday.

Determine weight based on desired repetitions. For example, if you are conducting two sets with goal repetitions of 8 to 15, you would set the weight so that volitional exhaustion occurs between 8 and 15 reps for both sets. This may take you a couple of workouts to determine. If you are able to conduct more than 15 repetitions, then increase the weight. If you cannot conduct at least 8 repetitions, then decrease the weight.

The next step is to choose the resistance exercises. Below are examples of exercises that you can implement into your resistance training program. Research has shown that improvements occur with lifting, plyometrics, body management exercises, and sports-specific exercises. I typically use a mixture of all of them. These are just a few exercise examples to get you started. If you are serious about your performance, consider hiring a strength-and-conditioning coach with a background in endurance performance.

Work your entire body, including the upper body, lower body, and core; avoid focusing on one area and ignoring others. Keep in mind that you have to control the bike with your upper body, and therefore you should not avoid upper body workouts. The lifts and exercises listed below supply a sufficient program to cover all the major muscle groups that are important to a mountain biker. You do not have to use all the resistance exercises listed below. Choose the ones that work best with your desired outcome. You can replace these lifts with others that work the same muscles, or focus more on a specific area by adding more lifts into your program. For example, you can replace squats with leg presses. If you are not familiar with the muscles involved with each specific lift, then I strongly recommend purchasing a book that shows the specific muscles used in each movement.

Resistance Training Exercises

Bench Press

The pectoralis major, anterior deltoids, and triceps brachii are the primary muscles used in the bench press (see fig. 3.2). Other muscles used in this lift are the serratus anterior and coracobrachialis. In order to conduct the bench press, lie flat on your back with both feet planted on the floor. Place your hands on the bar about shoulder-width apart with the palms facing away and fingers and thumbs wrapped around the bar. Begin by lowering the weight until it is about 1 inch from your chest. Do not bounce the weight off your chest. From the lowered position, push the weight back up to the start position.

Lat Pull-Down

The lat pull-down (see fig. 3.3) is designed to work the latissimus dorsi, teres major, and biceps brachii. Adjust the lat pull-down machine per the manufacturer's instruction. Grab the bar just wider than shoulder width so that your palms are facing away from you. Pull the bar down in front of your head, and then return to the start position.

Seated Row

The latissimus dorsi, trapezius, rhomboid (major and minor), teres major, posterior deltoids, and biceps brachii are worked during the seated row, as shown in fig. 3.4. Adjust the machine per the manufacturer's instructions. Begin by bringing the bar/handles to your chest and then returning to the start position. Maintain proper back posture throughout the movement.

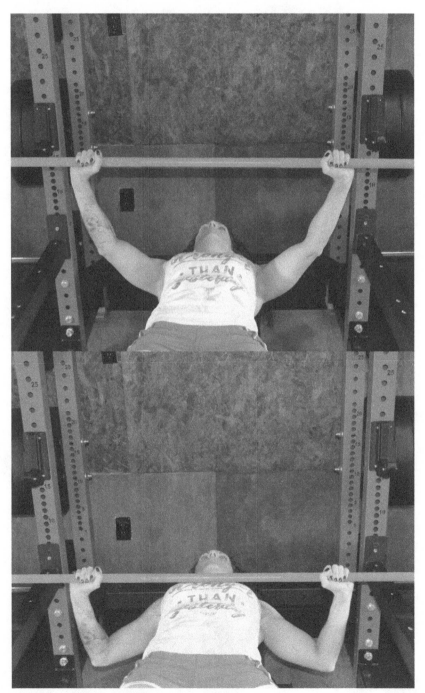

Figure 3.2.   Bench press. *Will and Renee Peveler.*

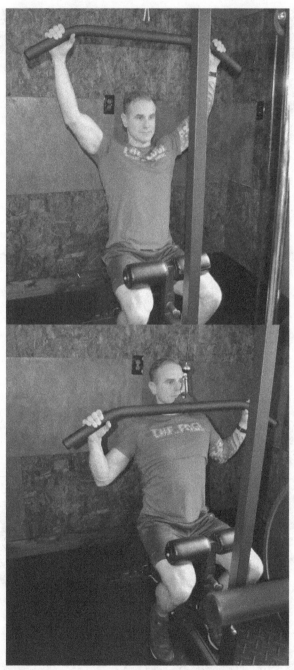

Figure 3.3.   Lat pulldown. *Will and Renee Peveler.*

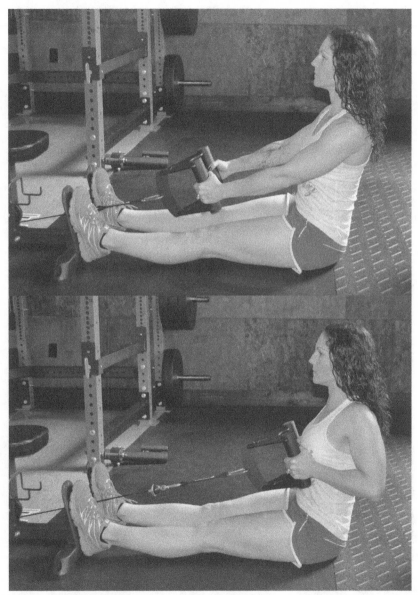

Figure 3.4.   Seated row. *Will and Renee Peveler.*

Overhead Press

The overhead press (see fig. 3.5) can be conducted either seated or standing. The deltoid, pectoralis major (clavicular head only), and triceps are the primary muscles used during this exercise. When conducted on a machine, follow the manufacturer's instructions. The overhead press can also be conducted using dumbbells. Grab the dumbbells in an overhand grip and place the dumbbells a little higher than shoulder level with the back of the hand facing you. This is the start position. Press up over the head and then return to the start position. Overhead press can also be conducted with a barbell, but I recommend beginners stick with dumbbells. Dumbbells allow more natural joint movement throughout the lift.

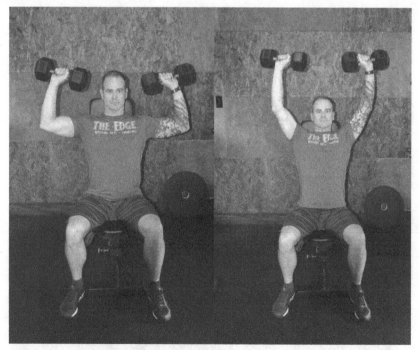

Figure 3.5.   Overhead press. *Will and Renee Peveler.*

Squats

The primary muscles used during the squat are the quadriceps, hamstrings, and gluteus maximus (see fig. 3.6). The first step in conducting the squat is to adjust the squat rack height so that you can easily take the bar off and put it back when the set is complete. When conducting the squat, center the bar across the back and shoulders and grab the bar with both hands. Choose a hand position that provides both comfort and control of the bar. Lift the bar off the rack and back up into position, making sure to stay over the safety bars. Place your feet shoulder-width apart. During the lowering phase, do not allow your knees to move forward beyond your feet. Lower into the squatted position until your thighs are parallel to the floor. Next push up with the legs, returning to the standing position. When pushing up, drive through your heels, keeping the weight centered. When you reach the top of the lift, do not lock your knees. In order to maintain proper posture, make sure that you do not look down with

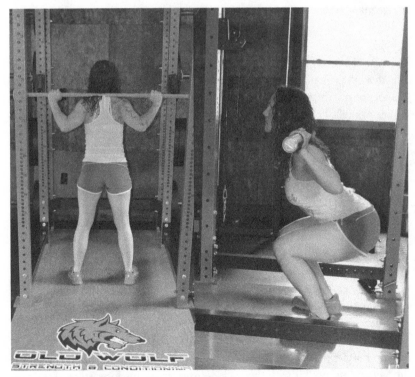

Figure 3.6.   Squats. *Will and Renee Peveler.*

your head as it will shift your center of gravity forward. Keep your head looking forward or slightly up, and drive with your heels.

Leg Extensions

Leg extensions focus on the muscles of the quadriceps (rectus femoris, vastus intermedius, vastus lateralis, and vastus medialis). Before beginning leg extensions, ensure that the machine you are working on is set up specifically for you. Do not lock your knees out at the top of the knee extension.

Leg Curls

Leg curls are designed to strengthen the hamstrings (semitenndinosus, semimembanosis, and biceps femoris). Because the gastrocnemius crosses the knee, it will be worked along with the hamstring muscles. Adjust the leg curl machine in accordance with the manufacturer's instructions. Leg curls (as well as leg extensions) are not typically recommended for sports performance because they are isolation exercises. However, cycling relies heavily on these muscles.

Deadlift

The deadlift primarily focuses on the gluteus maximus, hamstring, quadriceps, erector spinae, rhomboid, and trapezius muscles (see fig. 3.7). When conducting the deadlift, I recommend using a hex bar (trap bar) as opposed to a straight bar. When using a straight bar, you need to keep the bar as close to the shins as possible, which often leads to beat-up and gouged shins. The hex bar also puts your trunk in a more upright position and slightly reduces the risk of lower back injury. For those with lower back issues, most hex bars will have a higher handle that allows you to start from a higher position. Lastly, you are not competing in a power-lifting competition, and therefore a straight bar deadlift is not required. With the exception of slightly different knee angles and trunk angle, all other angles are the same and the work between a straight bar deadlift and a hex bar deadlift are the same (even though you can lift more with a hex bar). The center of gravity alters with a hex bar, and it allows for a more comfortable lift.

To conduct a hex bar deadlift, step into the hex bar with your feet about shoulder-width apart. Grab the bar and align it so that the center of the bar and center of the hands are at the midpoint of the ankle. When you grab the bar, do not bend at the waist and instead squat down. Drive the bar up from the feet and do not lift with the back. Thrust your hips forward as you come

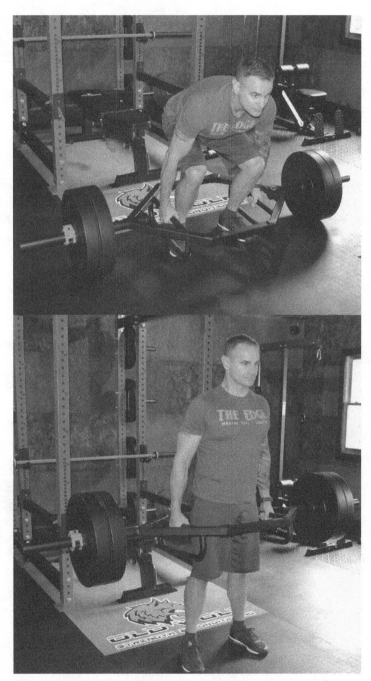

Figure 3.7. Deadlift. *Will and Renee Peveler.*

up (do not overexaggerate). During the eccentric phase (lowering back to the ground), make sure that the weights hit the floor evenly. If the weights touch the floor unevenly, you need to either slow down or drop weight in order to move smoothly through the motion so that both sides of the weight touch the floor at the same time.

Muscular Endurance Exercises

Pull-Ups

The pull-up is designed to improve the muscular endurance of the latissimus dorsi, teres major, and biceps brachii, as shown in fig. 3.8. The rhomboids are also worked when the shoulder blades are pulled together at the top of the pull-up. Grasp the pull-up bar a little wider than shoulder width with the hands facing away from you. In the start position, you will be hanging with your arms straight and no weight on the ground. Pull your body weight toward the bar until the chin clears the bar, and then return to the start position. Do not use a

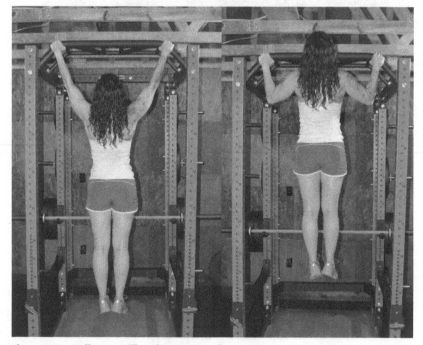

Figure 3.8. Pull-ups. *Will and Renee Peveler.*

swinging motion during this movement. If you want to improve grip strength, you can do dial rod pull-ups.

Push-Ups

Push-ups are designed to increase the muscular endurance of the pectoralis major, anterior deltoid, and triceps brachii (see fig. 3.9). Lie facedown on the floor, placing your hands just wider than the shoulders. From this position, push up until the arms are straight. This is the start position. From the start position, lower your body until the elbows are approximately at a 90-degree angle, and then return to the start position. The weight should be borne by your

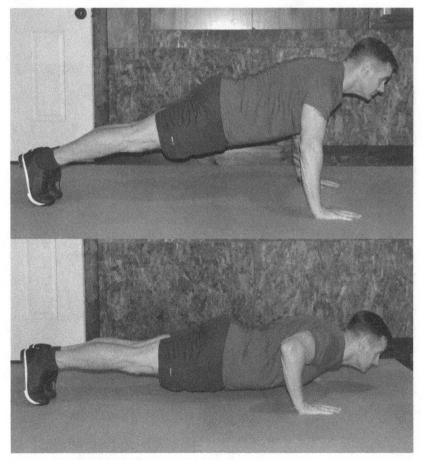

Figure 3.9. Push-ups. *Will and Renee Peveler.*

hands and toes throughout the movement, and your body should stay straight. If you are just beginning, you can conduct a modified push by changing the contact point from your toes to your knees.

Dips

Dips (see fig. 3.10) are designed to primarily work the pectoralis major, triceps, and anterior deltoid. This movement is typically conducted on dip bars. Start with your arms at your side and extended at the elbow. Lower your body until your chest is even with the dip bars, and then push back up. You can alter the percentage of activation of the pectoralis and triceps by leaning your body. The more vertical you are, the more the triceps will be activated, and the more you lean forward, the more the pectoralis major will be activated.

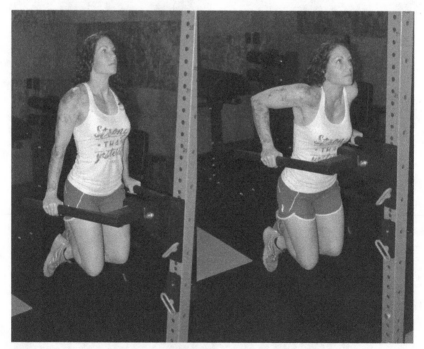

Figure 3.10. Dips. *Will and Renee Peveler.*

Horizontal Rows

The horizontal row (see fig. 3.11) primarily focuses on the latissimus dorsi, rhomboids, trapezius, posterior deltoid, and biceps brachii. To conduct this exercise, you will need a horizontal bar (power rack and barbell will work) and

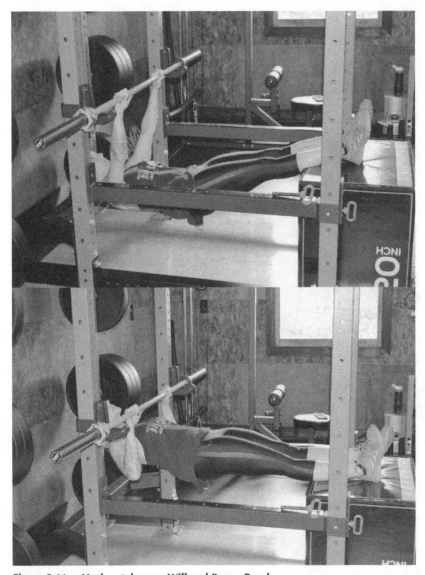

Figure 3.11.   Horizontal rows. *Will and Renee Peveler.*

a bench. From underneath, grab the bar with your hands a little wider than shoulder-width apart and place your feet on the bench. Keeping your body in a straight line, pull up on the bar until your chest touches and then lower back down until your arms are straight.

Lunges

The primary muscles involved in the lunge are the quadriceps, hamstrings, and gluteus maximus (see fig. 3.12). Lunges can be conducted weighted or unweighted. Beginners should start by conducting lunges with no weights and progress to weighted lunges only when ready.

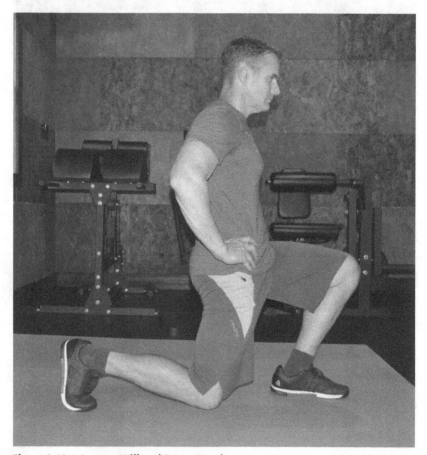

Figure 3.12. Lunges. *Will and Renee Peveler.*

Start by placing your feet about shoulder-width apart. Step forward with your right leg and lower your body until the thigh of the right leg is parallel to the floor and the knee of the left leg is almost touching the floor. Return to the standing position and repeat this process by stepping forward with the left leg. Lunges can also be conducted in a walking manner by leaving the lead foot planted and bringing the rear leg forward into a lunge.

Core Exercises

There is a common misconception that the core muscles are primarily just the abdominal muscles and erector spinae muscles. However, the core is correctly defined as the multitude of muscles (approximately 29) that are designed to stabilize the pelvis and spine. The core muscles are worked during all the previously described lifting movements to stabilize the spine and pelvis throughout the lift. I am, however, going to describe common exercises that focus on the abdominals and the erector spinae. Those truly interested in developing a workout to develop core muscular endurance can expand this portion of their workout by adding more exercises.

Crunches

Crunches are designed to focus on the rectus abdominis and the oblique abdominals. Lie with your back on the floor and place your legs in the air, bending at the hips and knees. You can also conduct the crunch by placing your heels on a bench. Place your arms across your chest and curl your body off the floor until the upper back is clear of the floor. Repeat for as many reps as possible. After completing a set of normal crunches, you can add a set of twisting crunches. From the same start position, curl up, twisting your right shoulder to your left knee, and then return to the start position. On the next rep, curl up twisting the left shoulder to the right knee, and then return to the start position. Repeat this sequence until exhaustion.

Leg Raises

The leg raise is designed to work the abdominal and hip flexor muscles, as shown in fig. 3.13. Lie on your back with your head off the floor, arms at your side, and feet just off the floor. Lift your legs just past 90 degrees of hip flexion and then return to the start position. Keep your legs straight throughout this process.

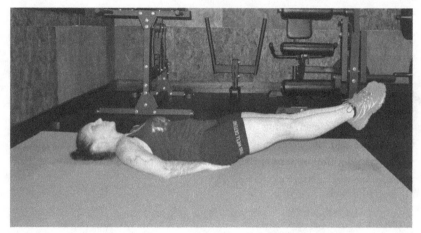

Figure 3.13.   Leg raises. *Will and Renee Peveler.*

Hanging Leg Raises

Hanging leg raises are designed to work the abdominal and the hip flexor muscles (see fig. 3.14). Hang from a bar or rings with your arms straight, and then curl up with your abdominal muscles as you bring your knees to your chest. You can twist to your left and right as you come up to focus more on the obliques.

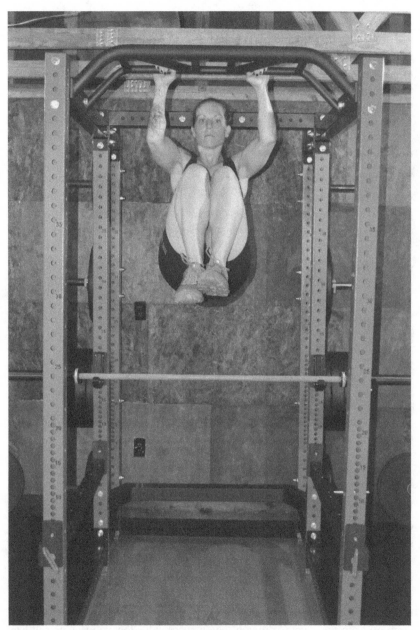

Figure 3.14.   Hanging leg raises. *Will and Renee Peveler.*

Back Extensions

Back extensions work the erector spinae muscles. Lie facedown on the floor with your toes pointed and place your hands behind your head or straight out in front of you. Begin by lifting your upper body off the floor and then return to the start position. You can either keep your lower body in contact with the floor or lift it from the floor in unison with the upper body to work glutes and hamstring muscles.

Roman Chair Back Extensions

The roman chair back extension works the erector spinae, glute, and hamstring muscles (see fig. 3.15). Adjust the roman chair so that the ankles are under the pad and the thighs are on the support pads. Place your hands on or by your ears and bend forward at the waist and then extend your back upward.

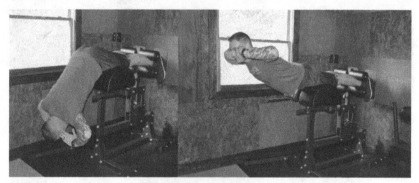

Figure 3.15.   Roman chair back extensions. *Will and Renee Peveler.*

Plyometrics

Plyometrics are a very important tool that will allow you to increase power upon completion of your strength-training phase. A plyometric exercise uses the stretch-shortening cycle to produce a more powerful movement. The stretch-shortening cycle involves an eccentric load that is stretched and then followed up by a powerful concentric contraction. An example of a plyometric movement is when you squat prior to a jump. When you squat down, you are stretching the eccentrically loaded muscles, and the concentric contraction occurs when you jump up from the squat. Adding in plyometrics will allow you to better utilize the stretch-shortening cycle to strike and move with greater power.

When adding in plyometrics, it is important to start slowly due to the heavy eccentric loads. As in all other workouts, make sure that you are using the correct techniques. Below I will discuss a few of the basic lower and upper body techniques that you can use in your training. There are many more valid plyometric exercises that can be used as well.

Box Jumps

When conducting box jumps (see fig. 3.16), choose a height that you can easily accomplish. While increasing height is how you will increase intensity, make sure that you can complete the desired number of repetitions prior to increasing height. Before beginning box jumps, I recommend conducting plyometric jumps from a flat surface. This will allow you to become accustomed to plyometrics before adding in the height of the box. Any jumps that you can do on the box, you can also do without a box. If you choose to purchase a plyometric jump box, I suggest buying a foam box as they are more forgiving on your shins compared to metal or wood boxes.

Begin by standing close enough to the box that you can easily make the jump, and place your feet about shoulder-width apart. Make sure that you have enough space so that you do not hit the box on the way up. Squat down,

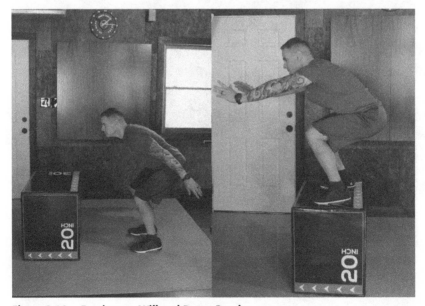

Figure 3.16.   Box jumps. *Will and Renee Peveler.*

moving your arms behind you (countermovement), and then jump up, landing with both feet in the center of the box. Next, jump down and then repeat. If you want to increase the workout, you can add a depth jump when you step off the box. To add the depth jump, step off the box, land on both feet, squat down, and jump again. Each of these movements should be completed in a controlled and fluid motion.

Lateral Box Jumps

Begin by standing next to the box so that your left side is facing the box. Make sure that you are close enough to the box to easily make the jump, but far enough away so that you do not hit the box on the way up. Squat down, moving your arms behind you (countermovement), then jump laterally, landing on the box. Step down on the opposite side, and then repeat the process going the other way. (See fig. 3.17.)

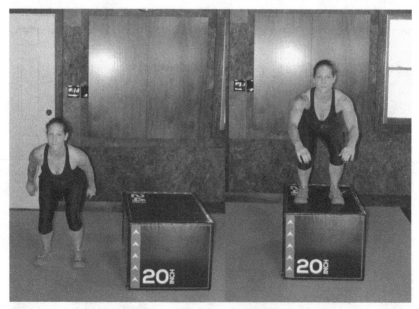

Figure 3.17.   Lateral box jumps. *Will and Renee Peveler.*

Chest Pass

When conducting upper body plyometrics, the use of a plyometric ball provides an optimal workout. Plyometric balls, also referred to as slam balls, wall balls,

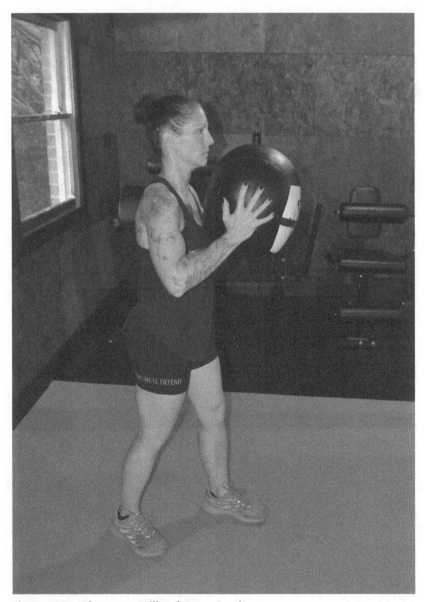

Figure 3.18.　Chest pass. *Will and Renee Peveler.*

and medicine balls, come in different weights and different styles. Some balls are made to bounce, while others are made to minimize bounce. All types work, and you will need to find which you prefer. Plyometric balls come in different weights, so choose a weight that allows you to complete the desired repetitions, while maintaining correct technique.

The chest pass (see fig. 3.18) can be conducted individually or with a partner. If you are conducting the chest pass individually, find a wall that will not be damaged when the ball makes contact. If working with a partner, your partner will catch the ball and then chest-pass it back to you. If the weight of the ball makes it difficult for your partner to safely catch, then take turns on a wall.

Begin by placing your feet about shoulder-width apart. Bring the ball to your chest, creating the eccentric load, and then push the ball away in a quick concentric contraction. If you are working with a partner, you will use the eccentric load from the catch in order to immediately pass the ball back to your partner.

Side Throw

Begin by standing in an athletic stance with your left foot forward and facing the wall. Hold the plyometric ball in both hands and twist to the right, creating the eccentric load. Follow up with a strong concentric contraction, and release the ball as you twist to the left. Repeat this process for the opposite side of the body. (See fig. 3.19.)

Overhead Slam

Begin by placing your feet about shoulder-width apart. Bring the ball above your head, creating the eccentric load. Next, contract concentrically to slam the ball into the floor. (See fig. 3.20.) You may want to choose a non-bouncing plyometric ball for this exercise. A plyometric ball that bounces can easily bounce up and hit you in the face. On the other hand, if you are careful, you can use a bouncing plyometric ball and catch it on the way back up as opposed to picking up a non-bouncing ball off the floor for every repetition.

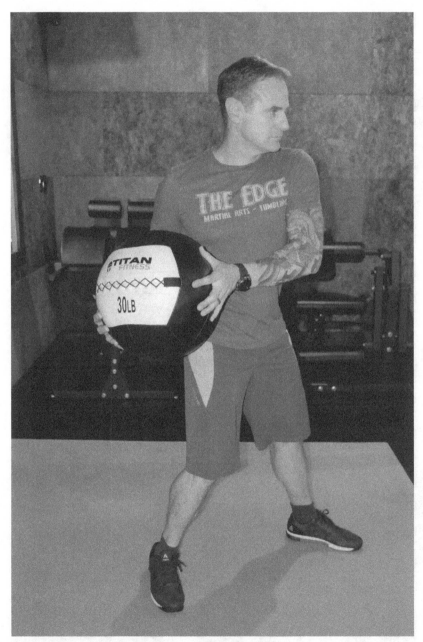

Figure 3.19.   Side throw. *Will and Renee Peveler.*

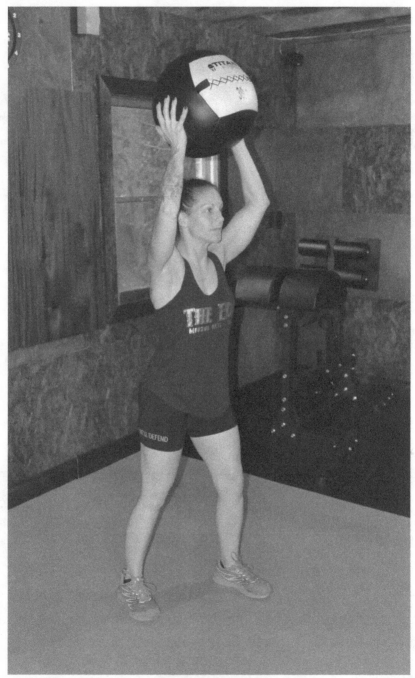

Figure 3.20.   Overhead slam. *Will and Renee Peveler.*

Squat Throw

Begin by placing your feet a little wider than shoulder-width apart. Squat down with a plyometric ball in both hands and between your legs, creating

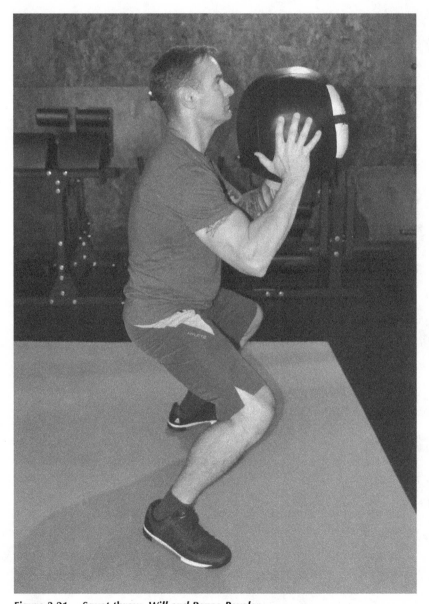

Figure 3.21.   Squat throw. *Will and Renee Peveler.*

the eccentric load. Drive through your heels and upward with your legs as you bring the ball up with your arms until your arms are above your head. Release the ball so that it is over your head and flying behind you after release. (See fig. 3.21.)

Stair Workouts

Stair workouts can be done to increase power, aerobic capacity, anaerobic capacity, or a combination of the three. If you choose to add a stair workout into your program, keep these factors in mind. When stairs are run at a slow pace that you can handle, it will be more of an aerobic workout. However, for most individuals, if you are running stairs, it will be at a higher intensity and therefore it will be an anaerobic workout. Keep in mind that plyometrics are still involved, but not optimized during the anaerobic workout. In order to make it a plyometric workout, decrease your speed and focus on the plyometric aspects; for example, instead of running, you could double leg hop, single leg hop, etc., at a slow pace.

When conducting stair workouts, there are a few things to keep in mind. The first is that stairs are constructed of hard material and are very unforgiving on the body. Always proceed carefully. Make sure that your shoes are tied securely prior to beginning your session, and check periodically throughout. Keep your focus on your technique throughout the exercise, and if you become too fatigued to maintain proper technique, then quit for the day. Most accidents occur because the athlete becomes too fatigued to conduct the movement, a foot catches, and they fall.

Sport-Specific Resistance

You can conduct sport-specific resistance training on your mountain bike by increasing the resistance. One example is over-geared hill repeats, in which hill repeats are performed in a harder gear than you would typically use to climb that specific grade. The increased resistance will force you out of the saddle, pedaling at a slower rate with greater power going into each pedal stroke. Do not add a sport-specific day on top of your off-season resistance training. Instead, use it as one of your resistance training days.

4

DEVELOPING A TRAINING PLAN

The previous chapters of this book discussed basic training principles, basic physiology, basic psychology, and areas of training for mountain biking. These chapters are important because they provide important foundational information that will help you to build a solid training program. Before you can build an optimal program, however, you must have a strong foundation of knowledge. In this chapter, I am going to discuss how to develop a strong training program built around the demands of your everyday life.

When developing your program, there are a few key points to remember. The first is that more than one road exists, and there are many different paths to your destination. Do not get too caught up on designing the perfect program in your first attempt. Design a sound program and make changes as you go based on marked improvements in performance and monitoring adaptation. Keep in mind that as long as you are not overtraining, you are fine. Do not be afraid of making a mistake when developing your program, because you will. Just learn from those mistakes and improve. Understand that your strength-and-conditioning program is an evolving and learning process.

Another key point is to stick with your program. While you do want the program to evolve with your progression, you do not want to move away from the key training principles, which are the foundation of program development. The key training principles will always remain true. One of the biggest mistakes beginners make is that they quit a program before the training has an opportunity to elicit a positive change, and then just jump from program to program with no real gains. Develop a sound program and stick with it. You will need to make alterations to volume and intensity based on how your body responds to the stimulus, but the program itself does not change.

Start small and work your way up to the appropriate volume. Trying to do too much too soon will lead to overuse injuries and maladaptation. Slowly add to your mileage, and only add intensity in when you have developed a sound endurance base. The two most common mistakes beginners make here are to train at race pace every time they ride and to train too often, not allowing time for recovery. It is important to develop a training program that integrates the hard and easy principle and to stay within the assigned intensity parameters for that particular training session. It is also vital that you incorporate dedicated recovery days into your training program.

The last key point is to write everything down as it avoids random disorganized training. This is especially true when trying to work a training program into your everyday life. If you do not schedule and make your training a priority, then things will get in the way and you will keep putting your training off and then have no time to complete it. Take the time and effort to write out your program as it provides a clear map toward your desired goals. When you write your training program down, you are more likely to follow the plan. It is also a good idea to record your progression as well, as this allows you to track your short-term goals.

There are three common approaches to developing a training program. The first involves hiring a coach to help you develop and implement a training program. The second is to use a boxed training plan from an online website or a book. The last approach involves making your own training program, which is what this book is designed to help you do.

COACHING

If you are serious about racing mountain bikes, I would recommend that you hire a qualified coach to help you achieve your goals. Look for a coach with documented coaching experience and a background in exercise science. You want a coach who can develop a sound program and understand the physiological mechanisms behind training and training adaptations. You should also consider the coach's experience as a racer. Coaches with race experience will have a better understanding of what it is like to race mountain bikes and therefore can provide meaningful feedback. However, it is important to note that how fast a coach was when he raced has no bearing on his ability to coach. I have come across great athletes who make horrible coaches.

If you are going to hire a coach, it is vital that you find a qualified coach. To better assess a coach's abilities, interview the athletes that he is currently coaching as well as athletes he has coached in the past. Look to see if the coach possesses any coaching certifications or formal education. USA Cycling has a coaching certification program, with three different coaching levels. The entry-level coaching certification starts at level 3, then moves to level 2, and then level 1. As the coaching progresses, the requirements and experience of the coach increase as well.

Often coaches will have certifications in strength and conditioning as well. The most widely respected strength-and-conditioning certification is the National Strength and Conditioning Association's Certified Strength and Conditioning Specialists (CSCS). This certification requires the coach to possess a four-year degree, pass a rigorous certification exam, and supply continuing education credits after obtaining the certification.

While hiring a coach is ideal, it will require an ongoing budget to pay coaching fees. Not only do you need to research the coaches' credentials, but it's also important to compare fees among different coaches to determine your cost-to-benefit ratio. Keep in mind that like most things in life, you get what you pay for. If you choose to hire a coach, it is one of those areas that you may not want to skimp on.

Online Coaching

Online coaching is another option and has become very popular in recent history. With current technology, a coach can work with you online and never even meet with you face-to-face. Many modern cycling computers contain GPS, heart rate monitoring, and power readings, which allow coaches to evaluate performance, mark adaptations, and prescribe training based on those adaptations. Modern technology makes online coaching a viable option. Prior to committing to an online program, examine all coaching level options, pricing, and reviews.

Online boxed training plans are another option. These training plans provide a day-to-day generic training plan without the interaction of a coach. Boxed plans use a "one size fits all" approach to training. There are no variations to these programs as everyone receives the exact same package. You will receive a weekly training plan to use to improve your mountain biking, but you will receive no coaching or advice on how to alter the program to elicit optimal adaptations.

These rigid programs are designed to provide lower volumes and intensities so that the average person can increase performance while ensuring overtraining does not occur. A boxed training program can be useful for beginners as it provides a safe, structured place to begin training. However, if you want to excel at mountain biking, you will need to make adaptations to the training plan based on your progression and how your body is adapting to the training volume and intensity.

DEVELOPING A TRAINING PROGRAM

This chapter is focused on helping you to develop your own training program. When developing a program, you must take into account your current fitness level, mountain bike experience, work schedule, and family schedule. Developing a program for the first time can seem overwhelming, and it can easily become frustrating. Just like anything else in life, it is important to start the journey by mapping it out and then taking your first step. If you follow the steps below, you will be able to develop your first program. The previous chapters of this book provide you with the foundations needed to develop a strong program. This chapter provides the necessary steps. The information below will give you a generic outline to use and adjust to your specific needs. As you become more advanced, you will need to alter the program to keep up with your advancements.

Determine Goals

The first step in this process is to determine your goals. It is important to set challenging but realistic goals based on your current fitness level, prioritization of mountain biking, and available time to train. If you have never raced before, make sure that you give yourself plenty of time to train prior to your first race. On a piece of paper, write out the following questions and answer them:

- What is my overall goal for mountain biking? (List all goals.)
- What is my current fitness level?
- What is my current mountain bike skill level?
- How much time can I devote to training?
- What are my logistical challenges?
- What budget am I working with?

After answering these questions, set both short- and long-term goals. Your original list of goals will most likely all be long-term goals. Examples of long-term goals may be to participate in a race, lose weight, or become healthier and more active. For each of those long-term goals, set short-term goals. Look at it like a ladder. If you only had the bottom and top rung of the ladder, you would be unable to climb to the top (your long-term goal). You need to add rungs to the ladder (short-term goals) in order to reach the top. Short-term goals give you easily reachable goals to strive for. If you have a long-term goal of racing a 50-mile mountain bike race but have never ridden before, then you should set short-term goals to help you reach the racing goal. Your first short-term goal may be to ride 5 miles of trail at a pace that is below threshold as it is a much easier goal to reach. You would then develop a program that slowly increases distance and intensity over time until you are able to reach your long-term goal of a 50-mile race.

Write down both your long- and short-term goals in your training log so that you have them for future reference. It is important to record your goals as writing them down makes it more likely that you will actively pursue them. Making a short list of goals and posting it somewhere you will see them on a regular basis will help keep you motivated as well.

Baseline Measures

At the start of your program you should be recording baseline measures. There are two primary reasons to conduct a baseline measure. The first is that it allows you to mark the start of your journey and then to measure improvements in performance. The second is that you can use the baseline measures to give you an unbiased look at your current fitness and skill levels. Numbers are impartial and do not lie.

Baseline measures can be either conducted in a laboratory setting or in a field setting. Lab-based measures are conducted in an environmentally controlled setting using precise measurement techniques and laboratory equipment. Some of the common lab-based tests are: $VO_{2\,max}$ testing, threshold testing, and body composition. While lab-based tests are excellent for providing baseline measures and for marking progression, they may not be readily available in your area and may not be cost-effective.

Often field-based methods are used in place of lab-based methods due to the ease of conducting the tests. Field-based tests do not require special training or expensive equipment and are extremely easy to conduct and analyze. Field-based tests can often be conducted at no charge as well.

Time trials are the most common field-based tests used to conduct baseline measures. A time trial requires that you cycle as fast as you can over a fixed distance. Treat the time trial as though it were a race. Make sure that you are well rested and well hydrated prior to conducting a time trial session. Also make sure that the weather is not too hot, too cold, or too windy when conducting your time trial.

You can repeat the time trial session periodically throughout your training season in order to determine whether your program is working. Conduct the time trial on the same course and under the same conditions. You cannot compare times from one mountain bike course to another as every mountain bike course is different. If your times continue to improve throughout the season, then you know that your program is working well. If there is no perceivable change or if times get worse, you need to examine your training program.

Determine Volume

Your training volume will be determined by the frequency and duration of your rides. Training volume can be calculated by a single session, as a weekly volume, or as a multiweek time period. Your actual training volume will be determined by the desired training goal of the training phase you are currently in.

Training volume will be determined by two primary concerns, the first of which involves how many days a week you can train and how many hours per day you can dedicate to training. Due to your individual responsibilities, you may be limited on the number of days a week you can dedicate to training. The second concern deals with the prescribed training volume for that particular training phase. The prescribed training volume will fluctuate throughout your training season.

In order to determine which days during the week you have available for training and the time slots available on those days, write out your weekly schedule. Include your work hours as well as any other recurring commitments. This process will give you a realistic idea of how much time you can devote to training. The allotted time slot should be large enough to not only accommodate actual training time but also logistics such as travel time and cleanup. You should train a minimum of three days per week. However, if you want to excel at mountain biking, then you should train at least five days per week. Advanced riders can train six to seven days per week if they correctly implement recovery training within the training schedule.

You must also determine the duration of each training session. The duration will be highly dependent on the goal of that day's training session and your current fitness level. For example, if it is a long, slow distance session, then the duration could be 40 miles if you are an advanced rider or 6 miles if you are a beginning rider. Due to the varying terrain of mountain bike trails, you may want to consider using time as opposed to distance in order to determine duration. You may be able to complete a 10-mile flat course faster than you could a 6-mile course that requires a lot of climbing.

Determine Intensity

Once you have determined your overall training volume, you will need to determine intensity. When determining training intensity, keep in mind the hard–easy principle, and make sure that you are not training too hard too often. Choose your training zone based on the training goal for that day (recovery, aerobic, threshold, or interval). Unless your periodization block requires multiple days of high intensity for that time period, do not conduct more than two high-intensity sessions per week. You can do more if you are in a specific periodization program that permits a higher level of volume and intensity followed by recovery. Low-intensity days (recovery, aerobic) should be monitored and controlled using a heart rate monitor and defined training zones.

Periodization

Periodization breaks up the training cycle into specific training periods, allowing the athlete to optimize performance. The human body is not designed to continually adapt to high-intensity levels and volumes without recovery. In other words, you cannot train at full speed year-round without allowing for recovery. By breaking your training into specific cycles, you can optimize both stimulus and recovery periods. The idea of periodization is to develop a training plan that allows the athlete to alter training intensity and volume in order to peak during the season with mini peaks throughout the season in order to optimize performance at key competitions. When looking at periodization, there are three primary levels: macrocycle, mesocycle, and microcycle. I will first discuss each level of periodization, and then I will provide example training plans.

Macrocycle

The largest of these cycles is called the macrocycle, and for most traditional sports it covers a year of training (preseason, in-season, and off-season). For mountain biking the macrocycle will be broken up into three distinct phases: preparation (often called preseason), in-season, and off-season. To develop your macrocycle, determine the dates of your first and last planned races for the upcoming year. In most areas of the United States, the mountain bike race season will run from March to October. After determining the length of your season, you will then divide the season into your three phases.

Preparation. The first of the three phases is the preparation phase, which is commonly known as the preseason. The preparation phase will typically last 9 to 12 weeks but can be longer or shorter depending on how important your first races are. During the preparation phase you will focus on increasing volume and intensity, building up to the competition phase. During this phase you will work on increasing your volume first in order to provide a strong base. Once volume has sufficiently increased, you will begin increasing intensity. The beginning, middle, and end of the preparation phase is a good time to conduct physiological testing (time trials, $VO_{2\,max}$, etc.) in order to ensure optimal training and adaptations.

In-season. The in-season phase is commonly referred to as the race season. You will need to establish all the races in which you would like to compete in order to develop your mesocycle (explained below) so that you peak optimally for your key races.

Off-season. The off-season phase serves two main purposes. First, it allows for a decrease in volume and intensity, which helps you to recover both physically and mentally from the race season. Racing places a heavy toll on your physical and mental capacities, and it is easy to become burned out if you do not plan a recovery period. Second, it allows you to not only decrease volume and intensity but to also alter training in order to perform better the following season. Implementing an off-season resistance program, while maintaining an aerobic base, is key to performance improvements the following season. Seasons can be won or lost depending on your off-season training program. The length of the off-season can vary between 6 and 10 weeks based on the length of the race season in your area and your desired length of the following preparation phase. A typical macrocycle for the in-season will go from April to October; the off-season will go from November to January; and the preparation phase will go from February to March.

Mesocycle

The mesocycle is a sub-cycle of the macrocycle and typically covers approximately a four-week period of training, but can range anywhere from one to eight weeks. There are multiple phases that can be used within a mesocycle, which can alter depending on the specific goals of that cycle. You will design your mesocycle so that the training program will alternate volume and intensity by increasing the stimulus to the point at which you will peak so that your performance peaks at the appropriate time. After the peak you will have a brief recovery period followed by increased stimulus toward another peak.

Common phases in a mesocycle are the preparation phase, build phase, peak/competition (taper occurs in this phase), recovery, and transition. You will need to develop mesocycles for your competition, off-season, and preparation macrocycle phases. During the preparation phase, more focus is placed on increasing volume as opposed to increasing intensity. The build phase is designed to increase intensity, which will in turn increase anaerobic threshold and improve race performance.

Tapering occurs after the build phase, allowing the body to recover from the previous stages in order to optimally perform for the upcoming race. Depending on the event, tapering can last one to two weeks. A one-week taper is sufficient for most events. Tapering for a race is often misunderstood and therefore conducted incorrectly. Often athletes will cut their volume and intensity too much or for too long a period of time, resulting in suboptimal performance. When tapering, slightly decrease overall volume seven days prior to the event as well as reduce training intensity and the number of high-intensity days. The two days before the race should be very easy training days, nothing hard or long.

Your training will peak at the competition phase. You can schedule your mesocycle to peak for one race or for multiple races. If you plan to peak for multiple races, do not attempt to hold that peak for more than two to three weeks before moving to a recovery phase.

A one- to two-week recovery phase will follow the competition phase. The recovery phase is vital as it permits your body to fully recover for competition and to move into the next preparation phase leading up to your next race. If it is the last competition phase of the race season, then you will transition into the off-season.

In order to set up your mesocycles effectively, first determine your race schedule for the upcoming season. Choose your races, and prioritize them as A (top priority), B (medium priority), or C (low priority). You should schedule your mesocycles so that you peak for all A races. Peaking for B races is nice but not a priority, and C races are typically considered training races. Now that you have your races scheduled and prioritized, develop your mesocycles to peak at the appropriate times.

If you can travel easily or if you have a number of races to choose from within your local area, you can actually do the reverse of this process. Set up your mesocycles evenly spaced and then pick races that occur when you naturally peak in your designed mesocycle.

Table 4.1 shows an example of a mesocycle where the first priority race occurs eight weeks into the race season. There are two C-level races and one B-level race prior to the first A race. You will treat the B and C races as training races. You can conduct a mini taper if you like or just incorporate the race into your training schedule as a hard day. Your training program for week 9 will depend on your race schedule. If you don't have another A race within the next three weeks, schedule a recovery week and go right back into another preparatory phase. If you have another A race within the next three weeks, schedule a couple days of recovery time and then maintain the peak until after the next A race. Then roll into another mesocycle.

Table 4.1. In-Season Mesocycle Example with B- and C-Level Races Prior to A-Level Race

April				May			
In-Season							
Week 1	Week 2 C Race	Week 3	Week 4 C Race	Week 5	Week 6 B Race	Week 7	Week 8 A Race
Preparation Phase				Build Phase			Taper and Race

The mesocycle for your preparation phase (preseason) will be slightly different than that of your in-season as you will most likely have no preseason races, and if you do, those races should be considered more for fun and training as opposed to placement. During the preseason, you will spend the first part of the season in the preparation mesocycle to focus on increasing your training volume. Remember that your training volume decreases significantly in the off-season. The second mesocycle in the preseason is the build phase where you will focus on increasing intensity while maintaining your volume built during the preparation phase.

Table 4.2. Off-Season Mesocycle Example for Increasing Intensity

February				March			
Preparation Phase (Preseason)							
Week 1	Week 2	Week 3	Week 4	Week 5	Week 6	Week 7	Week 8
Preparation Phase				Build Phase			

During the off-season you will decrease your volume and intensity in order to recover from the race season. The off-season is a good time to work on areas of weakness. For example, if you had trouble with steep climbs during the race season, tailor your off-season to increase your lower body muscular strength and muscular endurance.

Below is an example of your off-season mesocycles. While not shown, you would have a one- to two-week transition period in October. Use that transition period to recover physically and mentally from your race season. Keep in mind that the preparation phase will typically include increases in volume and the build phase will focus on increases in intensity. You will peak at the end of each phase in the off-season, but it will not be a performance peak. Instead, it will be a peak in volume or intensity for that portion of training. Off-season with four mesocycles is shown in table 4.3, and off-season with six mesocycles is shown in table 4.4. You can also have a phase that will focus on a specific area of training (see table 4.5). For example, you can focus a six-week preparation and six-week build phase on resistance training while maintaining your endurance volume and intensity at an off-season level.

Table 4.3. Off-Season Training with Four Mesocycles

November				December				January			
Off-Season											
Week 1	Week 2	Week 3	Week 4	Week 5	Week 6	Week 7	Week 8	Week 9	Week 10	Week 11	Week 12
Preparation Phase			Build Phase			Preparation Phase			Build Phase		

Table 4.4. Off-Season Training with Six Mesocycles

November				December				January			
Off-Season											
Week 1	Week 2	Week 3	Week 4	Week 5	Week 6	Week 7	Week 8	Week 9	Week 10	Week 11	Week 12
Preparation Phase		Build Phase		Preparation Phase		Build Phase		Preparation Phase		Build Phase	

Table 4.5. Off-Season Training with Focus on a Specific Area of Training

November				December				January			
Off-Season											
Week 1	Week 2	Week 3	Week 4	Week 5	Week 6	Week 7	Week 8	Week 9	Week 10	Week 11	Week 12
Preparation Phase						Build Phase					

Microcycle

Now that you know the overall training goals (macrocycle) and have broken those goals down into purposeful training periods (mesocycle), the next step is to determine your weekly training schedule. The microcycle is the weekly training program where you schedule the day-to-day training. While a microcycle typically covers the full week, you can break it down into smaller microcycles within a week time period when needed. For an in-season plan, see table 4.6. For a beginner weekly plan for three days a week, see table 4.7, and for an advanced weekly plan for six days a week, see table 4.8.

Table 4.6.   Example of In-Season Mesocycle Training

Day:	Monday	Tuesday	Wednesday	Thursday	Friday	Saturday	Sunday
Training:	Recovery	Recovery	Mid-Distance Ride, Zone 3	Recovery	Recovery	Long, Slow Distance, Zone 2	Long, Slow Distance, Zone 2

Table 4.7.   In-Season Beginner Weekly Mesocycle Training (Three Days a Week)

Day:	Monday	Tuesday	Wednesday	Thursday	Friday	Saturday	Sunday
Training:	Recovery	Medium Distance, Zone 2	Intervals	Recovery Ride, Zone 1	High-Intensity Ride, Zone 3	Long, Slow Distance, Zone 2	Recovery Ride, Zone 1

Table 4.8.   In-Season Advanced Weekly Mesocycle Training (Six Days a Week)

Day:	Monday	Tuesday	Wednesday	Thursday	Friday	Saturday	Sunday
Training:	Resistance Training	Medium Distance, Zone 2	Easy Ride and Resistance Training	Recovery Ride, Zone 1	Resistance Training	Long, Slow Distance, Zone 2	Recovery

Below are two examples of daily routines for off-season resistance training. The first (table 4.9) provides a minimal resistance plan, and the second (table 4.10) provides a more in-depth plan. You will see gains from either program, but will see slightly greater gains from the in-depth program. You can mix up different exercises for the same muscle groups. For example, you can replace squats with the leg press, or the bench press with the dumbbell press. The sets for most of the exercises are listed as two per exercise but can be increased to three sets per exercise if you choose. More than three would be overkill.

Table 4.9. Off-Season Minimal-Resistance Mesocycle Training Plan

Exercise	Sets	Repetitions
Bench Press	2	8–15
Lat Pull-Down	2	8–15
Squat	2	8–15
Crunches	3	Assigned Number or Volitional Exhaustion
Back Extensions	3	Assigned Number or Volitional Exhaustion

Table 4.10. Off-Season In-Depth Mesocycle Training Plan

Exercise	Sets	Repetitions
Bench Press	2	8–15
Overhead Press	2	8–15
Lat Pull-Down	2	8–15
Squats	2	8–15
Deadlift	2	8–15
Calf Raises	2	8–15
Crunches	3	Assigned Number or Volitional Exhaustion
Back Extensions	3	Assigned Number or Volitional Exhaustion

TRAINING LOG

Throughout the process of creating your training program, it is vital that you put your plan into writing by developing a training log. The training log has multiple purposes that will assist in your training and progression. The first purpose of a training log is to give you a detailed road map to follow. You will know exactly what the daily workout routine will be and will stay focused on your goal and not get sidetracked.

The second benefit is that it will keep you motivated. Research has shown that if you write out your plans in detail, you will be more likely to follow those plans. On days that you may not feel like working out, it will provide that little push to get you going. It helps with accountability.

The third major benefit is that recording your daily workouts allows you to monitor your progression. Improvements in performance occur slowly over time, and often we do not recognize these improvements. Looking back in your training log will help you to assess your progression in a quantitative and detailed manner.

Developing Your Training Log

As your training log will be specific to your individualized program, it would be difficult to find a printed training log that would specifically fit your needs. Luckily with today's technology, creating your own training log with all the specifics you need is very simple and affordable. I will provide key criteria to use when developing your training log. Do not put so much information in your log that it becomes overwhelming and useless. You will need the following information when developing your log:

Date and Time. Record the date and time of the workout for future reference to look for patterns in your training and progression.

Body Weight and Body Fat Percentage. Tracking body weight serves two main purposes: to monitor alterations to body weight over time and to track fluid loss when training in the heat in order to optimize rehydration. When possible, measure body weight before every training session and after a training session as well when training in the heat. Body fat percentage allows you to examine fat and fat-free mass over a period of time but does not need to be done every training session.

Morning Heart Rate. Check morning heart rate to determine readiness for training. An increased morning heart rate over consecutive days could indicate overtraining or dehydration. It also allows you to record adaptations to endurance training as morning heart rate will decrease over time with training.

Type of Training. State the type of training conducted: trail ride, road ride, resistance training, etc.

Volume. For cardiorespiratory training, record the distance and time of the session. For resistance training, record the sets and reps for each exercise. For anaerobic training, record the time, sets, and distances.

Intensity. Record all measures (HR, RPE, etc.) used to determine intensity during the training session. Record time in and time out of the desired training zones when appropriate.

General Comments on the Training Session. General comments provide an opportunity to include other pertinent information (weather, fatigue, injury, sleep, stress levels, etc.).

5

NUTRITION FOR
MOUNTAIN BIKING

O ne of the most important components of an athlete's training program is nutrition. Too often athletes will spend a large amount of time developing and implementing a training program and yet completely ignore any form of nutritional planning. Without the proper nutrition plan, you will not consume enough of the proper nutrients for recovery between bouts or enough to provide adequate fuel to train or compete effectively. The purpose of this chapter is to provide a basic introduction to nutrition in order to optimize mountain bike performance. The discussed guidelines are general in nature and designed for healthy individuals who do not have dietary restrictions. If you are regularly taking medication or have a known illness, check with your physician prior to altering your nutritional intake. If you have dietary restrictions, it is always a good idea to work with a registered dietitian who has a background in sports nutrition and can establish a detailed nutrition plan tailored to your specific needs and goals. Even if you have no dietary restrictions, working with a registered dietitian with a background in sports nutrition would be beneficial.

NUTRIENTS

There are six basic categories of nutrients that are important for an athlete: carbohydrates, fats, proteins, vitamins, minerals, and water. These nutrients are responsible for everything from energy transfer to anabolic processes. Each nutrient plays a specific role in normal body function. Knowing the specific nutrients, how they function, where they originate, and how they impact mountain bike performance will allow you to develop a rational and sustainable nutritional program.

Carbohydrates

Carbohydrates are one of the main fuel sources for the human body. Carbohydrates are ingested and then converted to glucose for transportation in the blood and glycogen for storage. Glycogen is not only important as fuel for athletic performance; it is also the only fuel source that the central nervous system and the brain can utilize. When glycogen stores become low during prolonged exercise, you become fatigued and confused. This is typically termed "bonking" and can be experienced during long hard rides. The human body is limited to roughly 2,000–2,500 kCals of stored glycogen.

The daily recommended intake of carbohydrates will differ depending on whether you are an athlete or nonathlete. For the nonathlete, roughly 50 percent of daily caloric intake should come from carbohydrates, whereas 60 to 70 percent of a mountain biker's daily intake should come from carbohydrates. To more precisely determine carbohydrate intake, the average individual should consume 5 to 6 grams of carbohydrates per kilogram of body mass per day, and endurance athletes should consume 7 to 10 grams per day. The range of 7 to 10 g/kg is highly dependent on the volume and intensity of training. As the training volume or intensity increases so too will the recommended intake.

For example, a 74.83-kg (165-lb) mountain biker would need to ingest between 523.81 and 748.30 grams of carbohydrates each day, depending on training volume and intensity. To give you an idea of what that looks like in food, a cup of plain oatmeal contains about 28 grams of carbohydrates, there are between 35 and 39 grams in a baked potato, and a small serving of pasta will contain about 40 to 50 grams. As you can see, it will take some planning to replenish your carbohydrate stores on a heavy training day.

Not only should you be concerned with the volume of carbohydrates ingested but also with the quality of ingested carbohydrates. Refined grains lose a significant amount of their nutrients during the refining process and should be avoided when possible. Whole grains, fruits, and vegetables are excellent sources of carbohydrates. Limit as many simple carbohydrates (simple sugars) from your diet as possible. Keep in mind that some simple carbohydrates are good, such as those found in fruit and milk. However, many simple sugars are not good, such as those found in ice cream, soda, and candy. Instead focus more on complex carbohydrates (whole grains, vegetables, etc.).

The glycemic index measures the effect of carbohydrate ingestion on blood glucose levels. Foods that are below 50 on the glycemic index have very little effect on blood glucose levels. However, foods that measure above 70 can cause a large increase in blood glucose levels, resulting in a significant spike in insulin (hyperinsulinemia), which in turn results in hypoglycemia (low blood sugar), and then fatigue. For this reason, it is recommended to stay away from foods that are high on the glycemic index. The one exception is during training sessions or when racing. Ingesting foods that are high on the glycemic index during a race or long training session will result in blood glucose spikes when you need them and in turn save the stored glycogen for later use.

Fats (Lipids)

Fats play many different roles in the body. They are used as a major source of energy, assist in thermoregulation, provide protection for vital organs, and assist in the transport of fat-soluble vitamins and the production of hormones. Fats provide a major source of energy during prolonged endurance activities, such as mountain biking. Once ingested, fats are stored as triacylglycerol in the body and provide a large amount of energy per molecule. Triacylglycerols are stored in muscle and in adipose tissue (around organs and just under the skin). The average individual stores approximately 70,000 to 80,000 kCals of fats. This number can obviously vary from individual to individual.

There are three categories of fats: saturated fats, unsaturated fats, and trans fats. Saturated fats can be found in foods such as meats, eggs, milk, and cheese. Unsaturated fats can be either monounsaturated (found in canola oil, sunflower oil, and almonds) or polyunsaturated (found in meats, eggs, nuts, fish, fruits, and vegetables). Trans fats are found naturally in small amounts within meats and dairy products and are not a great concern. However, trans fats that are artificially made through hydrogenation are unhealthy and found in processed foods such as cakes, snacks, and fast foods.

Approximately 30 percent of your daily intake should consist of fats, with the majority coming from unsaturated fats. Less than 10 percent of your dietary intake should come from saturated fats. Stay away from trans fats, as they are detrimental to your health. Also stay away from extremely low-fat diets (<15 percent of daily fat intake), as they can have a strong negative impact on health and performance.

Proteins

Proteins are primarily used for anabolic processes and provide very limited energy during exercise. Proteins are typically only relied on for energy production when glycogen stores are depleted. Proteins are vital in the recovery process as they help rebuild tissue. Excess ingested proteins are not stored in the body and are converted to either triacylglycerol or glycogen for storage. Meat, seafood, poultry, milk, cheese, eggs, and nuts are primary sources of protein in the diet.

As an athlete, you should ingest 1.2 to 2 grams per kilogram of body mass each day. The amount of protein that you need to ingest will be highly dependent on the volume and intensity of your training program. As volume or intensity increases, you will need to increase protein ingestion to support the necessary anabolic processes that are required after training. However, it is important to note that taking in very large amounts of protein can place a strain on the liver and result in dehydration and electrolyte imbalance. But this is typically not a concern for healthy individuals who are not ingesting more than 4 grams per kilogram of body mass per day.

VITAMINS

Vitamins do not provide energy directly. However, they are vital in many of the chemical processes that regularly occur in the human body. Here are some common examples: B vitamins and niacin are a significant part of the chemical process that ultimately results in the production of adenosine triphosphate (ATP); vitamin D is important for bone density; and vitamin C assists in iron absorption, to name only a few.

For most healthy mountain bikers who maintain a well-balanced diet, there is no need to supplement with vitamins. However, for those who may not be eating an adequate diet, vitamin supplementation may be beneficial.

MINERALS

Minerals are inorganic nutrients required for normal body function.

Calcium

The most abundant mineral in the human body is calcium, which plays a key role in many chemical processes in the body. Human bone mass is made up of 60 to 70 percent calcium, and therefore it is critical for maintaining a healthy bone density. Calcium is also stored in muscle and plays a major role in the chain of events that result in a muscle contraction. Calcium is primarily obtained by consuming dairy products.

Iron

Iron is another mineral that is necessary to maintain normal body function. It is used in the formation of hemoglobin and myoglobin. Iron is not required in large amounts and can easily be obtained through the ingestion of meat and some plant sources such as potatoes or beans. However, plants provide insufficient amounts of iron by themselves. Unless you are iron deficient or a vegetarian, there is no real need to take iron supplements. Supplementing with too much iron can also have a negative health impact.

Iron-deficient anemia results from low iron levels in the body and presents as a feeling of fatigue due to a decrease in hemoglobin. Certain populations are more prone to the development of iron-deficient anemia. Female athletes are susceptible due to iron loss occurring during the menstrual cycle, through heavy sweating during training, and through the high hemoglobin turnover rate associated with heavy training regimens. Vegetarians are also at risk due to the limited availability of iron in plants.

Phosphorus

Phosphorus is another mineral that is widely used in the body for various chemical processes. It binds with calcium to form calcium phosphate, which is vital for bone growth and development. Phosphorus is also important for protein synthesis and responsible for the formation of ATP. Phosphorus is consumed easily in most diets and can be found in meats, dairy products, and cereals.

Electrolytes

There are three primary minerals in the human body that are considered electrolytes: chlorine, sodium, and potassium. Electrolytes are electrically charged ions that are found within the fluids of the body. It is important to keep electrolytes balanced in the body as they help maintain homeostasis. Sodium and potassium are two electrolytes that athletes should be aware of when developing a sound nutrition plan. It is often stated that Americans ingest too much sodium within their diet, resulting in high blood pressure. While this is a true statement and you do not want to take in excess sodium, athletes need to ingest greater amounts of sodium in relation to the average sedentary individual. This is due to the excess sodium lost during training through sweat. The more you sweat, the more sodium you will lose. This is why ingestion of sodium after exercise in the heat is recommended and why many sports drinks will contain sodium. This is also why pickle juice is recommended for reducing muscle cramps in the heat. It isn't actually the "pickle" portion of the juice that is beneficial but is instead the high concentration of sodium found within pickle juice.

Potassium also helps maintain homeostasis through the electrical balance within the cells and is found in many common foods such as bananas, citrus fruits, and potatoes. A small amount of potassium is also found in fish. Individuals who maintain a healthy diet will acquire sufficient potassium without supplementation.

WATER

Water is vital for both sustaining life and sport performance as the human body is composed of approximately 60 to 70 percent water. Blood plasma consists of approximately 90 percent water and is responsible for the transportation of gasses, nutrients, and other compounds throughout the body. Blood plasma is also responsible for thermoregulation as water is an excellent conductor of heat. When exercising it is important to develop and maintain a sound hydration plan.

During exercise water is lost through sweating and through respiration. As you sweat, water moves from the interstitial space and exits the body through eccrine sweat glands in order to evaporate on the skin and cool the body. Water from plasma will move from the blood vessels into the interstitial space to replace the lost water and equalize pressure between the blood vessels and interstitial space. This action results in an overall decrease in plasma volume and a decreased ability to cool the body. Water loss during exercise can negatively impact both performance and health. A water loss that is equivalent to approximately a 2 percent decrease in body mass will negatively impact performance. As the water loss reaches a 5 percent decrease in body mass, there will be a negative impact on health. One of the primary health concerns with dehydration is the inability to properly dissipate heat, leading to heat-related illnesses.

Because of the high volume of fluid lost during prolonged exercise, the recommendations for daily water intake for average individuals (1.5 to 3 liters/day) cannot be applied to mountain bikers. Due to this fact, it is important to focus on replacing the volume of fluid that is lost during training or competition.

One of the best methods for determining water loss is to weigh yourself both before and after your training session. It is important to weigh unclothed before and after so that you are not measuring the volume of water retained in your clothes after the training session. The difference in weight between the before and after measures represents the volume of fluid lost during the session. The next step is to replace each pound lost with approximately 24 ounces of fluid. This rehydration recommendation assumes that you were properly hydrated prior to the exercise bout.

NUTRITION AND EXERCISE

To promote recovery, positive adaptations, and increased performance, you should spend some time developing a sound nutritional strategy. There are four basic areas to consider when developing a nutrition plan for exercise. The first is the type of nutrition, carbohydrates, lipids, proteins, etc., you will ingest. The second involves the quality of nutrition. Choose high-quality foods. The third involves the volume, or caloric intake, of your nutrition plan. Finally, the fourth consideration deals with the timing of the meals.

Before Cycling

When examining prerace/pretraining nutrition, the timing, quantity, and type of nutrition must be addressed. Meals should be eaten two to four hours prior to competition. Eat light foods that will provide adequate nutrition but that do not take a prolonged time to digest. For example, slow-cooked oatmeal, bagels, or fruits make an excellent breakfast, but stay away from the sausage, egg, and cheese sandwich.

Training or racing without eating prior can negatively impact performance and possibly health, especially on high-intensity days. Not eating prior to a workout can lead to low blood glucose levels, resulting in feelings of fatigue and dizziness. There is a larger effect at higher intensities due to an increased reliance on glycogen and glucose as primary energy sources. At race pace during a 15-mile mountain bike race, you will utilize 100 percent of your glucose and glycogen as a fuel source. Low blood glucose levels occur most commonly in individuals who skip breakfast for their morning training.

It is also not recommended to eat a large meal just prior to a training bout or race as it will often leave you feeling sluggish and with gastrointestinal distress. During exercise, blood flow will be directed to areas that need it most, such as the working muscles and the skin for cooling. It will also be redirected from areas that need it the least, such as the digestive tract. After eating a meal, blood is redirected to the digestive tract in order to properly digest the food. So, if a meal is eaten prior to exercise, these two systems are at odds. During exercise, inadequate blood flow will be redirected to the digestive system in an attempt to properly digest a meal, leading to gastrointestinal distress.

In general, it is recommended to avoid most foods that are high on the glycemic index. However, ingesting carbohydrates that are high on the index prior to the start of exercise will help spare glycogen during an endurance event lasting longer than an hour. Carbohydrates high on the glycemic index will increase blood glucose levels fairly quickly, which in turn will spare glycogen stored in the liver. Carbohydrates, such as sports gels, can be ingested approximately 5 to 10 minutes prior to the start of exercise. Supplementing with carbohydrates is only recommended for exercise lasting longer than an hour. Do not ingest sports gels more than 10 minutes prior to the start of the event, as this could cause an early blood glucose spike, leading to an overshoot of insulin, low blood sugar levels, and fatigue.

During Cycling

During training sessions and races that last longer than an hour, you will need to take in carbohydrates. Glycogen stores are topped off at around 2,000 to 2,500 kCals in the human body and therefore become a limiting factor for energy production through oxidative processes during prolonged exercise. As mentioned, ingesting carbohydrates increases blood glucose levels and therefore spares glycogen stores in the liver, offsetting glycogen depletion and the resulting fatigue. Keep in mind that glycogen is utilized at a much faster rate during high-intensity exercise.

When riding at high intensity for longer than an hour, you should ingest 30 to 60 grams of carbohydrates every 45 to 60 minutes of exercise. This is also true of cycling at lower intensities that last longer than 90 minutes. Choose carbohydrates that are easily digested and high on the glycemic index so as to enter the system quickly. Energy gels and sports drinks are typical choices. In comparison, sports bars enter the system at a slower rate. However, taking in solid foods on a long ride can help offset hunger as well as provide the needed carbohydrates.

When choosing what food source to use during training and racing, there are important aspects to consider. First, what is in the supplement? The nutrition label located on the package tells you how many carbohydrates are contained inside and what other supplements it may provide (protein, caffeine, etc.) as well. Another consideration is taste, which is especially true of sports drinks. If you do not like the taste, you will consume the substance less often, which will destroy your nutritional plan for that race and could result in greater dehydration. The last thing to consider is how your body reacts to the supplement. It is important to know how your body responds to a specific gel, bar, or drink, because the last thing you want to have to deal with is gastrointestinal distress during the race. Always try a new product on a training day prior to using it in a race.

It is vital to remain hydrated when training and racing. This rule is even more critical on hot and humid days as you will lose a greater amount of fluid on those days. As mentioned, dehydration results in a decrease in performance and leads to heat-related illnesses. You can hydrate with water, sports drinks, or a combination of both. Hydrating with water during sessions lasting less than an hour and a half will be sufficient in most cases. High-intensity activities lasting an hour and a half could benefit from supplementing fluid intake with a sports drink. However, in activities lasting longer than an hour and a half, it would be beneficial to use a sports drink to provide hydration, electrolyte replacement, and carbohydrates.

It is impossible to completely maintain hydration levels during a long training session or a race in the heat, resulting in dehydration. Therefore, it is vital that you develop a hydration plan and stick with it throughout the session. Thirst is a mechanism that lets us know that dehydration is setting in and that we need to drink. During exercise, if you wait until you are thirsty to drink, it is already too late and you have already begun a downward spiral that can lead to decreased performance and the development of a heat-related illness. Therefore it is vital to ingest fluids throughout the session.

Wearing a hydration pack when mountain biking is a great way to stay hydrated throughout the ride. Hydration packs allow you to drink easier when on a mountain bike, and therefore you will drink more often. All you have to do with a hydration pack is grab the tube, place the mouthpiece in your mouth, and drink. This does not require a great amount of coordination, and once the mouth piece is in your mouth, you can ride with both hands while you drink.

When you finish drinking, just drop the mouthpiece until you need it again. Using a water bottle takes more time and coordination, and therefore you will drink less often.

Hyponatremia, a fluid–electrolyte imbalance, is not typical in shorter races and is much more common in ultra-endurance events. So, unless you are doing longer mountain bike races (e.g., a 100-mile race), hyponatremia most likely will not be a concern. Hyponatremia occurs when electrolyte levels are extremely low, affecting the ratio of fluid and electrolytes. The imbalance created by a high concentration of water and low concentration of sodium can result in the following: headache, nausea, cramping, seizures, coma, heart attack, and death. Hyponatremia occurs during prolonged events where the athletes ingest large volumes of fluid without replenishing lost electrolytes, resulting in an electrolyte imbalance. Taking in electrolytes during prolonged exercise will help offset this imbalance.

After Cycling

Recovery is an important component of any training program, and nutrition is key in the recovery process. What you ingest after a workout is just as important as before and during a workout. Training applies the necessary stress for positive adaptations and eventual performance increases to occur. However, this stress results in catabolic responses during exercise. It is the anabolic process, which occurs after exercise, that ultimately results in improved performance. Post-exercise recovery not only helps with the anabolic processes but also begins the refueling process.

You must start refueling within one to two hours after completion of exercise. The typical recommendation to optimize recovery is within 45 to 60 minutes. The four primary nutrients to ingest are water, electrolytes, carbohydrates, and proteins. Replace each pound of fluid lost through sweating with approximately 24 ounces of fluid. Use of a sports drink can be beneficial for both fluid and electrolyte replacement.

Carbohydrates and proteins should be ingested using a 4:1 ratio (4 grams of carbohydrates to 1 gram of proteins). Carbohydrates are necessary for replenishing glycogen stores, and proteins are vital for supporting the anabolic processes after exercise. You cannot completely replenish glycogen stores directly after a workout; it will be an ongoing process throughout the rest of the day. Ingesting protein after exercise also assists in glucose and amino acid uptake into the muscles as well as influencing insulin levels. These factors are why the 4:1 ratio has been so successful during the recovery process. Recovery sports drink mixes that provide the necessary 4:1 ratio have been shown to be very effective at aiding recovery. Research has demonstrated that chocolate milk provides the same ratio and the same benefits.

BODY COMPOSITION

Body composition is the composition of the body in relation to fat and fat-free mass (muscle, bone, tissue, etc.). One of the most accurate and most used methods for determining body composition is body fat percentage, which examines the percentage of fat to fat-free mass. For example, a body fat recording of 15 percent indicates that the individual's body mass is 15 percent fat and 85 percent fat-free mass. Monitoring body fat percentage is an excellent way to track changes in your body composition.

For General Health

Many people begin mountain biking for health reasons and the desire to get into better shape. Currently in America, more than 65 percent of people are classified as overweight and more than 30 percent are classified as obese. Being overweight or obese can result in various negative health conditions, such as hypertension, high cholesterol (LDL) levels, type II diabetes, cardiovascular disease, certain types of cancer, gall bladder disease, joint problems, breathing problems, and all-cause mortality. Keep in mind that overweight individuals who are physically active are less likely to develop cardiovascular disease than individuals who are thin but sedentary.

If you are participating in mountain biking for health reasons or because you enjoy the activity, you need not worry too much about body composition. By training and eating right, body composition will take care of itself over time. The recommended body fat percentage range is 8 to 19 percent for males and 17 to 28 percent for females. Maintaining a healthy body composition within these recommended ranges is ideal for promoting optimal health. Classification of overweight begins at a body fat percentage greater than 20 percent for men and 30 percent for women. As body fat percentage increases beyond the initial classification of overweight, health risk increases significantly. It is important to note again that individuals who are overweight but routinely physically active are four times less likely to develop cardiovascular disease compared to thin individuals who do not participate in physical activity. Remember that having too little body fat can also have a negative impact on health. The essential body fat percentage for normal bodily functions is 4 percent for males and 12 percent for females.

For Competition

If you wish to race mountain bikes, you will need to be a little more concerned with body composition. Overall body mass, regardless of body composition, affects mountain bike performance. The greater the mass, the greater the power requirements for climbing hills on a bike. As an athlete you do not want to decrease your overall mass by decreasing lean muscle mass. Instead, you want to decrease overall mass by decreasing body fat.

The recommended body fat ranges for body composition for competitive mountain bikers are 4 to 10 percent for males and 12 to 20 percent for females. While a low body fat percentage may be desirable for competition, there are a few factors you must consider. The first is that a low body fat composition is very difficult to achieve and maintain. The closer an athlete gets to the lower end of the recommended athletic range, the greater the risk of decreased performance and compromised health. The second consideration is that not everyone will respond in the same manner to decreased body fat percentages. I have worked with elite-level cyclists whose performance dropped when their body fat percentage became too low, even though it was above the recommendations for an elite-level racer. When or if you get down to the lower range, make sure that you carefully monitor both performance and health. The goal is to be as light as possible without negatively impacting health or performance.

Measuring Body Composition

If you are serious about performance, you will want to track changes in body composition over time. Different methods for determining body composition are described in this section, along with the advantages and disadvantages of each. Choose a method that is both accurate and feasible.

Body Mass Index

Body mass index (BMI) is solely based on height and weight. It provides a simple and easy way to determine if an individual is underweight, normal, overweight, or obese and can be calculated using either the metric or the English/imperial system. Formulas for both systems have been provided below.

English $BMI = 703 \times weight\ (lb) \div height^2\ (inches^2)$

Metric $BMI = weight\ (kg) \div height^2\ (M^2)$

If your BMI is <18.5, you are considered underweight; normal BMI falls between 18.5 and 24.9; overweight is considered to be between 25 and 29.9; and obese is classified as a BMI ≥ 30.

Body mass index is an excellent tool for estimating body composition for large-scale populations, but not so much for the individual athlete. The reason for this is the fact that muscle is denser than fat and therefore weighs more. At the time of this writing, I weigh 194 pounds and my height is 71.75 inches. This would make my BMI 26.49, classifying me as overweight. However, my body fat is at 8 percent and I am not overweight. This demonstrates the primary disadvantage of relying on BMI to determine body composition when working with athletes.

Bioelectrical Impedance

Bioelectrical impedance systems use electrical currents in order to estimate body fat percentage. These systems require contact with either the hands or the feet. Once contact is made, the system passes an electrical current through the body to measure resistance to flow. Lean body tissue contains high concentrations of water, and therefore the electrical current passes easily. Fat contains little water and therefore provides resistance to flow. As fat stores increase, resistance to flow also increases. It is a fast and easy method for determining body composition. However, bioelectrical impedance systems are neither reliable nor accurate.

Bioelectrical impedance systems rely heavily on the ability of the electrical current to easily flow through water, therefore hydration levels significantly impact body fat percentage estimates. Your hydration levels during training will continuously fluctuate, especially in the hotter months, resulting in large fluctuations of bioelectrical impedance readings. Due to the large fluctuations in hydration levels and the inherent variability in these machines, I do not recommend them for measuring and tracking body composition.

Hydrostatic Weighing

Hydrostatic weighing (underwater weighing) has long been considered the gold standard for determining body composition. This method is based on Archimedes' principle, which states that the weight of water displaced by the body is equivalent to the buoyant forces acting on that body. Lean body mass (muscles, bones, organs, etc.) has greater density than water and therefore sinks, and fat is less dense than water and therefore floats. The amount of lean mass and fat mass will determine how buoyant an individual is in water.

While hydrostatic weighing is considered the gold standard, the process requires large specialized equipment and trained professionals. This method involves the use of a water tank large enough for a human to completely submerge under water without touching the sides or bottom of the tank. The athlete must also be physically able to completely submerge, exhale as much air as possible, and remain still long enough to obtain a steady measure of underwater weight. This process makes it difficult for those who are uncomfortable underwater.

Dual-Energy X-Ray Absorptiometry

Dual-energy X-ray absorptiometry (DXA) determines body composition through the use of two low-energy X-ray beams and has the ability to accurately measure density and distinguish between fat and fat-free mass. Due to this method's accuracy and reliability, it is now often considered the best way to determine body composition. However, the DXA system is extremely expensive and requires very specialized skill to operate.

Calipers

More than any of the methods previously mentioned, I recommend the use of skin-fold calipers for determining body composition. Skin-fold calipers are accurate, inexpensive, easy to learn to use, and far more accessible and affordable than the other methods. Skin-fold calipers work by pinching a fold of skin and fat and measuring the thickness of the fold. From the skin-fold measurements, total fat stores are estimated using simple formulas. Skin-fold calipers cost anywhere from $25 to $200. The major differences between a lower- and higher-cost caliper are accuracy and durability.

Conducting skin-fold testing is relatively simple but does take some practice to master. There are different tests used to measure skin folds, but the three-site test is the most widely used. The most common body sites used for men are the chest, abdomen, and thigh. The three most common sites for females are the triceps, iliac, and thigh.

When conducting skin-fold measures, it is important to accurately measure each site as described: Position the hand so that the fingers point down, and fold the skin between the thumb and index finger as shown in figure 5.1. Once your fingers are positioned over the correct spot, pinch the skin, bringing it up into a fold. For an accurate measurement, pinch skin and fat only. Too large a pinch typically results in getting muscle, which produces inaccurate measurements. Next, place the caliper pincers directly below your thumb and index finger with the gauge facing up so that you can read it. Once the caliper is in position, allow the calipers to close on the fold by slowly releasing the lever. Do not release the skin fold with your fingers until you record the measurement and remove the calipers. If you release the skin fold prior to the calipers, it can be slightly painful. Take three to four measurements at each site to ensure consistent readings. It is important to measure precisely where described in order to obtain valid measurements. It is also important to be consistent with your measurements. Figure 5.1 and the following instructions will provide you the necessary information to conduct a simple three-site test.

Chest

The chest site is located along the outer edge of the pectoralis major at the midpoint of the muscle. The skin fold should be in line with the outer edge of the muscle (see fig. 5.1).

Abdomen

The abdomen site is located in line with the navel and one inch toward the side. Fold the skin vertically, not horizontally.

Iliac

The iliac site is located just above the hip bone. Fold the skin in line with the natural crease at the hip bone.

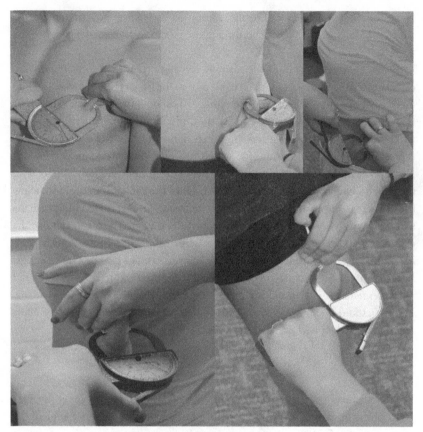

Figure 5.1. Skin folds. *Will Peveler.*

Triceps

The triceps sites are located at the back of the arm, centered and halfway between the shoulder and elbow. Fold the skin vertically.

Thigh

The thigh site is located on the center line of the thigh halfway between the hip and the patella. Fold the skin vertically. When working with athletic women, it can be difficult to properly obtain the correct measurements. As the thigh is a primary storage location for fat in women and athletic women have significant muscle mass in the legs, it may take a little harder pinch in order to accurately measure.

Once you have recorded all three sites, take the sum of the readings and plug the necessary data into the following equations:

Men   Body Density = 1.10938 – (.0008267 × sum of skin folds) + (.0000016 × [sum of skin folds]^2) – (.0002574 × age)

Women   Body Density = 1.0994921 – (.0009929 × sum of skin folds) + (.0000023 × [sum of skin folds]^2) – (.0001392 × age)

This first step gives you the estimated body density for the three-site skin-fold test. Once body density has been established, the next step is to determine body fat percentage using the following formula:

Body Fat% = (4.95 ÷ Body Density) – 4.50 × 100

Example Equation

Male: Age = 25; Chest = 5, Abdominal = 9, Thigh = 4 (Total = 18)
Body Density = 1.10938 – (.0008267 × 18) + (.0000016 × [18]^2) – (.0002574 × 25)
BD = 1.088
Body Fat% = (4.95 ÷1.088) – 4.50 × 100 = 4.96 percent

WEIGHT MANAGEMENT

One of the reasons, even if it is not the main reason, that people become involved in mountain biking is to get in shape and lose weight. There are a few important concepts to keep in mind when pursuing your goal of weight loss. The first and foremost is patience. No one puts on excess weight overnight, and therefore it is unrealistic to believe that you can lose it overnight. Remain patient, avoid undue frustration, and stick with the plan. It is very common to become frustrated with your progression. When things get frustrating, ask yourself: Do I want to be standing here a year from now having lost weight, or do I want to be standing here a year from now saying I wish I would have stuck with it and lost weight? Tracking your weight loss over time will help you become less frustrated.

Second, recognize that weight loss is not an easy process. You must be prepared for hard, physical work in order to achieve your goal. Additionally, you will need to implement a healthy diet to accomplish your goal in a safe and productive manner. Ignoring these simple facts will result in frustration and failure.

Finally, it is important to understand that not everyone responds to weight loss in the same manner. Do not compare your weight loss to another's. This is unrealistic and counterproductive. However, it does not mean that you cannot work in a group toward the same goal. As a matter of fact, working with a support group can be very beneficial. Just do not compare your journey with other members of the group.

Factors that Affect Weight Management

Genetics

Genetics play a major role when it comes to body composition. Research shows that children of overweight parents are much more likely to be overweight than children of non-overweight parents. How body fat is distributed in the body is also strongly affected by genetics. It is easier for some people to lose weight while others continuously struggle. However, this does not mean that you are fated to be overweight just because you have a genetic predisposition toward weight gain. All it means is that you need to be more careful of how you eat and that you need to exercise on a regular basis.

Lifestyle

While genetics is one of the key factors in determining body composition, it is lifestyle choices that have the greatest effect on body composition. Lifestyle is defined as the daily choices we make every day that affect how we live our lives. The two key lifestyle choices that affect body composition are physical activity and diet.

Eating out often is one of the common mistakes people make. Food offered at sit-down and fast-food restaurants typically provides more calories in one meal than most people need in one day. At this point, I am only focusing on the caloric content and not the nutritional value of the food. Also, keep in mind that this is a generic statement that covers the vast majority of restaurants and that there are restaurants that provide good portion sizes and healthy options.

It would be unrealistic to never eat out or grab something from a fast-food restaurant. Here are a few guidelines that can help you when you do choose to eat out. The first recommendation requires a little preplanning on your part. Determine the caloric content of the foods that are offered at the restaurant you plan to visit. Many restaurants provide this information on their online menu.

Another option is to decrease your portion size. Many restaurants will have different options when it comes to portion size, which allows you to order the portion size that best suits your needs. If there is only one option for portion size and it is too large for you, simply do not eat it all. Just because you order the meal does not mean that you have to eat all of it in one sitting. Too often I have ordered a meal, eaten the entire thing, and then felt miserable afterward. One way to avoid this scenario is to portion your meal when you receive it, only eat the prescribed portion, and take the rest home for another meal. At one of my favorite restaurants I will order a pasta dish and divide it into three servings and get three large meals out of it. If you do not have the willpower to stop eating when you are full, then ask for a "to go" box at the beginning of the meal and place the portion that you do not plan to eat in the box to take home. If you are eating with someone who has similar taste, you can also consider sharing a meal.

Preparing and eating meals at home, if done correctly, is the best option when it comes to managing body composition. Ideally, you want to prepare meals from fresh foods that are not excessively processed. Eating healthy at home is not as expensive as one might think, and you will discover that it is much less expensive than eating out. Another misconception is that you have to spend hours in the kitchen in order to cook healthy meals. While the time to cook a meal does vary, depending on what you are cooking, there are many healthy meals that can be prepared quickly. If you are not familiar with healthy cooking, consider buying a cookbook that focuses on the subject. You will soon find healthy, tasty meals that are easy to prepare.

Even when eating healthy at home, be aware of portion sizes. Modern dishware has gotten larger over time, and if you fill your plate you will probably take in more calories than you need. Most of us were raised on "cleaning" our plate before leaving the table in order not to waste food. While the logic behind this practice is understandable, it is much better to listen to your stomach and stop eating when you are full.

Meal planning is one method that will save you time and effort and allow for healthy meals. The first step to eating healthy begins when you make your grocery list. Making a healthy grocery list and sticking to that list will help eliminate unhealthy eating, and prevent those impulse buys just because something looks good. If you do not buy junk food, you can't eat junk food. It is also not a good idea to grocery shop after a hard workout when you are tired and hungry. Whenever I shop when I am hungry, my grocery basket always seems to be fuller and filled with some less-than-healthy choices.

Always read the nutrition label when purchasing foods in order to determine amounts of cholesterol, sodium, sugar, calories, etc. When examining the caloric content, it is important to determine how many calories per serving as well as serving size. For example, a serving size may be a half cup and a caloric content of 80 calories per serving. But if you ingest a full cup, then the caloric content would be 160 calories.

Another valuable tool for weight management is a nutritional log. Keeping a nutritional log of everything you eat for the day will allow you to determine the volume of calories consumed. This is an eye opener for many individuals who do not realize how many calories they ingest in a single day, and can be a very effective tool for demonstrating the need for a lifestyle change. When keeping a nutritional log, record everything that you ingest and the calorie content of each. Keep in mind this includes everything you eat, including snacks, and everything you drink. Keeping a nutrition log is tedious work and may not be something that you want to maintain on a permanent basis, but try to keep a log until you have made the proper adjustments to your eating habits.

Goals for Weight Management

Setting goals for your weight management program is an important part of the process of losing weight. Weight loss will be challenging for everyone, and therefore it is important to set realistic long- and short-term goals. Setting a weight-loss goal of 10 pounds over an 8- to 10-week period would be realistic for most individuals, whereas setting a goal of losing 10 pounds in a week would be very unrealistic. Setting unrealistic goals will negatively impact your weight-management program and lead to serious discouragement. As mentioned previously, losing weight takes a long period of time and you must remain patient. Setting short-term goals in conjunction with your long-term goal will allow you to monitor small steps in progression over time and help limit discouragement.

Safe, effective, and sustainable weight loss is considered to be roughly a loss of one pound per week. There will be weeks when you lose more and others when you lose less. There may even be times when you gain a little. Understand that weight will fluctuate, and do not become discouraged.

In order to optimally set weight-management goals, know what your current body composition is as well as your desired body composition. The first step in this process is to determine your current body weight and body fat percentage, discussed previously in this chapter. The next step is to determine your desired body composition. While elite-level mountain bikers have very low body fat percentages (males as low as 4 percent and females as low as 11 percent), this is an unrealistic goal for many. Typically, the goal of 8 to 19 percent for males and 17 to 28 percent for females is a good and achievable goal. I understand that I have provided a wide range of body fat percentages for both male and female mountain bikers. However, where you would like to be in that range is a personal choice. Once you have determined your current weight, current body fat percentage, and desired body fat percentage, use the formulas below to determine weight loss.

> (Current Weight) × (Current Body Fat Percentage) = Weight of Fat in the Body
> Current Weight – Weight of Fat in the Body = Weight of Fat-Free Mass
> 1 – Desired Body Fat Percentage = Percent Fat-Free Mass
> Weight of Fat-Free Mass ÷ Percent Fat-Free Mass = Desired Body Weight
> Current Body Weight – Desired Body Weight = Desired Weight Loss

Example Equation

> Male: 210 lbs: Currently 22% Body Fat; Desires 12% Body Fat
> (210 lbs) × (.22) = 46.2 lbs
> 210 lbs – 46.2 lbs = 163.8 lbs
> 1 – .12 = .88
> 163.8 lbs ÷ .88 = 186.14 lbs
> 210 lbs – 186.14 lbs = 23.86 lbs

In the example above, a 210-pound male with a body fat percentage of 22 was able to determine that his desired body weight would be 186.14 pounds and that he would need to lose 23.86 pounds to reach the goal of 10 percent body fat. Remember, the goal is really about body composition and not weight. Because muscle is denser than fat, it weighs more. As you train and improve, muscle will hypertrophy over time and increase the weight of your lean body mass. Therefore, you will need to periodically rework the equations and adjust your weight-management goals.

Caloric Balance

In its most simplistic form, weight management is all about caloric balance. When your caloric consumption is equivalent to your caloric expenditure, your body composition will remain at a near constant. If you consume more calories than you expend, you will gain weight. If you consume less calories than you expend, then weight will decrease over time. It would be extremely difficult to count the precise number of calories consumed and expended during a single day. However, counting calories in and calories out as precisely as possible will give you a good place to start. Some days you will take in slightly more than you use and others you will take in slightly less than you use. However, an overall deficit will balance out over time, resulting in weight loss. Keep in mind that if caloric intake remains too low for too long, metabolism can decrease, which is counterproductive to weight management. Extremely low caloric intake can also lead to catabolism of lean tissue, primarily muscle, in the body, which is also counterproductive.

It is commonly recommended that males consume between 2,000 and 2,500 calories per day and that females take in between 1,500 to 1,800 calories per day. It is important to keep in mind that these recommendations are for the average male and female who do not participate in regular athletic training, and therefore would represent insufficient calories for most mountain bikers. A cross-country mountain bike race can burn more calories than the average recommended calories per day. In order to optimally determine calorie requirements, you must first estimate how much you utilize on any given day.

The first step in determining caloric balance is to measure basal metabolic rate (BMR) or resting metabolic rate (RMR), which is the minimum energy required to properly maintain normal body function at rest. Both BMR and RMR will provide similar numbers, but differ in methodology of measurement. Resting metabolic rate typically provides numbers that are slightly higher than BMR, but the terms are often used interchangeably. For the purpose of this book and to eliminate confusion, I will use the term "basal metabolic rate." Basal metabolic rate generally ranges from around 1,100 kCals to 2,100 kCals per day. It is the minimum energy required just to exist, and any physical activity conducted throughout the day will add to basal metabolic rate. This is why the typical daily caloric recommendations for individuals range from 1,600 kCals/day for females to 2,500 kCals/day for males. These numbers go up for physically active males and females.

A linear relationship exists between heart rate and increased metabolism (typically estimated by VO_2), and therefore heart rate can be used to estimate basal metabolic rate. In order to estimate BMR using heart rate, you will need a heart rate monitor that estimates kCals at rest. Record caloric expenditure at rest for 10 minutes and multiply by 6 to determine caloric expenditure for an hour. The resultant number is then multiplied by 24 to determine caloric expenditure for an entire day (BMR).

Laboratory testing for BMR and RMR is time consuming and expensive. Therefore, formulas are often used to estimate both. While formulas are not as accurate as direct measures, they can provide a fairly accurate estimation and a great place to begin.

Male   kCals/day = 66 + (13.7 × body weight in kg) + (5 × height in cm) – (6.9 × age)

Female   kCals/day = 665 + (9.6 × body weight in kg) + (1.7 × height in cm) – (4.7 × age)

Example Equation

Male: 180 lbs (81.63 kg), 72 in tall (182.88 cm), age 25
kCals/day = 66 + (13.7 × 81.63) + (5 × 182.88) – (6.9 × 25) = 1,926.23 kCals

After basal metabolic rate has been determined, add caloric expenditure due to activity to the equation. If you had a morning bike outing that used 600 kCals, then went for a short hike with your kids and used 200 kCals, you would then add 800 kCals to your basal metabolic rate. Any physical activity (mowing the lawn, cleaning the house, etc.) above resting needs to be added to BMR. Keep in mind that his methodology is not 100 percent accurate and only gives you a ballpark number. This is why counting calories ingested, counting calories utilized, and measuring changes in body mass are all important components of weight management. If you lose or gain too much weight, adjust caloric intake accordingly.

Most heart rate monitors can estimate energy expenditure for endurance activities based on heart rate. The estimations provided by most heart rate monitors will be decently accurate for endurance activities. However, heart rate monitors cannot provide an accurate estimation of caloric expenditure for activities such as interval training or resistance training. For these activities you can use metabolic equivalents (METs) to help you determine energy expenditure for your specific activities. One MET is equal to 3.5 ml/kg/min, which represents a resting state. So, each MET you go above 1 is an activity level above your resting state.

The first thing to determine when using METs to calculate energy expenditure is the particular METs for the activity that you are conducting. If you are lifting weights, the METs will range from 3 (very light) to 6 (vigorous). Determine where your overall intensity was for that session. An example of a 3 would be when you first start lifting and you are working on technique, not pushing a lot of weight and stopping at a set number of reps before volitional exhaustion. An example of a 6 would be when you are lifting at high intensity to volitional exhaustion with every set. You can also use METs to estimate energy expenditure for endurance activities as well. The metabolic equivalent for mountain biking can range from 8 to 14 METs, depending on intensity.

To calculate energy expenditure from METs, you will need your current body mass in kilograms for the equation I provide below, the time spent conducting the activity, and the METs for that activity. When looking at time for running, it is fairly simple: know your start and stop times. When looking at something such as a resistance training session, it is not as straightforward. If you conduct your resistance training and stay on task, you can count your entire session as time. However, if you instead spend a lot of time talking and extend an hour session into an hour and a half, then you only count the hour. Keep in mind that these are estimations, but you want to be as accurate as possible. Following is the formula and an example problem:

(METs)(Body mass in kilograms)/60 = kCals/min
An 81.63-kg male athlete completed a mountain bike race in an hour and a half (90 minutes) at a vigorous intensity.
(14 METs)(81.63 kg)/60 = 19.04 kCals/min
(19.04 kCals/min)(90 min) = 1,713.6 kCals

As you can see in the example above, this individual's caloric expenditure for the race would be 1,713.6 kCals. I used the same numbers from the previous example where I calculated basal metabolic rate. So, at this point in the day this individual would have expended 3,639.83 kCals (BMR of 1,926.23 kCals + mountain bike race of 1,713.6 kCals). You would add in any other significant energy expenditure throughout the day to get a total for the day. You would then subtract energy consumed during the day to determine your net caloric balance.

When training for mountain biking, make sure to replenish the calories used throughout the day. This process is vital for energy replenishment as well as for driving anabolic processes for recovery. As mentioned previously, it is all about manipulating caloric balance in order to reach your specific weight-management goals. If you know how many calories you burned throughout the day, you know how many you need to replace. This is where your nutrition log can be helpful. By reading the caloric content of the food you consume and keeping track of the totals, you can compare caloric expenditure to caloric intake. Keep in mind that it is not just about the volume of nutrients but the quality of the nutrients as well.

Fad Diets

One of the biggest mistakes that people make in the pursuit of their desired body mass is that they look for shortcuts. Unfortunately, there are no safe or sustainable shortcuts to weight management. This tendency for individuals to look for the fastest and easiest way to lose weight has resulted in a market for fad diets. There is no short, fast, easy, or magical way to weight loss. It is a long and gradual process that requires dedication and work. Stay away from fad diets—they do not work. When it comes to weight loss, if it sounds too good to be true, then it is. Fad diet programs result in no change in body composition at best and lead to health-related problems at worst.

In recent history, low-carbohydrate and no-carbohydrate diets have been pushed as a healthy and fast way to lose weight. However, there is nothing healthy about a low-carb or no-carb diet. This is doubly true for an endurance athlete. There are three primary reasons to stay away from a low-carb diet. The first and foremost is that the only source of fuel that the central nervous system and the brain can use is glycogen (the storage form of carbohydrates). Inadequate supplies of glycogen result in mental confusion and fatigue. As a survival mechanism, the body will produce glycogen by breaking down protein in the body. Excess protein is not stored in the body, and therefore muscle is degraded in order to provide the protein required for conversion to glycogen.

Use of lipids as a fuel will also be compromised due to low glycogen stores. As stated previously, lipids require glycogen in order to be completely catabolized for energy. Low glycogen stores and compromised lipid catabolism results in a decrease in pH (i.e., increased acidity). Other common complications of a low-carb diet are dehydration, electrolyte imbalance, strain on the liver, and strain on the kidneys.

A low-carbohydrate diet will negatively impact mountain bike training and performance. Glycogen stores are extremely important when training or racing at high intensities. Because glycogen stores are limited to around 2,000 kCals, you do not want to begin a training session or race with low glycogen stores. You will fatigue early and to a greater extent, and you will have trouble thinking clearly.

It would be untrue to state that you cannot lose weight through a low-carbohydrate diet. However, the weight that is lost is not entirely due to decreased lipid stores and instead will be a result of significant lean tissue loss, water loss, and lipid loss. Loss of muscle mass will have a strong negative impact on sport performance. There is also no need to take in excess carbohydrates, as excess carbohydrates will be converted to and stored as lipids.

Another commonly used fad diet for weight management is diet pills. Diet pills are considered a supplement and therefore fall outside FDA regulations. This allows companies to make blatantly false claims without fear of prosecution. The combination of no FDA oversight and people being desperate to lose weight has resulted in the development of a multibillion-dollar diet pill industry. Diet pills do not work as advertised and can lead to health complications.

Because of this risk, it is not recommended to use diet pills as a source of weight management. Not all, but most diet pills contain stimulants that increase metabolism, which in turn greatly increases resting heart rate and can cause heart palpitations and other medical complications. Because exercise naturally increases heart rate, diet pills can elevate that increase. On hot, humid days when blood plasma volume drops significantly due to sweating, the use of diet pills can apply excess strain on the heart.

It would be impractical to list and discuss all the fad diets that are currently being pushed, and therefore I will just give you some basic advice here. First, as mentioned previously, if it sounds too good to be true, then it most likely is. Weight loss requires time and effort, and there is no substitute. Weight management requires that you increase caloric expenditure through physical activity and that you eat a well-balanced diet that meets all your nutritional needs. And second, you cannot "target" fat. Fat is fat, and there is no "special" type of fat in the body. Nor can you "target" specific storage locations of fat. There is not a special exercise or diet that will target belly or hip fat. With increases in physical activity, you will see an increase in fat stored in muscle, needed for increased energy availability during exercise, and a decrease in adipose storage.

ERGOGENIC AIDS

The word "ergogenic" means work enhancing. In the arena of sports performance, ergogenic aids are any aids that increase performance. Typically, ergogenic aids do this in three basic ways. The first is that they directly increase performance during an event. The second is that they promote recovery between bouts. The third is that they allow for better training in order to improve later performance. When considering ergogenic aids, it is important to examine their effectiveness, known and possible side effects, ethics, and legality.

Ethics, Legality, and Regulations

Athletes are very focused on finding ways to improve performance, and ergogenic aids can provide a pathway for such improvement. However, when choosing ergogenic aids, the legality and ethics of specific ergogenic aids must be considered. Ethics can be very subjective and are typically based on an individual's morals and sense of right and wrong. What one person may see as ethical, others may not. However, there is no such gray area when looking at rules and laws. Every sport has a set of rules that competitors must adhere to in order to compete. USA Cycling has a list of banned substances that they test for, which will be discussed in greater detail below. There are also laws that prohibit certain substances, such as steroids.

In sports there is a basic premise that all competition is conducted on an even playing field and that there are no unfair advantages. Any differences in performance should be based strictly on genetics, training, tactics, and ergogenic aids that are permitted by the sport's governing body. If an ergogenic aid is illegal, such as steroids, then it is also against regulations and hopefully counter to the established ethical guidelines of the athlete.

Mountain biking's governing body, USA Cycling, takes decisive steps in the effort to keep the sport clean. The International Olympic Committee created the World Anti-Doping Agency (WADA) in order to regulate the use of ergogenic aids in sports. The charge of this committee is to create a list of banned substances, develop rules, test for banned substances, and enforce rules. The United States Anti-Doping Agency (USADA) has joined WADA and is responsible for implementing WADA regulations in this country, and USA Cycling has signed on to the USADA for testing.

When determining whether a substance should be banned or not, WADA examines three main areas during deliberation: (1) Is the substance illegal? (2) Does the substance pose a serious health risk? (3) Does the substance give the athlete an unfair advantage over their competitors? An answer of yes to one or more of these questions can result in the substance being placed on the banned-substance list.

You are ultimately responsible for knowing what is on the banned-substance list and ensuring that you are not taking a supplement or medication that contains any of the banned substances. USA Cycling keeps an updated list on what is currently banned by the sport. If you are prescribed a medication that contains a banned substance, you can file for a therapeutic use exemption.

Supplements

The Dietary Supplement Health and Education Act of 1994 (DSHEA) defined a supplement as a nonfood, a nonfood additive, and a nondrug, so that supplements would not fall under the same stringent restrictions as foods. While the FDA has the ability to remove products that have been shown to cause health issues, there are no strict guidelines for production, quality, and content. This act also allows supplement companies to make claims without scientific proof and to be intentionally vague. As long as supplement companies do not claim to cure or mitigate a disease, they can make any unsubstantiated claim they desire. The DSHEA allows supplements to remain outside of good manufacturing practices (GMP), which require that all drugs be within a very strict limit (typically within 1 to 2 percent) of what is stated on the label. Because supplements are not regulated by the FDA for content, many products do not contain the precise amount of the specific ingredient stated on the product label. Scientific studies have examined supplements and found that some have exactly what is stated on the package while others have little to none of the advertised product.

Due to the way supplements are marketed, it can be difficult to know what works and what does not. This makes it difficult to determine if a specific product will work as advertised, and it is important to look to other sources for information. Sometimes the testimonies of professional athletes are sought out as sources. But beware, often professional athletes are paid by the supplement companies to advertise products. The athlete may or may not actually use the product in training, however, and may even just believe that the supplement works when it truly has no effect on performance.

Magazines are also not a valid source for information on the effects of ergogenic aids. The magazine may be reluctant to print an article that a supplement does not work when that company is paying for advertising in its pages. It is not uncommon to see a supplement advertisement appearing as an article and then in tiny print somewhere on the page stating that it is a paid advertisement.

Peer-reviewed scientific journal articles are the best sources of information because the reviewed studies are conducted under strictly controlled settings and in an unbiased manner. This can be difficult at times due to not having free access to all journals, and they are often written in such a way that you need a strong understanding of chemistry to know what is stated in the article. Textbooks are often a good source as they have condensed the information from various scientific articles into an understandable review of the ergogenic aid.

If you decide to try a specific ergogenic aid, ensure that you know the possible side effects, and pay attention to how your body reacts to the supplement.

Most supplements are expensive, and it would be illogical to spend money on a product that has little or no effect on your performance. Calculate a cost benefit ratio for yourself.

There are a few ergogenic aids that can be beneficial for mountain biking. Some were mentioned at the beginning of the chapter (water, carbohydrates, proteins, and sports drinks). If you do not think water is an ergogenic aid, try cycling on a hot day without it and see what happens to your performance (joking, don't do that). Protein is also a vital ergogenic aid as it greatly assists in the anabolic process in the body, aiding in recovery. Carbohydrate ingestion during competition has been shown to improve performance during sustained endurance events and is vital for refueling during recovery. Electrolyte replacement is also vital during long events and for recovery.

Caffeine

Believe it or not, caffeine is also an ergogenic aid and is the most widely used supplement in the world. It is a naturally occurring stimulant found in plants (coffee beans, tea leaves, cocoa nuts, etc.). Caffeine is also found naturally in many products we use daily, such as coffee, tea, and soda, but it is often added to other products as a stimulant. Research strongly supports the use of caffeine for improving human performance during endurance sports.

Caffeine can improve performance in three basic ways. The first is that it can easily cross the blood/brain barrier, acting as an ergogenic aid by decreasing feelings of pain and fatigue during exercise, resulting in the ability to race or train at a higher intensity level. The second is that caffeine both stimulates and increases the mobilization of free fatty acids into the blood, resulting in an increased availability for energy production and, thus, conserving glycogen stores. And finally, caffeine increases the muscles' ability to contract by also increasing activity at the neuromuscular junction and increasing motor unit recruitment.

While caffeine is widely used by a large portion of the population, there are potential side effects. The most common include muscle tremors, gastrointestinal distress, headache, nervousness, elevated heart rate, arrhythmia, and high blood pressure. Side effects are more likely to develop at high levels of ingestion and in individuals who do not normally consume caffeine. While it is commonly stated that caffeine acts as a diuretic, research has shown that this is not true during exercise, primarily due to the release of antidiuretic hormone and aldosterone that occurs during exercise in order to retain water. The risk of dehydration and thermoregulatory complications is more likely to occur with caffeine ingestion in a hot environment.

It is important to know how your body reacts to caffeine prior to using it as an ergogenic aid, and it should never be used in high dosages. A key point to caffeine use is that it does not have to be taken in large doses to increase endurance performance. Caffeine ingestion equivalent to 2.5 cups of coffee has been found to be sufficient to improve performance. Caffeine peaks in the system around one hour after ingestion and therefore should be taken an hour prior to competition. Also be aware that some organizations consider caffeine a banned substance. The NCAA bans caffeine usage equivalent to about six to nine 8-ounce cups of coffee. The number of cups will vary depending on the athlete's body mass and timing of ingestion. Do not take caffeine pills as the quantity of caffeine within a pill is suspect. Anecdotally, I have worked with athletes who were habitual coffee drinkers that experienced negative health consequences when using caffeine pills as an ergogenic aid.

Habitual use of caffeine actually diminishes its ergogenic effect. For those who ingest caffeine (coffee, soda, etc.) on a regular basis, it is recommended to cease caffeine ingestion seven days prior to competition in order to optimize the effects of caffeine for sports performance.

Anabolic Steroids

Two illegal ergogenic aids that are commonly used in mountain biking are anabolic steroids and blood doping. The next two sections will discuss these ergogenic aids to give a better understanding of how they work and why you should avoid their use. It is also important to educate yourself on these topics as they are often discussed in relation to training and competing in elite-level sports.

Anabolic steroids (synthetic testosterone) are unfortunately prevalent in all sports. Steroids promote the anabolic process in the body and improve performance by increasing the speed of recovery, repairing damaged tissue, creating greater hypertrophy, and reducing the catabolic effects of exercise. The ability to recover faster between training bouts allows an athlete to train harder more often, which in turn leads to improved performance. Steroids are typically administered through injection, oral doses, patches, or cream.

There are reversible and irreversible side effects that occur with steroid use. Reversible side effects include acne, depression, increased rage, infections at injection sites, and high cholesterol. These side effects dissipate once steroid use has stopped.

The irreversible side effects of steroids occur due to prolonged and heavy use and are typically more serious. They include cancer, liver disease, cardiovascular disease, and baldness. Side effects that are specific to males are testicular atrophy, impotence, developing mammary glands (breasts), and a permanent decrease in natural testosterone production. Women run the risk of developing facial hair and a deeper voice. Steroid use in pregnant women can also lead to birth defects. Due to the lack of strong scientific research studies in humans, it is not possible to truly know all the negative impacts steroid use has on health.

Blood Doping

The term "blood doping" covers any method used to increase red blood cell count. Red blood cells are responsible for transport of oxygen, which is a key component for endurance sports. If red blood cells increase, then your ability to transport oxygen to the working muscles also increases, and therefore performance increases. There are three primary methods used for blood doping: autologous, homologous, and erythropoietin. Autologous blood doping involves removing blood from the athlete and spinning the blood in order to separate plasma from hemoglobin. The plasma is then injected back into the athlete and the red blood cells are stored for later use. It takes approximately four to six weeks for hemoglobin levels to return to normal. The hemoglobin is then reinfused prior to competition in order to increase red blood cell count. The downside to this method is that the athlete will be weak for a period of time, which affects training.

To prevent the period of weakness following blood removal during autologous blood doping, some athletes choose to use homologous blood doping instead. Homologous blood doping involves infusing red blood cells from a matched donor just prior to racing. This method carries a high risk of disease transmission and infection, and it is possible that the athlete's body may reject the donor blood. Antigens found in blood differ significantly between individuals, making this method of blood doping easy to detect.

Erythropoietin is a naturally occurring hormone that is produced in the kidneys and is responsible for stimulating red blood cell production in the bone marrow. Epoetin (synthetic erythropoietin) is injected in order to increase red blood cell production. A negative side effect of epoetin is that it can drastically increase red blood cell production, resulting in a large increase in hematocrit, which can negatively impact health. The use of epoetin also requires iron supplementation in order to provide the excess iron needed to create hemoglobin.

Blood doping is banned not only because it gives the athlete an unfair advantage but also due to the serious health complications that can occur when implementing this process. All three of these methods significantly increase hematocrit levels. If hematocrit gets too high, it will result in an increase in blood viscosity, which in turn could lead to a stroke or heart attack. Mountain biking requires endurance performance over a prolonged period, and on a hot day dehydration can easily occur. When an athlete becomes dehydrated, plasma volumes are significantly decreased, which increases blood viscosity. Blood doping combined with dehydration is a deadly formula.

6

COMPETITION

RACES

As mentioned previously, the first step in developing your training plan is to determine your race schedule. In this section I am going to discuss where and how to find races. Your local bike shop and cycling club are great places to look for upcoming races. Local riders are a great source of information in regard to which local races are the best to compete in and which you may want to avoid.

USA Cycling is another excellent source for finding races as most mountain bike races are sanctioned by them. You can find the mountain bike race schedule for the year on the USA Cycling web page (https://usacycling.org). The organization provides insurance coverage, race publicity, USA Cycling ranking for the racers, safety requirements, and other benefits.

Active.com is another internet source for mountain bike race information. While USA Cycling provides information on sanctioned races, Active.com provides information for both sanctioned and non-sanctioned races. On Active .com you will need to choose mountain biking from a drop-down menu as they are a registration site for many different sports.

Mountain bike races are held at varying distances and on varying terrain, and it is important to know both in order to make a decision on whether or not to add the race to your schedule. If you are new to mountain biking, keep the distances lower and pick terrain that is not above your skill level. Most races will have varying distances based on racers' skill levels and race categories. Many races will have a beginner-level race distance. USA Cycling–sanctioned events will have category 3 (beginner), category 2 (intermediate), category 1 (advanced) and professional category races. Distances often vary based on category. For example, category 3 racers may race two laps, while category 1 racers may race six. Some mountain bike races will still use the old mountain bike category designations of beginner, sport, expert, and pro (USA Cycling replaced this system with categories 1 through 3 in 2009).

When choosing a race, make sure that your technical skills are up to the challenge of that particular course. Mountain bike race terrain can be a smooth, rolling, and nontechnical trail where you can race at a fast pace with no strong technical challenges, or the course can be extremely technical, requiring a high level of skill to ride or race. Choosing to race a course that is beyond your skill level can result in a greater number of crashes and can be discouraging to new racers. As your bike-handling skills increase, you will be able to race more technical courses. If it is a local race, you can always ride the trails prior to registering for the race so that you can get a feel for the technical requirements.

The size of the race may be something you want to consider as well. Some racers prefer smaller events with less crowds and fewer racers. Whereas other competitors prefer large crowds and a large race field. Both have their advantages and disadvantages. The smaller races have fewer people and therefore are typically less crowded on the trail. A smaller group of people racing may also be less intimidating for those just starting out. The downside to smaller races is that they may not be as well supported on the course. For example, large races have a big wow factor that brings with it a lot of excitement and energy. When you have 1,000-plus mountain bikers competing in an event, it creates a festive atmosphere that takes on a life of its own, providing a great experience for everyone involved.

Registration

You can save money by registering early for races. At times these savings can be very substantial. Make sure to note the fee-increase dates so that you do not miss the lower early-entry costs. Early registration also guarantees you a spot in races that are more popular or have limited registration. Some races fill up quickly, and if you wait too long you will not be able to obtain a spot. A downside to early registration is that very few races will refund registration fees if you find it necessary to back out for any reason.

USA Cycling requires that you have a race license to participate in any of their sanctioned events. When purchasing a race license, you have two options: either an annual license or a one-day license. If you plan on participating in more than one race, it makes more sense to purchase the annual license. To make things easy, purchase your license prior to race registration so that you have your USA Cycling number.

Logistics

When choosing a race, also consider the logistical requirements (scheduling, travel, and lodging). Ensure that the date will fit within your current family schedule, work schedule, and training schedule. Always double-check your calendar prior to registration so that you do not double book. As mentioned, most registration fees are nonrefundable.

Next, determine the distance you will have to travel in order to compete. Local travel is usually very easy as you can arrive at the race in the morning, compete, and then return home. The farther the race is from your home, the more planning you must do. You may need to travel a day or two prior to the race and will need to decide if you are driving or flying, as well as make hotel and bike transport arrangements. Local races are typically less expensive (no lodging and minimal travel), require less planning, and are typically less stressful overall. Local races are also held on trails that you are most likely already familiar with or a trail that you can easily become familiar with prior to the race.

If you choose to fly to the race, consider how you will transport your bike to and from the competition. Flying with your bike has become expensive, and there is a heavy risk of a lost or damaged bike in the process. If you decide to fly, it is important to pack your bike correctly (described below) and to know the total round-trip cost of flying with your bike. You will also want to know the bike policy for the airline you choose to book your flight with. Another option is to ship your bike to the race using a mail carrier service or your local bike shop. Most local bike shops have a packing and shipping service that they provide. If you choose this route, make sure to contact the local bike shop where you plan to race to make return shipping arrangements as well. This option may be more expensive than doing the shipping yourself, but it does save you some headaches.

The last option is to rent a mountain bike from a local bike shop at the race location. If you choose this option, make sure you are familiar with the bike you will be renting and that you reserve the correct size. If you choose to rent, I advise bringing your own pedals and cycling shoes. Measure your current bike setup and take those measurements with you so that you can set the rental bike up in the same manner.

Prior to race weekend, review the race schedule and plan your weekend based on the schedule. Determine when and where packet pickup will occur, and schedule accordingly. Most races have packet pickup the morning of the race near the start. However, some races require packet pickup the day prior to the race, which may or may not be at the race site. Most races will have packet pickup both on the day prior and on race day. Picking up your packet the day before the race allows you to make sure everything is good with your registration and to place your race number on your bike early. Take the time to read through the race material for any specialized information concerning the race.

It is important to know the trails prior to racing or riding an area. Most places will have maps of the trail system that you can download and print. Place the printout of the map in a Ziplock bag and keep it in your hydration pack for referencing on the trail. While most all races will have the trail visibly marked, it is still possible to miss a turn and become lost.

Plan a prerace ride in order to become familiar with the race course so that you can best determine how to traverse the course on race day. It will make you aware of any technical obstacles that you may encounter and let you know at what speeds you can take certain sections. Even if you know the course, it is still a good idea to conduct a pre-ride as some sections of the trail will be cut off in order to make a specific course.

Race Budget

Develop a budget for your registration fees, travel, and lodging. Race fees are not inexpensive and can add up quickly as the race season progresses. Entry fees for mountain bike races range from $35 to around $100 with the average cost of a race being about $50. Make a list of your chosen races with the cost for each. Then add travel, lodging, and food costs into your budget for each race. This will give you an outline for your race season budget. Once you know how much you will spend in the upcoming race season, you can then develop a plan to meet the budget requirements for racing.

Equipment Check

The night before you leave for a race, conduct an equipment check to ensure you have everything you need. You do not want to show up to a mountain bike race minus your cycling shoes. I have forgotten my shoes before, and it is no fun racing in running shoes on clipless pedals. Be meticulous about your equipment check. Create a checklist with everything you will need before, during, and after the race. The next step is to lay out all your gear and visually mark everything off the list. Below is a basic checklist of the equipment you will need for most mountain bike races. Adjust the checklist to fit your specific needs.

- bike
- helmet
- cycling shoes
- hydration pack
- tire pump
- bike tools
- spare tubes
- cycling clothes (shorts, jersey, socks, etc.)
- gloves
- sunglasses
- nutrition
- towel
- shoes for before or after the race (Crocs are great for this)
- foul-weather requirements (rain jacket, etc.)

If you are going to be gone for more than one day, you may want to consider packing two bags. The first bag is your race bag for all your racing gear and tools. The second bag will contain clothing, travel supplies, and anything else you may need. If you are flying, however, you may not want two separate bags due to cost.

Packing Your Bike

If you are traveling by plane or shipping your bike to the race, you will need to pack it carefully to ensure that it arrives to the race undamaged. You have two basic options when it comes to choosing a bike case. The first is to use a cardboard bike box that bike manufacturers ship their bikes in. You can find these at any local bike shop. The cardboard is thick and does provide protection, but it is still just cardboard. Your second option is a plastic hard case designed specifically for bike transport. These cases provide greater protection than cardboard boxes, but they do cost substantially more.

If you are unsure of how to pack your bike within a box, you can pay a local bike shop to pack your bike for you. If you are going to pack your bike yourself and are new to this process, you will want to practice packing and unpacking your bike from the box so that you are confident you can do it on race day. It is better to make a mistake before the race when you still have time to get your bike to your local shop than it is to try this process for the first time on race day.

Following are the basic steps for packing your bike properly. Keep in mind there may be steps that you will need to add or remove based on your specific bike and bike box. Also, if you purchased a plastic bike box, the manufacturer will have specific instructions for packing your bike using their box.

1. Remove the front and rear wheel from the bike. Some boxes allow you to leave the rear wheel attached when packing.
2. Remove the skewers from both wheels.
3. Place plastic protectors into the front fork and rear stay drop-outs to help prevent damage.
4. Remove the stem from the fork steer tube, and zip-tie the handlebars along the side of the frame. Place padding between the handlebars and the frame to prevent damage.
5. Remove the pedals from the bike.
6. Remove the rear derailleur and attach it to the rear stay with a zip tie.
7. Remove the seat post and seat from the bike (no need to remove the seat from the seat post).
8. Pack everything securely and safely into your bike box.

Make sure that you have enough time to rebuild and test your bike once you arrive at your race destination. This step should be a priority. The sooner you realize there is an issue, the more time you will have to correct the issue prior to your race. You do not want to spend all that time, effort, and money on a race and then not be able to compete because there is a problem with your bike.

Race Day

On race day get up early enough to eat, go to the bathroom, and arrive at the race venue with plenty of time to line up for the start of the race. Get to the race venue early enough to find parking, ensure your bike is operating correctly, conduct your warm-up, and line up at the start line on time. Getting there early allows you to prepare for the race without the extra anxiety of rushing and worrying about missing your start time.

If you were unable to pick up your race packet prior to race day, this should be your first stop of the morning to ensure that there are no unforeseen complications and because the lines can be long. Once you receive your race packet, place your number on your bike and your timing chip on your body. Timing chips will typically go on your wrist or ankle. I prefer the wrist so that there is less worry about it coming loose while pedaling. Double-check the start time and start location of your specific race. Often start times are dependent upon race category. In large races they will also split up start times based on age and gender as well as category.

Next, go through your final prerace bike check to ensure that everything on your bike is functioning correctly. You should check your tire pressure, your suspension pressure, and your skewers, and run through all your gears and make sure all bolts are tight.

Now that you have everything set up to race, you will most likely need to find the bathroom prior to beginning your warm-up. Unfortunately, when you are nervous about the race it is inevitable that you will require another bathroom stop. As there are always many more racers and spectators than bathrooms, it is a good idea to get that out of the way early as well. Don't make the mistake of having to decide whether to remain in the bathroom line or start the race.

Next is your warm-up. Make sure that you time your warm-up early enough that you are ready to go at your appropriate start time. Do not warm up for too long or too early if you have a later start time. The actual race course will most likely be closed prior to the start, and you may have to warm up on the road or on an alternate trail. At large races it may be advisable to bring a stationary trainer to warm up on as the trails will be closed and the roads may be congested with people coming into the race area.

MOUNTAIN BIKE SKILLS

There are certain basic mountain bike skills you will need to have mastered prior to your first race. The more practice you have, the better you will become at each of these skills. Therefore, it is important that you adhere to dedicated practice times. As your skills improve, so too will your speed as you will be able to traverse rough terrain at a faster rate.

Improved skills will also decrease the risk of acute injury. This is mountain biking and you will crash; unfortunately, there is no way around this fact. As you become more skilled, you will crash less, but even professional mountain bikers will occasionally experience a crash.

Improved skills will result in less walking through obstacles with your bike, and more riding. In the beginning you will walk your bike down intimidating hills, up steep bumpy climbs, and over challenging obstacles. This is perfectly normal and is what you should be doing as a beginner. As your skills improve, though, you will find that obstacles that previously required you to get off your bike and walk are now easy to ride through.

Pedaling

Believe it or not, pedaling is a skill that will take some riding before you perfect it. The good thing about cycling is that you do not have to perfect pedaling in order to ride. As a matter of fact, you most likely will not notice the changes in your pedal stroke as you become better at it. As you cycle, you will develop neuromuscular recruitment patterns that result in smoother and more efficient pedaling.

If you examine your crank arms and pedals while riding, you will notice that your feet will always be directly opposite each other. As one leg is pushing down, the other leg is pulling up. The leg that is pulling up is not applying a great amount of force to the pedal cycle, but instead is applying force to unweight the pedal and make it easier to push down with the other leg. This cycle requires coordinated muscle recruitment patterns by both legs simultaneously and opposite in direction.

To examine the pedal stroke, look at it as though it is a clock face. The majority of force produced by the cyclist will occur from the 12 o'clock position to just prior to the 6 o'clock position. I will start the discussion from the 12 o'clock to 3 o'clock positions where the leg applies forces in the forward and downward direction. The actions during this motion are hip extension, knee extension, and plantar flexion at the ankle. The primary muscles involved in this movement are the gluteus maximus, hamstring, quadricep, gastrocnemius, and soleus muscles.

From the three o'clock to the six o'clock positions, force is applied down and back. The actions during this motion are hip extension, knee extension, and plantar flexion at the ankle. The primary muscles involved in this movement are the gluteus maximus, hamstring, slight quadricep, gastrocnemius, and soleus muscles.

As you are going from the 6 o'clock position to the 12 o'clock position, you are using minimal force and just unweighting the leg to reduce the amount of energy used by the opposite leg as it pushes downward. From the 6 o'clock to 9 o'clock positions, the force is applied up and back. The actions during this motion are hip flexion, knee flexion, and slight plantar flexion at the ankle. The primary muscles involved in this movement are the rectus femoris, hamstring, and slight gastrocnemius muscles.

From the 9 o'clock to 12 o'clock positions, the force is applied up and forward. The actions during this motion are hip flexion, knee flexion turning over to knee extension, and dorsi flexion at the ankle. The primary muscles involved are the rectus femoris, hamstring (knee flexion), quadricep (knee extension), and tibialis anterior muscles.

As stated earlier, as you develop neuromuscular recruitment patterns for optimal pedaling, you will become a more efficient cyclist. It is important to produce equal power output between both legs during the pedal cycle. There are two common methods you can use to determine whether you are pedaling smoothly or in an uncoordinated manner. The first is the use of a power meter or computer-driven trainer that provides pedaling analysis. These tools have the ability to measure how smoothly you are pedaling and will provide data for you to adjust your pedaling. Some systems provide instantaneous feedback between the left and right pedals and allow you to adjust your pedaling until both sides are even.

A less expensive method is to place your bike in a stationary trainer and listen for smooth pedaling. Smooth pedaling will sound like an uninterrupted spinning of the wheel across the training roller. A non-smooth pedal stroke will have a very distinct sound. You will hear the wheel significantly speed up with every downstroke of the pedal as opposed to a smooth, noninterrupted sound. The greater the sound difference, the greater the discrepancy.

Cadence

Cadence is your pedaling rate and is measured in revolutions per minute (RPM). The most efficient cadence for cycling is 90–100 revolutions per minute. Beginning cyclists usually stay at a lower cadence (70–90 RPM), which is ultimately inefficient. The reason beginners start off at a lower cadence is due to the greater aerobic demand of a higher cadence. As you increase your aerobic capacity, you will find that a higher cadence is more efficient and that you will fatigue at a slower rate at any given speed.

When climbing steep hills, you will have to decrease cadence, especially if you have to climb out of the saddle. Steep climbs require a reduction in cadence that will correspond to the steepness of the grade, your current aerobic capacity, and the combined weight of you and your bike. Whenever possible, it is more efficient to climb seated and at a higher cadence. However, in mountain biking you will often find climbs that are steep enough to require a decrease in cadence.

Shifting

Learning how to shift and when to shift is very important in order to make your cycling smooth and enjoyable. It starts with carefully choosing the combination of front chainring and rear derailleur cog (referred to as gear selection) you want to use when riding as your speed will solely be determined by your cadence and gear selection (the number of teeth on the front chainring and the number of teeth on the rear cog). Determine the gears you want in the front chainring and those you want on the rear cog. This is simplified if you have a mountain bike with only one front chainring as you will only be shifting on the rear cogs.

The left shifter (if you have more than one chainring) operates the front derailleur, and the right shifter operates the rear derailleur. One of the most important rules is that you must be pedaling in order to shift gears. If you shift and then pedal, it will put the chain in a bind and can damage the drive train.

It is also important not to have too much force going into the pedals when shifting gears. Slightly decrease power when shifting in order to allow for a smooth shift from one gear to another. If you are applying a lot of power during a climb and need to shift, you will need to significantly back off the torque prior to shifting. You will lose momentum, but there is no other way around it. If you attempt to shift under high torque, you will bind up and possibly damage the drive train.

It is important to learn to anticipate the need to shift gears. When approaching a climb or a steep descent, coming to a complete stop, or hitting a sharp curve, you should anticipate your gear shift and not wait until it becomes necessary to shift with the pedal under pressure. When you come to a complete stop, anticipate what gear you will want to be in when you start to pedal again. For example, if you are on a flat section and then stop just before a climb, shift to an easier gear prior to stopping.

When approaching a climb, switch gears in anticipation of the climb. If you know you will have to use a smaller chainring on the front crankset, do that first and then adjust the rear gears as the climb progressively steepens. Try to avoid shifting the front chainring while on a steep climb. Do not attempt to grind up a climb without changing gears as it is better to spin at a higher cadence. There will be times when the climb is short enough to ascend without changing gears or having to excessively grind, and still not lose momentum. You will be able to gauge those climbs as you become a more experienced rider. There is nothing worse than getting halfway up a climb and realizing that you are over-geared and unsure of how much more force you can apply to the pedals.

Braking Techniques

You will need to learn how and when to apply the brakes properly when mountain biking. The trick is to keep your speed under control and learn how to feather your brakes. Ride at a speed that is equivalent to your current skill level and equal to your knowledge of the trail. If you are not familiar with the trail, it is easy to be going too fast on a downhill and hit a sharp corner with no time to scrub off speed. As you become familiar with the trail, you will learn where to pick up speed and where to slow down.

Learning to feather your brakes is important. To do this, gently apply pressure so that the pads make contact, slowing the wheel slightly. As you apply more pressure, the wheel rotation will decrease further. Through trial and error, you will learn how much force to apply to the brakes so that you only scrub off the desired speed. There is hardly ever an instance where you want to lock up the brakes as once the wheels stop rotating, you lose the ability to control your bike.

It is important to note that the front brake has considerably more stopping power than the rear brake due to the inertial properties of both the bike and the rider. When you apply the brakes, your body mass will shift toward the front of the bike, and the bike mass rotates forward as well. When you and the bike shift forward, less weight is applied to the back of the bike and therefore less stopping power. If you slam on the front brakes, you will fly over the handlebars. This phenomenon has been experienced by many beginning riders. When stopping, apply pressure equally to both brake levers and shift your weight back on the saddle. How far back on the saddle will depend on how quickly you need to stop and whether or not you are going down a hill. When braking downhill, significantly shift your weight to the back of the saddle. Through practice you will learn how to feather the front and back brakes to elicit the desired outcome.

As mentioned, avoid locking up the wheels when braking as that makes it very difficult to control the bike. If you are in a situation where you have to lock the brakes up and you lose control of the bike, ease up on the brakes to regain control, and then apply more force. Momentarily allowing the wheels to turn will allow you to regain control of the bike, but it will then require a longer distance to stop. You will have to decide which is most important at that particular time.

When cornering, it is important to scrub off speed prior to entering the curve and then lean into it. You can even speed out of a curve if you time it right. Hitting the brakes during a curve can be problematic. It is okay to feather the brakes if you need to, but never lock up the wheels during a curve as that will stop the wheels from turning and you will find yourself going straight, not following the curve. Through trial and error, you will be able to learn how to adjust speed through curves.

Finding the Best Path

When mountain biking, learn to read the trail and pick the best course to travel. On single track there may be only one path to follow as the trail is very narrow. On wider trails you can choose to go down the left side, the right side, or even the middle. You may also need to switch sides as the route changes along the trail. Often, but not always, the best path of travel is the worn path that many cyclists have taken before. Choose the smoothest, fastest route along the trail. As you progress in mountain biking, your ability to read a trail and pick a path along that trail will increase.

Always remember that your bike will travel in the direction you are looking. Many times when mountain biking you will have a very narrow path that you would like the bike to follow in order to optimize performance and prevent crashing, for example, if riding a narrow single-track trail with a small drop into a ditch on your left. It would be important to focus on the narrow trail and guide your bike along the trail as you pedal. Where many beginning cyclists make a mistake is when they focus their attention on where they do not want to go as opposed to where they do want to. For example, in the narrow single-track trail scenario, you might focus your attention on the ditch because you are afraid to steer into the ditch. Because you are focused on the ditch, that is the direction your bike will travel. When riding, work on focusing your attention on where you would like the bike to travel.

Downhill

When traversing downhill sections (see fig. 6.1), it is important that you ride within your skill level. Do not attempt downhill sections that you are not comfortable with. There is nothing wrong with walking your bike downhill if you believe it is beyond your current skill level. You will find that as your skills improve, there will be very little you cannot ride down. When descending, keep your speed under control and do not ride faster than you can currently handle. However, keep in mind that having your wheels rolling at speed will keep you upright more easily than riding too slowly or with the brakes locked up.

When riding downhill it is important to shift your weight toward the back of the bike. If your weight is shifted toward the front, it is much more likely that

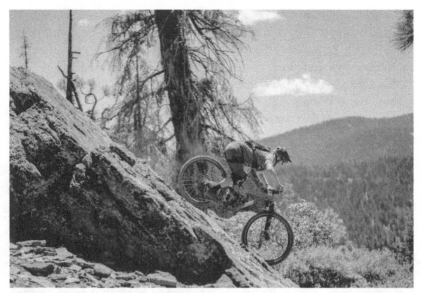

Figure 6.1. Downhill. *Fuji.*

you will fly over the handlebars. During steep downhills you may even need to shift your weight behind the saddle to keep the back end of the bike in contact with the ground while keeping your center of gravity low as well.

Learn how to feather your brakes to optimize speed while controlling your descent. Improper braking will not only cause you to go slower (not necessarily a problem) but may result in you taking an unnecessary flight over the handlebars. You must find a balance between the steepness of the trail, the roughness and technical level of the trail, your abilities, and how much you apply the brakes given the specific scenario.

Choose a path that allows for the fastest descent with the least number of obstacles. As you become more experienced, you will learn to pick the best path down in order to optimize performance and limit crashes.

Uphill

Climbing hills in mountain biking can be challenging and not just because of the grade. The trick to climbing while mountain biking is to keep strong traction between the rear wheel and the trail. Therefore, it is important that you keep your weight shifted over the back wheel to increase friction and improve climbing. Keep in mind that you are on an incline and that shifting your weight back on the saddle can place your weight too far back, which is counterproductive. The goal is to align your weight to push the tire into the ground. Too far forward or too far back and you will feel the rear tire slip as you pedal. Leaning too far back on a steep climb can result in you toppling backward.

When climbing, it is important that you pick a path up the trail that maximizes traction. When possible, avoid climbing over roots, loose gravel, slick mud, and any obstacles that you may not be able to traverse easily. Pick the path of least resistance.

Cornering

Cornering (see fig. 6.2) is a lot of fun, but you must make sure that your skill level is up to the speed you are cornering, or it can get ugly quickly. In the beginning, take the corners slowly and pick up speed as your skill level and confidence increase.

When entering a turn, it is important to pick the path that allows you to travel through the turn, losing as little speed as possible. Look well ahead along your path of travel so you know what is coming and can plan accordingly. An ideal path is to go to the outside and then cut toward the middle of the trail as you exit the turn as this will give you a smoother curve. However, with mountain

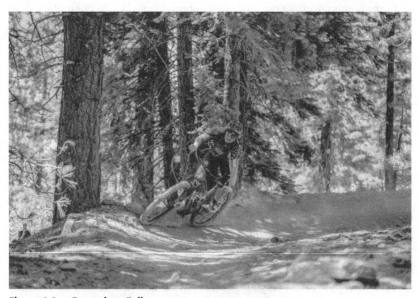

Figure 6.2. Cornering. *Fuji.*

biking it may not be that simple due to obstacles in the trail (rocks, roots, fallen limbs, ruts, etc.).

As you approach the turn, scrub off the necessary speed. How much speed you will need to drop will be dependent on the sharpness of the turn and your skill level. Wide, sweeping turns allow you to corner through the turn with scrubbing little to no speed. Whereas a switchback will require you to slow to a crawl in order to make the turn. Ideally you do not want to be in a situation where you must scrub off a lot of speed during the turn. If you find yourself needing to slow down in the turn, then rely on the rear brake and not the front. Keeping the front tire rolling allows you to better corner through the turn. As mentioned earlier, if you lock up your breaks and the wheels stop turning, you will then travel in a straight line and not follow the curve.

As you enter the curve, you will lean your bike into the curve while maintaining a balanced upper body. In most all cases, you want more lean with the bike and less with the body. However, there are instances, such as riding banked curves, where the body will lean more with the bike but still not be in line with the bike. Keep your upper body relaxed and allow the bike to move underneath you. You will learn how much to lean your bike the more you ride and practice. During this process, keep your center of gravity low as you corner.

Depending on how much you must lean the bike into the curve, you will either want your pedals so that your feet are in the 3 o'clock and 9 o'clock positions or with the inside pedal to the top of the stroke to give you ground clearance on the inside. If you have to lean your bike substantially, pull the inside pedal up to the 12 o'clock position in order to keep it from hitting the ground. I personally prefer to pull my inside pedal up to the 12 o'clock position any time that I have to lean the bike at all. Hit your inside pedal on the ground once while cornering and you will understand the importance of keeping it up and out of the way. As you lean the bike into the curve, place your weight on the outside pedal. Be sure to keep your center of gravity low throughout the turn.

You can gain speed coming out of a curve by pedaling as you begin to exit. You will need to be at a point in the curve where you are not substantially leaning the bike and the pedal will clear the ground as you begin to apply pressure to it. Through practice you will learn when you can begin pedaling as you exit a turn.

Switchbacks are sharp turns that you often find as you wind your way up or down a hill or mountain. These turns are typically somewhere close to 180 degrees in angle and can be rounded out in the curve or very sharp. To negotiate sharp switchbacks, slow down and steer more with your handlebars as opposed to leaning the bike. Do not slow down too much as it will be more difficult to keep your bike upright.

Riding Over or Through Obstacles

When mountain biking, you will often need to ride over or through obstacles that cross the trail. When approaching an obstacle, decide if you are going to ride over it, jump it (discussed below), carry your bike over it, or walk your bike around it. Many branches, rocks, and ruts can easily be ridden over without difficulty. First decide if the object is small enough so that you do not hit your crankset on it while riding over it. If the chainring or your crankset will hit the object, then either jump it or walk it. You will learn to estimate the correct clearance height through trial and error. If you see a lot of gouges across a fallen log, be cautious as the log is tall enough for your chainring to hit it.

To ride over an object, pull up on the front wheel as you approach the obstacle and ride on the back wheel. Once your front wheel clears the object, lower the front wheel to the ground and slightly unweight the back wheel as it rolls over the object. It is important to time the front wheel so that it does not catch on the object, which could result in you flying over the handlebars. Throughout this process you should have your pedals in the three o'clock and nine o'clock positions. If you have a pedal in the six o'clock position, it will hit the obstacle, resulting in a quick visit dirtside. If the obstacle you are traversing is a rut or depression, then pick up your front wheel prior to the depression and allow your back wheel to drop into the depression as you ride through it. The speed at which you approach these obstacles will be highly dependent upon the height of the object and your current skill level.

As your skills improve, you will be able to ride over larger logs or rocks using a slightly different method. As you approach a log, lift your front tire so that it lands on top of the log and can easily roll over. You will use the front wheel as your pivot point. Once the front wheel makes contact with the log, you will lift the back wheel so that as the front drops off the other side of the log the back wheel will cross right over the top. This method requires great timing and coordination but becomes easy with adequate practice.

Jumping Obstacles

You can also bunny hop (jump) obstacles that are across the trail. As you approach an obstacle, judge the height and width of the obstacle for clearance. If it is beyond your current level to jump, simply ride over the obstacle or walk your bike. While there are steps in the jumping process and it is a little more complicated than the following explanation, a bunny hop is when you jump into the air and bring your bike with you.

The first step to a bunny hop is to get your front wheel off the ground. Most beginners attempt to get the wheel off the ground by simply jerking up on the handlebars. In order to correctly and effectively lift the front wheel off the ground, however, you will need to crouch down into the bike, pushing the handlebars downward, and then pull up and back on the bar as you push forward with your feet while shifting your weight. Do not lean too far back as this will be counterproductive to getting the back wheel off the ground. Next comes the jump or bunny hop. When the front wheel is off the ground, spring up with your legs and push the bike forward as you lift the back wheel off the ground.

Timing is very important when jumping over an object. You must time it so that the front wheel is off the ground prior to reaching the object and the back tire leaves the ground before it strikes the object. If your front tire catches on the approach, you can fly over the handlebars. If your back tire catches, it will either slam the front of your bike down or simply roll over the obstacle.

When learning to bunny hop, begin by practicing without an obstacle to jump over and at a slower speed. As your jumps improve and you gain confidence, start adding small obstacles and then pick up speed. Slowly increase height and speed as you are able.

Clipless pedals will assist with bunny hops as they keep you in contact with your bike and give you more control during the jump. I have found that beginning mountain bikers learn to control their bikes and jump better when using clipless pedals and shoes as opposed to shoes and flat pedals. You can easily bunny hop on flats and shoes; it is just more difficult for beginners.

Jumps

There will be many places on a single-track trail where you will be able to catch some air (see fig. 6.3). You will have two basic types of jumps on a trail. The first has an incline, a crest, and a rideable decline on the other side. These jumps can be taken at slower speeds that allow you to just ride down the back side. The second is an incline ramp with a vertical drop on the other side or a gap you must clear before landing on the other side. This type of jump will require you to jump the width of the gap as you cannot ride down the vertical drop. However, most all jumps have an option to ride around so that you can bypass the jump if you are not comfortable.

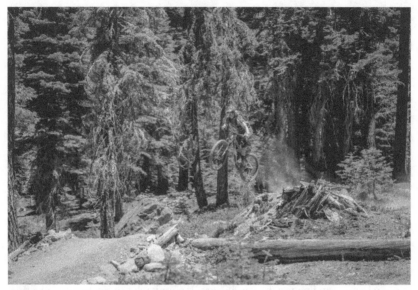

Figure 6.3. Jump. *Fuji.*

As you progress up the ramp, shift your weight back to the rear wheel as you lift the front, similar to the bunny hop I described. As you are already on an incline with the front wheel higher than the rear, you will not have to use much force. Then lift with the back legs, again similar to the bunny hop. Do not pull up too hard with your legs as you will force the nose of the bike down.

Once you leave the incline and are in the air, make sure that you are relaxed. The biggest mistake beginners make is to tense up while in the air. When landing on flat ground, attempt to land both wheels at the same time or the back wheel slightly prior to the front. It is okay to land with the front wheel slightly before the back as long as you are still landing decently level. Never land with your front wheel too far down as you may go over the handlebars. Landing with too much weight in the back can be very jarring. When landing on a decline, however, it is okay if your front wheel lands slightly before the back wheel.

As mentioned previously, timing is important when jumping. Do not jump early as you are just hopping over the crest. Let the incline do the work for you. Jumping too late can cause the nose of your bike to drop and that can be disastrous as well.

Speed on the jump is also important as you do not want too much or too little. If it is a roller, then too little is not an issue as you can just roll through the jump. Too little speed on a jump with a vertical drop can also be okay as long as you do not have to clear the gap. Just keep your front wheel up and drop down. When there is a gap that you have to clear, going too slow can be a problem as you will need enough speed to make it across the gap.

Too much speed can also be a problem if the trail is not straight or there are other obstacles. You cannot change direction or speed while in the air. Make sure that you have plenty of room to land and maneuver prior to any turns or obstacles. If it is a high jump with a landing ramp, it is important that you land correctly on the decline on the opposite side. Going too fast and overshooting the decline can result in a hard landing on flat ground, depending on the height of the jump.

Water Crossings

When coming to a water crossing, first scope out the depth, obstacles, and current before attempting to cross. Keep in mind there are large differences between crossing a 4-foot-wide creek and a river. If in doubt, just walk across. When examining a water crossing, look for the shallowest route across with the least number of obstacles. Most small rivers will have shallow areas for crossing, which is why the trail leads to that area. However, with mountain biking you will generally just deal with creek crossings and will rarely encounter river crossings. If you cannot see the bottom of the creek or river, assume that it is deeper than you think. Also understand that after heavy rains, all of the above can easily change on a trail you ride frequently. I was racing in Alabama during a heavy downpour and the creek crossing that was barely covering the bottom of my wheels on the first lap was above the bottom bracket by the third lap and flowing swiftly.

Look for obstacles that can catch your wheels or pedals. Clear flowing water makes this easy. However, muddy water makes it nearly impossible to see anything that is submerged or any drop-offs. Stay away from algae-covered rocks as they are very slick. It doesn't matter how technically skilled you are, riding across algae-covered rocks will take down the best rider.

When crossing water, maintain your momentum as it will help you get over obstacles and keep you upright. Naturally, if there are a lot of large rocks to maneuver through, you will have to slow down and ride more technically.

When crossing shallow creeks with few to no obstacles, coast across with your pedals at three o'clock and nine o'clock to avoid hitting submerged rocks with your pedals and to keep your shoes and pedals from submerging. You will need to approach with enough momentum to get you across without pedaling.

If the creek is too wide or too deep to coast across or the path is too technical, you will need to pedal through the crossing.

Avoid going deeper than your hubs. Modern hubs and bottom brackets are sealed fairly well, but water has a way of seeping in where you do not want it. Any time I submerge my hubs or bottom bracket, I always perform maintenance afterward to ensure that all the water is out. However, creek crossings are a lot of fun. So, before going in too deep, you will have to weigh the cost benefit of water crossings and maintenance.

It is important to keep safety in mind at all times. You should avoid fast-moving water as it can sweep you and your bike downstream before you know it. Water can be more powerful than you think. If you are not a strong swimmer, avoid large bodies of water where you are unsure of the depth or swiftness of the water.

7

SPECIAL CONSIDERATIONS FOR TRAINING AND COMPETITION

Previous chapters discussed how the body responds and adapts to exercise, information that applies to everyone in general but may need to be modified based on factors such as age, gender, disease state, or disability. This chapter covers special considerations for specific populations that require adaptation to their training program in order to be successful. Due to gender differences, males and females respond slightly differently to training. As we age, the body alters and will not adapt to training in the same manner, and therefore training programs must adapt. Specific disease states alter the body's ability to adapt and may require special care and consideration. And finally, certain biomechanical and physiological adaptations must be made when working with disabled athletes as well.

WOMEN

In recent history female participation in sports has increased dramatically. When developing a training program for females, the same training principles discussed earlier can be applied without alterations. Women adapt to training stimuli in ways that are very similar to male athletes. However, there are some distinct differences, and there are a few key factors that should be taken into consideration when developing a training program.

Sex Differences

We should begin by acknowledging that there are key physiological differences between males and females. One of the main differences involves hormones, primarily testosterone and estrogen. Males naturally produce 10 times more testosterone compared to females. Greater volumes of testosterone result in greater anabolic processes and therefore a significantly larger increase in muscle mass. Men can produce a faster contraction than women due to a greater speed of signaling, resulting in greater power. Muscle mass distribution also differs between males and females. A greater percentage of muscle mass is distributed in the upper body in males. It is important to note that there are no physiological differences between male and female muscle tissue and that the main difference in muscle mass is directly related to hormone levels. When looking at absolute strength, men are on average 30–60 percent stronger than females. These numbers are based on the average population. When looking at peer groups (mountain bike racers of the same level and weight), the percentage differences are on the lower end. However, when you make the comparison based on weight lifted in relation to lean body mass, the differences diminish but remain significant.

Often women are concerned with becoming "bulky" or "looking like a guy" due to resistance training and therefore will avoid it. This is an unfounded concern as women do not produce the volume of testosterone that men do and therefore will not bulk up with off-season resistance training designed for mountain biking. A female would have to develop a resistance-training program designed to specifically bulk up in order to achieve that goal. Due to hormonal differences, it is much more difficult for females to put on muscle mass. Also, keep in mind that lifting occurs in the off-season and that even male mountain bikers will not see significant increases in size during an off-season resistance program.

While females do not produce large amounts of testosterone, they do produce a large volume of estrogen, which affects the way females develop physiologically. One of the key roles of estrogen is increased lipid storage, particularly in the thighs and hips. This is the reason that essential body fat in females is 12 percent as opposed to 4 percent in males. Increased lipid storage is essential for the reproductive process. This is also why you can have a female cyclist and male cyclist of the same weight, yet the male is stronger because a greater percentage of his weight will be from lean muscle mass. Keep in mind that this statement is assuming both cyclists are of the same competitive level. Estrogen also plays an important part in female bone growth, as it increases calcium storage and retention.

Females also have a lower aerobic capacity in relation to their male counterparts. There are several factors that contribute to this phenomenon. The first is that males possess a larger overall blood volume and increased hemoglobin count per milliliter of blood compared to females. A greater hemoglobin count increases oxygen-carrying capacity, which in turn increases performance. To help offset lower levels of hemoglobin, females typically have higher levels of 2,3-DPG, which helps release oxygen into the tissue more easily. However, this does not completely compensate for the gender differences. Women also tend to have a smaller heart size, which in turn decreases stroke volume. All of these factors lead to a lower aerobic capacity, resulting in lower $VO_{2\,max}$ measures. At any given fitness level, females will produce $VO_{2\,max}$ scores that will be 5 to 10 ml/kg/min lower than their male counterparts.

While sex differences are scientifically verified, it does not mean that all males can outperform all females. The key is that males possess a higher aerobic capacity, greater lean muscle mass, and faster activation at any given level of competition. A pro female mountain bike racer could beat an amateur-level male racer; however, she would have difficulty with a pro male cyclist.

Female Athlete Triad

One of the common concerns for female athletes is the female athlete triad. As the name suggests, the triad consists of three distinct but interlocking components: inadequate caloric intake, amenorrhea, and osteoporosis. The process begins with inadequate caloric intake. Athletes expend a lot of calories, and when caloric expenditure consistently and excessively exceeds caloric intake, it creates a negative balance resulting in an unhealthy body composition. As mentioned earlier, 12 percent body fat is considered essential in females. Those who drop below this percentage run the risk of developing the female athlete triad as well as other health discrepancies. This caloric imbalance is commonly brought on by the desire to optimize performance as well as concerns with body image.

Often the desire to optimize body composition for performance and body image can become an obsession and lead to eating disorders such as anorexia nervosa and bulimia. Over half of female athletes have been diagnosed with eating disorders. However, you do not have to have an eating disorder to be in a constant negative caloric balance. Mountain biking has a high caloric cost and therefore requires a high caloric intake. A female mountain biker may appear to eat normally but still be in a negative caloric balance. When eating disorders are present, there is a strong psychological aversion to food or what food represents to that individual. In this case, the psychological aversion does not exist; they are just not eating adequately. It is a good idea to monitor caloric expenditure as well as caloric intake. Another way is to monitor body composition to ensure that you maintain essential body fat.

The next component of the female athlete triad is the development of abnormalities in the menstrual cycle, ultimately leading to amenorrhea (cessation of the menstrual cycle). Prolonged negative caloric balance and unhealthy body composition have a negative impact on the hypothalamus, reducing the release of gonadotropic hormones, which in turn impacts estrogen production and the menstrual cycle. An unhealthy body composition does not have to exist for amenorrhea to occur, however. High-intensity training has also been shown to lead to amenorrhea.

The final component of the female athlete triad is the development of osteoporosis, where bone density decreases resulting in bones becoming brittle and easily fractured. Estrogen is responsible for the absorption and retention of calcium. When estrogen production greatly decreases with the cessation of the menstrual cycle, calcium absorption and retention greatly diminish, leading to a decrease in bone density. While the female athlete triad is a serious concern for women of all ages, special attention should be paid to those in their developmental years when bone growth is paramount.

Female Biomechanics

One of the main structural differences between males and females is the pelvic girdle. Women have a wider pelvic girdle and a wider sacrum, and the pelvis is shaped slightly differently. These differences are necessary to accommodate the birth process. These factors also lead to altered lower extremity biomechanics and a greater risk of lower extremity injuries compared to males. Knee injuries (primarily ACL ruptures) are more prevalent in female athletes. Female athletes are six to eight times more likely to rupture an ACL than male athletes of the same sport. One method for decreasing the risk of injury is to strengthen the knee extensors (quadriceps) and the knee flexors (hamstrings). Typically, the quadriceps muscles will be significantly stronger than the hamstring muscles. Research supports that the less there is of a strength difference between the extensors and flexors, the less likely an injury will occur.

Pregnancy

Research has demonstrated that there are many benefits for women who exercise during pregnancy. Some of the proposed benefits are a decrease in excessive weight gain, decreased labor pains, a decreased risk of developing gestational diabetes, and an easier return to pre-pregnancy weight and fitness level after birth. Exercise during pregnancy should only be conducted by women who are experiencing a normal pregnancy and have their doctor's permission. Remember, only your doctor can determine if you are healthy enough to exercise and at what level you can train.

If you become pregnant, sit down and have an honest and detailed conversation with your doctor concerning exercise. When it has been established that you are experiencing a normal, healthy pregnancy, then discuss your goals and training plan with your doctor. The doctor will establish your training limitations, which you should follow precisely. Throughout the pregnancy, continue to maintain an open dialogue regarding your training.

When pregnant, your training goals will need to be altered. You will need to eliminate risk of impact from your training. As pregnancy progresses, balance becomes compromised. As the baby grows and the belly protrudes, the body's center of gravity shifts. While you can still train, mountain biking is not recommended during pregnancy due to the risk of impact during a crash. As long as it is cleared by your doctor, riding a stationary bike to reduce the risk of falling is recommended.

During pregnancy, a hormone, relaxin, is released in order to relax the pelvis to prepare for birth. Unfortunately, relaxin also causes other joints in the lower extremities to loosen too, which leads to decreased stability and balance.

Your training intensity will also need to be lowered. Blood flow is redirected during exercise to the working muscles and to the skin for cooling, which in turn reduces blood flow to the fetus. At mild to moderate intensity, reduced blood flow does not impact fetus health. However, as intensity increases, a greater amount of blood is redirected from the uterus. It is for this reason that vigorous high-intensity exercise should be avoided during pregnancy. When training, it is okay to exercise until you feel slightly fatigued, but never exercise to exhaustion while pregnant. Due to alterations in blood flow during pregnancy, heart rate becomes an unreliable tool for determining exercise intensity. Instead, use perceived exertion to determine intensity.

Due to reduced blood flow to the skin and increased insulation, your ability to dissipate heat is greatly compromised during pregnancy. A significant increase in the fetus's core temperature can negatively impact development. Do not train in the heat, stay well hydrated, and be mindful of any significant increase in core temperature. Train during a cooler part of the day or inside to avoid overheating.

Exercising in a supine position, on your back, is also not recommended during pregnancy, as it lowers cardiac output and can restrict blood flow to the fetus. Find alternate exercises to replace those that you typically conduct in a supine position.

AGING

Aging has a strong impact on our ability to adapt to training. We are all on a theoretical curve where physical abilities increase through life until they peak somewhere between the ages of 25 and 30 years old. We can briefly maintain that peak until our physical abilities begin to gradually decline around the ages of about 35 to 40. This curve remains true for all healthy individuals. Naturally, someone who trains will have a higher performance level at any point in the curve when compared to a sedentary individual.

Fitness level along this curve can be altered by increasing or decreasing physical activity. If a collegiate athlete who has been active his entire life stopped training after college, his fitness level would drop down to the level of someone who is sedentary. The reverse is true for someone who has been sedentary his whole life and then decides to start training. However, the basic principle still remains true in that your ability to adapt to training will begin to diminish around the age of 35 with a significant decline starting around 45 years of age.

Aerobic capacity also decreases significantly with age. It is estimated that there is a reduction in $VO_{2\,max}$ of approximately 1 ml/kg/min a year. Much of the age-related decrease in $VO_{2\,max}$ is due to a significant reduction in physical activity, which occurs as an individual ages. Those who remain active throughout life can offset the loss in $VO_{2\,max}$. While not as steep a decline, those who remain active will still see a reduction in aerobic capacity due to a reduction in cardiovascular function and an age-related decrease in muscle mass (sarcopenia).

Sarcopenia is a common component of aging. However, the extent of the decline in muscle mass is highly dependent on the individual's fitness level. For those who remain active throughout life, the decrease is lessened. While physical activity goes a long way toward preventing loss of muscle mass, it cannot completely offset sarcopenia. The aging process results in a large decrease in hormone production, resulting in a decrease in protein synthesis and, therefore, a decrease in muscle mass.

With age there is a naturally occurring decrease in bone density. There are two distinct stages: osteopenia and osteoporosis. Osteopenia is a decrease in bone density that occurs prior to the development of osteoporosis and is much less severe. Bones at this stage are more susceptible to damage compared to normal bones, but less susceptible in relation to bones in an osteoporotic state.

Osteoporosis is a severe decrease in bone density, resulting in a greater susceptibility to fractures. Both states occur due to age-related decreases in hormones. In males there is a link between an age-related decrease in testosterone production and a decrease in bone density. In females there is a strong relationship between estrogen levels and bone density. This leaves postmenopausal women strongly susceptible to the development of osteoporosis due to a significant decrease in estrogen production. Estrogen is a key hormone in the absorption and retention of calcium in females. Since estrogen production is greatly diminished with age, the absorption and retention of calcium decrease, leading to a reduction of bone density.

There are two main things that you can do to help prevent a decrease in bone density. First, consistently maintain a healthy, well-balanced diet. Second, participate in weight-bearing activities. Bones respond to stress in the same basic manner that muscles do. If you apply adequate mechanical stress to the bone, then bone density increases. If inadequate mechanical stress is applied to bone, then bone density decreases. Weight-bearing activity is the only way to increase bone density. Examples of weight-bearing activities are running, lifting, plyometrics, and heavy bag workouts. Road cycling has been shown to be non–weight bearing, resulting in no significant increase in bone density. However, mountain biking has been shown to be weight bearing with significant increases in bone density due to the rough terrain. Off-season resistance training is weight bearing and provides adequate stress throughout the entire body that will result in an increase in bone density.

These recommendations are not guaranteed protection against the development of osteopenia and osteoporosis, however. There is also a genetic component for the development of these disorders. But maintaining a proper diet and including weight-bearing activities in your training are vital steps toward maintaining proper bone density.

A significant decrease in cardiac output occurs with aging. This decrease is a result of a diminished stroke volume and maximal heart rate. The age-related decrease in stroke volume occurs due to a reduction in the left ventricle's ability to expand and contract, resulting in less blood ejected from the heart each beat. At the same time, there is an estimated decrease in maximal heart rate by one beat per minute (bpm) each year. The decrease in maximal heart rate is believed to be attributed to age-related changes to the cardiac-conduction system (electrical signaling for contraction) combined with decreased sensitivity of the myocardium to specific hormones, primarily epinephrine and norepinephrine. A decrease in cardiac output results in a corresponding decrease in aerobic performance.

Another key factor in an age-related decline in performance is the lessened ability to recover between training bouts, resulting in a decrease in an individual's ability to handle higher volumes and intensities. Monitor your response to training as you age, and adapt the training program accordingly. There will come a point when both intensity and volume will need to be adjusted to allow time for adequate recovery. The exact timing is variable and will be highly dependent on your age, training status, health, and training goals.

There is a decrease in neuromuscular response as you age. You will notice diminished performance in reaction times, neuromuscular recruitment patterns, and speed of contraction. The greatest impact is seen in voluntary muscle responses to a stimulus. An example would be a decrease in your ability to make a quick adjustment when riding rough terrain. Staying physically active will offset this decline, but it will not completely negate it.

Flexibility also decreases as we age. There are various reasons that flexibility decreases with age, for example, problems at the joints, decrease in elasticity of the muscle, etc. But the primary reason for such a decrease is directly related to a lack of flexibility training. If you want to stay flexible as you age, then you need to maintain a flexibility program.

Do not let age-related decreases in performance discourage you from pursuing your goal. Use this information to help develop a training program that will optimize your increases in performance. Keep in mind that increases in performance can occur at any age and therefore should not hinder anyone from starting a program. It is important to note that fitness gains for someone beginning a training program at age 45 will not occur as quickly or be as large as an individual who started a program at 20, assuming both are utilizing the same program. Training can lead to increases in muscle mass, decreases in body fat, increases in bone density, and lower blood pressure, and can positively impact cholesterol levels and provide many other health benefits. While medical clearance is important for all ages, it is vitally important that older individuals consult a physician prior to beginning an exercise program.

CHILDREN AND ADOLESCENTS

For the purpose of this section, childhood is defined as age 6 to puberty, and adolescence is defined as the time period from puberty to 18 years of age. Getting our youth involved in physical activity at an early age is extremely important, and mountain biking is an excellent way to do it.

Children and adolescents differ from adults both physiologically and psychologically. It is important to understand these differences as children should not be trained as small adults. The main physiological difference involves hormone levels. Prior to puberty, children produce very small amounts of hormones and therefore cannot adapt to training as effectively as adults. Research has demonstrated that performance gains in prepubescent children occur in areas of aerobic performance, anaerobic performance, muscular endurance, and muscular strength. However, the mechanisms behind these improvements occur through physiological pathways that are slightly, but importantly, different than adults.

With endurance training, children can experience significant gains in aerobic performance. However, with these gains there is little to no change in their aerobic capacity or $VO_{2\,max}$ measurements. Instead, increases in aerobic performance are attributed to improved neuromuscular recruitment patterns. As the child's technique improves, he becomes more economical and his aerobic performance improves dramatically with no alteration to aerobic capacity.

This same basic concept applies to resistance training as well. With resistance training children can see an increase in both muscular strength and muscular endurance. This increase in strength is not due to muscle hypertrophy, but instead occurs due to neuromuscular adaptations that occur through training. Children under the age of 13 should only be doing bodily muscular endurance resistance training and should not be lifting heavy weight.

The overall key message is that training for children should not focus on attempting to alter aerobic capacity or strength. Instead the training programs should focus on producing proper technique, leading to optimizing recruitment patterns.

Training for kids should focus on having fun while learning. At this stage, training should not feel like a chore, and children should look forward to it. The biggest mistake people make here is forcing training on children and working them too hard. Watch and listen to your child, and she will let you know when she is tired and needs a break.

During puberty, hormone levels begin to increase. As a child reaches adolescence, the ability to adapt to training, beyond just neuromuscular, improves dramatically. During puberty, male testosterone production increases to about 10 times that of prepubescent levels, resulting in a substantially increased rate of growth. During this period, joints may not be as stable, which may result in pain and possible injury during sports. Once puberty is reached, both volume and intensity can increase, but not yet to the level of an adult. An adolescent can begin an entry-level adult program at the age of 16. This is an average age, and programs should be individualized as some adolescents mature faster or slower than others.

Another aspect to consider when working with youth is that they are still developing psychologically. Children and adolescents may not be able to readily grasp complicated concepts. So keep the explanations simple and expressed in terms they can understand. This will not only get the concept across to them but will also prevent them from becoming frustrated.

Avoid training intensities and training volumes that are too high. In recent history, sports-related injuries have drastically increased in children due to improper training volumes. Children are developing overuse injuries that typically do not occur in athletes until their collegiate or professional careers. One of the primary reasons for this is that adult training programs are being applied to children and adolescents. Another reason is that kids are now playing sports at a high volume and intensity year-round. It is highly recommended that children stay active year-round, however, and mountain biking is an excellent way to stay active. But it is important to keep track of the overall training volume and intensity to prevent overtraining and overuse injuries. Not every training session needs to be high intensity. It is also important to account for your child's other sports when considering overall training load.

WEIGHT AND OBESITY

Mountain biking is an excellent way to improve health and lose weight, and many become involved in the sport for this reason. Research shows that individuals who are overweight and physically active are significantly less likely to develop cardiovascular disease than thin, inactive people. You do not have to look like a model on the front of a magazine to be fit and healthy. There are certain key points you should consider when mountain biking while overweight or obese, however.

If you are overweight, you are much more susceptible to the development of heat-related injuries as fat storage acts as insulation, reducing the body's ability to effectively dissipate heat. While this can be beneficial on cold days, it is counterproductive on hot, humid days. When training in the heat, be cognizant of the signs and symptoms of heat-related illness (discussed in chapter 8).

DIABETES

Diagnosed diabetics are typically well versed on their disease, treatment, and symptoms. While you may be confident that you can manage your diabetes, you should still consult with your doctor when beginning mountain biking. This section is not intended to provide medical advice, but instead to discuss a few key considerations that you may wish to discuss with your doctor. When developing a plan with your doctor, discuss how to alter diet and insulin injections, if needed, to accommodate your current level of training.

Another reason for obtaining a physician's clearance prior to starting a training program is that diabetes can result in the development of other health complications. Some of the common comorbidities are high blood pressure, cardiovascular disease, compromised peripheral vascularization, and peripheral neuropathy. While exercise is recommended for individuals with diabetes, it is important that diabetes is under control prior to starting a program and that control is maintained throughout training. Once cleared to participate in physical activity, you must monitor blood glucose levels before, during, and after training and adjust accordingly.

Diabetics are also well versed in the pathophysiology of the disease and its related factors. The following information is more for the coaches and trainers who may be working with diabetics. While there are other pathologies, I will discuss the two basic pathologies for the occurrence of diabetes. The first occurs when the insulin-producing cells located on the pancreas are damaged, which ultimately limits insulin production. This is usually due to an autoimmune dysfunction where the body's immune system attacks the cells. Because the pancreas cannot produce adequate amounts of insulin, many diabetics will need to inject insulin into their system. This type of diabetes is typically referred to as type I or early onset diabetes.

Whereas type I diabetes is a result of a decrease in insulin production, type II diabetes is a result of a decrease in insulin sensitivity at the insulin receptor sites. Insulin receptor sites are down regulated (reduction in hormone receptor sites) in response to chronic high levels of insulin being released into the system. This commonly occurs due to consumption of an overabundance of foods that are high on the glycemic index, resulting in regular insulin spikes in order to offset spikes in blood glucose. However, the two primary risk factors for the development of type II diabetes are being sedentary and being overweight.

Both exercise and proper diet have a strong effect on type I and type II diabetes. Due to the permanent damage to the islet beta cells of the pancreas, exercise and proper diet do not provide a cure for type I diabetes. However, a combination of exercise and diet can positively impact it by helping keep the disease under better control. Proper diet and exercise have a much stronger impact on type II diabetes as they increase insulin sensitivity.

If you have diabetes, work with a registered dietitian who is familiar with sport performance. It is unlikely that the average coach would have sufficient knowledge to adequately assess and prescribe proper nutrition to a diabetic, and some state regulations even prohibit giving nutritional advice to those with a disease state such as diabetes.

Low blood sugar (hypoglycemia) is of great concern for diabetic athletes, which is why it is important to monitor blood glucose levels before, during, and after exercise. Glycogen (the storage form of blood sugar) and glucose are the only sources of energy the brain can utilize. Therefore, when blood glucose levels are low, the brain and central nervous system are negatively impacted. The initial response to low blood sugar is the release of epinephrine (commonly referred to as adrenaline) in an attempt to increase blood sugar. The release of epinephrine results in a significant increase in heart rate, the development of muscle tremors, anxiety, and an increased appetite. These are the most common early warning symptoms of hypoglycemia. As hypoglycemia begins to affect the brain, symptoms of hypoglycemia worsen, resulting in headache, dizziness, fatigue, irritability, slurred speech, blurred vision, confusion, lack of coordination, and unconsciousness. In severe cases hypoglycemia could even result in coma or death.

Hypoglycemia can progress very quickly, and training should cease instantly upon presentation of symptoms. The athlete should then immediately measure blood glucose and respond accordingly. Diabetic athletes will typically keep foods high on the glycemic index available to help counteract a hypoglycemic episode. The athlete should eat, recheck blood sugar levels, and then make an educated decision on whether or not to continue training. If blood sugar levels are not within the normal limits or the athlete does not feel well, the training session should be canceled.

Mountain biking places a heavy strain on glycogen stores and blood glucose levels, and therefore adjustments to both diet and insulin may need to be considered. It is important to remember that blood glucose is released from the liver and into the blood at a much higher rate during exercise. Insulin-dependent mountain bikers may need to adjust insulin timing and dosage. It is very important, however, that you not make any alteration to your diet or timing, delivery system, and dosage of insulin before thoroughly discussing it with your physician prior to implementation.

ASTHMA

Asthma is characterized by difficulty breathing and is one of the most common chronic diseases that affects athletes. During an asthma attack, the air passage constricts and mucus builds up, interfering with normal breathing. The severity of asthma attacks varies and ranges from slight discomfort while breathing to a life-threatening blockage. For some athletes, asthma only occurs in relation to physical exertion, where an episode will occur only during or shortly after exercise, and is known as exercise-induced asthma. It is important to note that asthmatic symptoms can present 5 to 10 minutes after the cessation of exercise. Any asthma trigger (pollen, carbon monoxide, etc.) can increase the risk of exercise-induced asthma. Environmental factors also play a role. Cold, dry environments greatly increase the risk of an incident, whereas warm, humid environments reduce the risk.

A slow, gradual, and longer warm-up is recommended for those diagnosed with asthma. If you have frequent or severe asthma, pay close attention to your warm-up protocol. If prescribed by a physician, an inhaler can be used prior to competition in order to help prevent an occurrence. Never train without your inhaler physically present. As a coach it is always a good idea to have the athlete show their inhaler prior to the start of any session. Inhalers contain banned substances (primarily albuterol), and therefore use of an inhaler requires a medical waiver.

DISABLED ATHLETES

I believe that participating in mountain biking is an excellent idea for everyone, and I do not believe that disabilities should discourage or eliminate anyone from participation. For the context of this discussion, "disabilities" will be an all-encompassing term, covering everything from physical and intellectual disabilities to neuromuscular diseases. Mountain biking and strength-and-conditioning techniques can be adapted to accommodate an athlete's individual disability. You can find numerous examples of disabled athletes who have been very successful competing in mountain biking. It is beyond the scope of this section to give detailed advice for specific disabilities, so instead I will focus on general advice.

The first important step is to know and understand your specific disability as it relates to physical activity. Adjustments in bike setup and technique may be required to accommodate for your specific disability. Do not get stuck in the trap of trying to precisely follow the taught techniques when your disability pre-vents you from doing so. It will be frustrating and nonproductive. Instead, focus on the idea of the technique and what that technique is supposed to accom-plish. Once you understand the desired outcome, the next step is to develop a technique to accommodate for your disability that produces the same desired outcome. This may require mechanical alterations to the bike.

There is not a sport that does not have a related risk of injury. Some sports do possess greater risk than others, and there is risk involved when competing in mountain biking. Depending on your disability, you may or may not be at greater risk than the average cyclist. Therefore, it is important to understand your specific disability-related risks when it comes to participating in moun-tain biking. Speak with your doctor about your desire to become involved in mountain biking and discuss any specific concerns for participation, increased risks of participation, and adaptations that need to be made in order for you to safely and effectively participate. After speaking with your doctor, make a list of all concerns, risks, and necessary adaptations, and develop a strong training and racing plan.

If you have a coach, educate your coach about your disability. They may have never coached an athlete with your specific disability before and the more knowledge they have, the better they can assist you in reaching your goals. It is not only important to educate them about your specific disability but also to let them know you are not made of glass and that you are there to participate to the fullest of your ability and want to be challenged, to learn, and to grow just like anyone else they coach.

Lastly, there are many organizations that work with disabled athletes. The International Paralympic Committee is a great resource for disabled athletes (https://www.paralympic.org/). While mountain bike racing is not currently a Paralympic sport, road and track cycling are. These two sports are similar enough to mountain biking that many of the training and equipment ideas can cross over to mountain biking. There are many other organizations that provide training and information for disabled athletes. These organizations not only provide information but also provide an opportunity for you to connect with other athletes who have similar disabilities and are willing to share their expe-riences. Reach out and find an organization that fits best with your personal situation.

8

INJURY AND INJURY PREVENTION

This chapter is designed to provide basic information on injury and injury prevention for mountain biking. Mountain biking is a moderate-risk sport, where injuries are not uncommon in both training and competition. This chapter will focus on injuries where preventable measures exist. I will discuss both the mechanism of the injury and any possible injury-prevention strategies. The following is not meant to be medical advice, and you should always be evaluated by a doctor when any injury occurs.

PHYSICAL EXAM

Prior to beginning a mountain bike program, it is important that you get a physical exam to ensure that you are healthy enough to participate. If you have been inactive up to this point, it is even more important to have a physical exam prior to starting as being sedentary is a major risk factor for the development of cardiovascular disease, type II diabetes, high cholesterol, high blood pressure, and other medical problems. A physical exam will catch medical conditions that you may not be aware you have.

If you have a diagnosed disease state, doctors will often recommend physical activity as a method for improving overall health. If you are currently under the care of a doctor for a specific disease state, it is important that you consult with your doctor prior to participating in mountain biking. A physician is in the best position to advise you on your involvement in the sport.

It is recommended that older individuals (males over age 45 and females over 55) seek medical clearance prior to beginning any exercise program. As we age, we become more susceptible to the development of specific disease states, such as cardiovascular disease. As mountain biking can place a heavy demand on your cardiovascular system, it is vital that older individuals, and anyone showing signs or symptoms of cardiovascular disease, obtain medical clearance prior to beginning.

Below is a list of the common signs and symptoms associated with cardiovascular disease. The following list is not all inclusive and these symptoms only indicate the possibility of the disease. Only your physician can diagnose it or rule it out. Also, keep in mind that cardiovascular disease can be asymptomatic.

- chest pain at rest or during exercise
- pain in the arms, shoulder, neck, or jaw region
- abnormal shortness of breath
- irregular heartbeat (speed or rhythm)
- edema in the ankles
- cramping in the calf muscles
- unusual fatigue
- dizziness
- fainting
- difficulty breathing when lying down

When looking for a primary physician, I always recommend finding a sports-specific doctor or at least a physician who understands athletes. They will have a better understanding of the stress you will be putting your body through, how the body responds to training, and the mind-set that goes along with being an athlete.

When suffering from muscular injuries, connective tissue damage, or bone damage, I recommend seeking medical advice from an orthopedic sports-medicine specialist. These practitioners have a strong background in sports medicine, giving them insight into the mechanisms behind the injury and what it will take to optimally get you back to training and competing. They can make better decisions on your training load and what you can and cannot currently handle given your specific situation.

ILLNESS

Overall, exercise is good for the body and results in improved immune function in healthy individuals. However, a hard training session actually challenges the immune system, making you more susceptible to developing an illness just after completion of training. In addition, athletes who are frequently overtrained often develop compromised immune function. Frequent or persistent illness is a common sign of overtraining.

There are a few general guidelines to follow for training when ill. In most cases, training should be avoided when you do not feel well as your illness may become worse or last longer than it would have otherwise. Training should be avoided if you feel nauseous, have a fever, a headache, or body aches, or are experiencing severe fatigue. In most cases, you are okay to train with a cold as long as you do not have a fever or body aches and you have no chest congestion.

When your immune system is already fighting an illness, training will further suppress it, decreasing your ability to fight off the illness. Missing a few days of training to recover from an illness will not completely derail your training program, whereas attempting to push through illness could make it worse and result in an increased time off from training.

When taking over-the-counter or prescribed medication, know how it can interact with exercise. For example, decongestants can act as a stimulant, resulting in a significant increase in resting and submaximal heart rates. While this may not be harmful, it can result in alteration to training zones while on decongestants. Decongestants can also cause dehydration and drowsiness. Always ask your doctor how your medication can affect exercise.

CHAFING

Chafing is a common problem for all cyclists due to friction occurring between the bike saddle and the cyclist. Chafing presents as broken, sore, and red skin. In severe cases, chafing can result in bleeding. Infection can occur when bacteria interacts with the abrasions from chafing, resulting in a saddle sore. Saddle sores often present as small pimples but can develop into cysts that must be surgically lanced.

To prevent chafing, make sure that you have a good pair of bike shorts as they provide a layer of protection between you and the bike saddle. Bike shorts contain a chamois (pad) that covers the area of skin that commonly comes in contact with the saddle. The chamois is designed to reduce chafing and provide a little extra cushioning. You can also rub chamois cream into the chamois of the cycling shorts to add lubrication and decrease friction.

Another common cause of chafing is an improper bike fit. If the saddle is adjusted too high, it will result in you rocking back and forth across the saddle. This motion will increase friction and result in chafing. When the saddle is tilted nose down, it causes you to continually slide down the saddle. Every time you slide down the saddle you automatically push your bottom back up the saddle in order to maintain your riding position, resulting in chafing.

As mentioned previously, saddle sores are created through a combination of chafing and bacteria. Therefore, it is important to address the issue of bacteria as well. During a ride, your cycling shorts will become warm from generated heat and wet from sweat, providing an excellent breeding ground for bacteria. When you complete your training session, it is a good idea to get out of your cycling shorts as soon as possible. Always wash your riding shorts between rides in order to eliminate bacteria.

URINARY TRACT INFECTIONS

Urinary tract infections (UTI) are a common problem for females and even more so in female cyclists. The same scenarios that lead to chafing and saddle sores can result in a UTI as well. The constant moving on the saddle coupled with bacteria in the shorts can result in a urinary tract infection. It is important to get out of your wet cycling shorts and shower as soon as possible. Wash your shorts immediately after a ride and always ride in clean cycling shorts. These simple steps will go a long way toward reducing your risk of developing a urinary tract infection.

NUMBNESS

When cycling you have three primary points of contact: handlebars, saddle, and pedals. While you spend time in and out of the saddle when mountain biking, the majority of the time you will be in contact with the saddle. While in the saddle there is a lot of weight placed on the groin region, putting pressure on nerves, which can result in penile numbness in male mountain bikers. While groin region numbness is more common in males, it can also occur in female cyclists. Numbness will typically dissipate once pressure is relieved from the groin area. If numbness persists upon completion of your ride, you should seek medical attention. Three are three basic methods used to rectify this issue: altering bike setup, changing saddles, or purchasing new shorts.

The first thing to do is to make sure that your saddle is horizontal and not positioned nose up or nose down. A nose-up position will push the nose of the saddle into your groin area, causing numbness, whereas a nose-down position will cause you to slide forward in the saddle where the narrow part of the saddle will push into your groin area. If placing the saddle horizontally does not alleviate the problem, the next steps are to examine your shorts and your saddle. If you do not have a good pair of shorts, you will need to do some shopping as a good pair of shorts makes a huge difference. If your saddle is horizontal, your bike fit is correct, and you have a good pair of cycling shorts, then your saddle is most likely the culprit. This is where things get a little tricky as saddles are not one style fits all. You will have to try different saddles until you find one that alleviates your numbness issues.

Your feet and toes can also become numb during rides, especially long rides. There are two main areas that can cause foot numbness: shoe fit and the pedal shoe interaction. Shoes that are too small or secured too tightly can result in foot numbness. Mountain bike shoes should have a snug but not tight fit. When buying mountain bike shoes, try different brands and styles to see what fits best. Often, cycling shoes are narrow in the toe box. If your shoes fit as they should, and your foot is still feeling numbness, you may have the closures too tight (Velcro, shoe laces, ratchet straps, etc). Loosen the straps and see if that helps.

The second possible cause of foot numbness could be the shoe and pedal interaction. If the sole of your mountain bike shoe is not stiff enough and gives as you apply force downward, the pedal can push up, creating pressure on the foot. Too narrow a pedal can add to this problem. The worst combination would be a thin clipless pedal and a thin-soled mountain bike shoe. Cleat placement can also apply pressure to the foot, resulting in numbness. Make sure that your setup is correct and that the cleat is placed on the shoe so that when you are locked into the pedal, the pedal axle is centered on the ball of the foot.

If all these issues have been addressed and your feet still go numb, it may just be that particular shoe. I had a pair of shoes that felt as though they fit correctly and were not closed too tightly, and my feet would still go numb during longer rides. I bought a different pair of shoes and the problem went away. So, if you have tried everything else, it may just be time for a new pair of shoes.

Hand numbness can also occur when riding for extended periods of time. As stated previously, the body contacts the bike in three places: the pedals, the saddle, and the handlebars. The hands support the weight of the upper body and help absorb the vibrations from the uneven terrain. Your hand position on the narrow handlebar places pressure on the ulnar nerve located in the palm of the hand, which can result in numbness over a longer ride. The numbness typically presents in the fourth and fifth fingers. While hand numbness is common in all cycling, it is often amplified in mountain biking due to the vibrations sent up the fork from the uneven terrain. A good front-suspension fork will assist in eliminating the worst of the shocks, but your hands will still have to absorb some of them. Another way to reduce vibrations and help with hand numbness is to add a layer of padding between your hands and the handlebars with a good pair of padded cycling gloves. The last thing to check is your bike fit. Your bike should be set up so that you do not have too much of your weight distributed forward onto the handlebars.

It is important that you address any reoccurring numbness to an area as it could result in permanent damage. If you cannot determine a remedy on your own, seek help from a professional bike fitter. You may also need to seek medical advice if the numbness is persistent.

OVERUSE INJURIES

Unfortunately, overuse injuries are quite common in mountain biking. Mountain biking requires repetitive motion in a relatively fixed position and places stress on the muscles, connective tissues, bones, and joint structures. An overuse injury presents as chronic pain in a specific area that is directly related to training. An overuse injury can hurt before, during, and after training. Some overuse injuries may feel fine during training but then hurt after training or the next day when getting out of bed (plantar fasciitis is an example). The pain can range from mild and annoying to excruciating. If not addressed appropriately, the damage and pain can increase with continued training. Persistent pain should be evaluated by a doctor.

There are many factors that can contribute to overuse injuries. Many of these factors relate to improper training. One of the common mistakes made by beginning mountain bikers is increasing training volume or intensity too quickly. Remember to progress your training in a controlled and correctly paced manner. Always increase your volume first and then increase your intensity once you establish a solid base.

Another common cause of overuse injury is overtraining. It is important to allow adequate recovery time between training bouts. When you ignore necessary recovery time, it leaves the body in a weakened state that is susceptible to the development of an overuse injury. Be as diligent about your recovery as you are about your training.

Lack of flexibility is another leading cause of overuse injuries. I cannot count the number of athletes I have worked with whose overuse injury was the result of lack of flexibility. Once the flexibility issues were addressed, the overuse injury subsided. When joints are not able to easily go through their full range of motion during exercise, it can result in strain in that area and the development of an overuse injury.

Muscular strength around a joint can also play a factor in the development of overuse injuries. The weaker the muscles around a joint, the less stable that joint is and the more susceptible to the development of an overuse injury. Muscular imbalances can also lead to the development of an overuse injury. For example, if the quadriceps muscles are significantly stronger than the hamstring muscles, it will result in an anterior pull at the knee, resulting in static and dynamic instability. The closer the match in strength between the hamstring and quadriceps muscles, the more stable the joint will be. Not only should you work on increasing strength but also on ensuring muscular balance.

The last primary cause of overuse injuries is improper biomechanics or technique. In mountain biking, improper bike fit results in poor biomechanics, which can often result in the development of overuse injuries. When cycling, the human body and the machine work together in order to produce motion. As the human body cannot be adjusted, the bike must be adjusted to fit the particular anthropometrics of the cyclist. While you do move on the bike a lot more during mountain biking than you do in road riding, you are still cycling in a relatively fixed position with very little movement. Due to the rough terrain, pedaling cadence does vary for mountain biking throughout a ride. However, cadence will still remain anchored around 90 rpm. If you maintained an average of 85 rpm for a 90-minute trail ride, you would have pedaled 7,650 revolutions. This is a high-volume repetitive load. If your bike fit is not correct, it can easily result in an overuse injury. An improperly adjusted saddle (too far forward, too far back, too high, or too low) can result in knee pain.

In the following sections, I will list and briefly discuss the most common overuse injuries in cycling. I will discuss the mechanism behind each of the overuse injuries. Keep in mind that the pain you might experience could be due to something other than an overuse injury, and it is important to always consult a doctor when you are experiencing sharp or persistent pain.

Knee Pain

Knee pain when cycling can present anteriorly (front of the knee) or posteriorly (back of the knee). The location of the pain can provide clues as to what could be occurring. Anterior knee pain will typically occur at the patella (kneecap) or just below at the patellar tendon (tendon leading off the patella that attaches to the tibia at the tibial tuberosity). Patellar tendonitis occurs when excess stress is placed on the patellar tendon during the pedal cycle. Anterior knee pain is typically a result of cycling in too high a gear, large increases in training volume or intensity, or when the saddle height is set too low. While not as common as anterior knee pain, posterior knee pain can occur due to the stress of cycling. The most common cause for posterior knee pain is a saddle height that is too high.

Achilles Tendonitis

When pushing down during the pedal cycle, the foot has to plantar flex so that the force generated through the hips and legs can be applied to the pedal. The foot acts as a lever and the triceps surae (gastrocnemius and soleus) must contract heavily during this process. The triceps surae attaches to the posterior surface of the calcaneus via the Achilles tendon. These repetitive forces can place a lot of stress on the Achilles tendon, resulting in damage and inflammation. Achilles tendonitis usually occurs due to riding in too large a gear, increasing intensity too quickly, or if the overall training volume is too high.

Plantar Fasciitis

Plantar fasciitis presents as pain along the bottom of the foot located at the heel. Plantar fasciitis can be very painful. The plantar fascia is the connective tissue that runs along the bottom of the foot from the calcaneus of the heel to the toes and is responsible for maintaining the longitudinal arch of the foot. Plantar fasciitis occurs when the plantar fascia becomes damaged and inflamed. While damage can occur acutely, it often occurs due to repeated stress. Pain typically occurs after the ride but can also occur during. Plantar fasciitis can be very painful when getting out of bed in the morning. This occurs due to the plantar fascia shortening and tightening overnight. It is not uncommon for the pain to decrease throughout the day as the fascia loosens up as you move around. It is often recommended to sleep in a night splint as it keeps the foot in a neutral position and keeps the fascia from shortening and tightening too much during the night. There is a large amount of force placed on the foot as you push downward on the pedal. Due to this large force, it is important to use mountain bike shoes with a stiff sole that can alleviate some of the force placed on the plantar fascia. Plantar fasciitis can also occur due to the pedal axle being located too far forward on the ball of the foot, which effectively increases the movement of that foot.

It is important to address overuse injuries early in order to prevent greater damage. Too often athletes will ignore overuse injuries until they develop into an injury that requires a large amount of downtime or surgery. If you develop an overuse injury, it is important to address it seriously. If the pain is sharp or persistent, have it evaluated by a doctor. A common practice with most overuse injuries is to use rest, ice, and elevation. When approved by your doctor, over-the-counter anti-inflammatory medications can help decrease swelling and alleviate pain.

ABRASIONS

As crashing when mountain biking is very common, so too are skin abrasions. Skin abrasions occur as your skin travels across a surface, creating friction burns and lacerations. Abrasions are open wounds and should be treated as such. If the abrasion is serious, seek medical attention immediately. If lacerations are present, those should be addressed by a doctor as well. In most cases, abrasions are small enough to address at home. When sliding across the trail, small rocks, dirt, and other debris can become embedded in the wound and will need to be cleaned out in order to decrease the risk of infection. Make sure to clean the wound of all debris with a medical scrub brush. After the wound has been cleaned, coat it with ointment. Depending on the location and seriousness of the wound, you can keep it covered during the oozing stage. If you suspect infection, seek medical attention. Common signs of infection are listed below:

- swelling
- increased pain
- wound enlarging
- spreading redness around the wound
- fever
- puss and drainage

EXERCISING IN THE HEAT

Training in the heat places a great amount of strain on the human body. Heat is generated as a byproduct of metabolism. As intensity increases, so too does metabolism, resulting in an increase in internal temperature. This internal heat generation during exercise, coupled with environmental heat, creates a very precarious situation.

The two forms of heat entering the body from the environment during training are radiation and conduction. Radiation is the primary method and is the transfer of heat through electromagnetic waves. The sun provides radiant heat and is the most common form of heat. Radiation from the sun can either be direct or reflected off objects, such as asphalt. During the summer, thermal ground heat will radiate upward and can be transferred to the body during training. Conduction is not experienced to a large degree during training as it requires direct molecular contact in order for heat to transfer. The most common form of conduction during training is when the foot makes contact with the hot ground.

In order to prevent a heat-related illness, it is important to dissipate heat effectively from the body. In order for the body to dispel heat through radiation, the body temperature must be higher than the environmental temperature, not always an option. Conduction is not an effective method for heat dissipation during exercise either. Therefore, the two main sources for heat dissipation during exercise are convection and evaporation. Convection is the transfer of heat through a fluid medium. As the air travels across the body, the boundary layer of air next to the skin is continuously replaced with cooler air. The faster the boundary layer is replaced, the faster the body can dissipate heat. This is how fans work to help keep the body cool during exercise.

Evaporation of sweat on the skin transfers heat to the environment and is the primary method of heat dissipation during exercise. In order for the cooling process to occur, the sweat must evaporate on the skin. Relative humidity (the ratio of water contained in the air compared to the amount the air could contain) affects the ability of the human body to cool through the use of evaporation. If the relative humidity is 60 percent, then 40 percent of the air can accept the water. If the relative humidity is 90 percent, then only 10 percent of the air can absorb water, leaving little room for evaporation to occur and negatively impacting evaporative cooling during exercise. Windy days are beneficial as air moving across the skin will continually replace the boundary layer with less-saturated air to aid in cooling.

During exercise, heat is generated by the working muscles, increasing both muscle temperature and core temperature. In order for cooling to occur, the heat must be transferred from the muscles and core to the skin so that it may be dissipated into the surrounding environment. Blood makes an excellent transporter of heat as roughly 50 to 55 percent of blood consists of water. Autoregulation of blood flow allows for the redirection of blood flow to the skin in order to dissipate heat through evaporation, convection, and radiation. The cooled blood will then recirculate through the body to pick up more heat, and the process repeats. Keep in mind that as heat increases, a greater amount of blood flow will be redirected to the skin. This lowers the volume of blood flow to the working muscles and reduces performance.

As you can see, blood is vital in the process of heat dissipation. As blood is made up of predominantly water, hydration status strongly impacts the body's ability to cool. When you become dehydrated, your ability to cool the body is strongly impacted. To make a long story short, sweat is filtered plasma, and as you sweat, plasma volume decreases. The decrease in plasma volume results in dehydration and impaired cooling. As your ability to dissipate heat becomes compromised, the core temperature begins to steadily rise, resulting in the development of a heat-related illness. Water loss equivalent to 2 to 3 percent of body mass will negatively impact performance, whereas a loss equivalent to 5 percent or greater will negatively impact health. These numbers assume that you began the session fully hydrated.

Heat-Related Illness

Heat-related illness occurs when the body's ability to dissipate heat has been compromised due to high internal and external temperatures and dehydration. Heat-related illnesses are of serious concern and can result in death if untreated. As a mountain biker, there are many discomforts or pains that you can push through (I do not advise this course of action). However, a heat-related illness is not one of them. The primary heat-related illnesses are heat cramps, heat exhaustion, and heat stroke.

Cramps

Cramps present as very strong and painful muscle contractions, and they can occur due to dehydration and sodium loss. The best way to counter heat cramps is to stop exercising, get to a cool environment, rehydrate, and ingest electrolytes.

193

Heat Exhaustion

As your ability to dissipate heat continues to diminish, the thermoregulatory system is unable to effectively dissipate heat. The primary symptoms of heat exhaustion are as follows:

- headache
- dizziness
- nausea
- feeling of weakness
- tingling sensation in the skin
- chills
- pale, moist skin
- rapid, weak pulse

Heat Stroke

As you progress beyond heat exhaustion, your ability to dissipate heat is further impacted, resulting in heat stroke. Of the three heat-related illnesses, heat stroke is the worst as it can cause serious health issues, including death. Some of the heat stroke symptoms are the same as those found in heat exhaustion. There are a few key symptoms that differ, however, the most important of which is the development of a core temperature of 104 degrees (F) or higher. The other differing symptoms are cessation of sweating and hot, red, dry skin; these are signs that you have moved from heat exhaustion to heat stroke. The full list of the symptoms of heat stroke are:

- core temperature greater than or equal to 104 degrees F
- hot, red, dry skin
- cessation of sweating
- rapid, strong pulse
- headache
- dizziness
- nausea
- feeling of weakness
- tingling sensation in the skin
- confusion
- chills

At the first sign of a heat-related illness, you should stop exercising immediately, cool the body down as quickly as possible, and drink plenty of fluids. As heat-related injuries can escalate in severity in a very quick progression, it is important to cease activity immediately upon the first signs. Once core temperature starts to increase beyond the body's ability to control it, it will continue to rise as long as you exercise and generate metabolic heat in a hot environment.

Once you have ceased activity and have moved into a cooler environment, continue working to bring the core temperature down. There are methods you can use to lower core temperature to normal levels, such as taking a cool shower or bath, applying cold towels, or using ice packs. As dehydration is a key component of heat-related illnesses, it is also very important to ingest fluids. Rehydration can become problematic when you are nauseous and cannot keep fluids down. If this is the case, a trip to the doctor and an IV will most likely be required. If you suspect that you have heat stroke, seek medical attention immediately.

Prevention

The best way to prevent a heat-related illness is to not have an event in the first place. Here are a few basic prevention strategies that will help you avoid heat-related illnesses. When training outside, avoid the hottest part of the day and instead train early before the temperatures get too high. If training indoors, try to keep the temperature as cool as possible and use fans.

Choose appropriate clothing when training in the heat. Clothing should be breathable so that sweat is able to evaporate on the skin in order to cool the body. When training outside, do not wear dark colors as they will absorb radiation from the sun to a much greater extent than lighter colors.

As stated previously, proper hydration is important for dissipating heat and maintaining a functioning core temperature. Unfortunately, most athletes are chronically dehydrated during the summertime due to long hours training and inadequate hydration strategies. Keep track of water loss and water ingestion in order to help maintain proper hydration levels. Check your weight before and after training to determine water loss, and replace each pound lost with approximately 24 ounces of fluid.

Acclimatization is the strongest step that you can take to help prevent a heat-related illness. It will take approximately two weeks of training in the heat for significant physiological changes to occur during the acclimatization process. As the body adapts to the heat, more blood will be directed to the skin for cooling and there will be a more efficient distribution of blood throughout the body.

There will be significant alterations to sweating; you will begin to sweat more, sweat will start at a lower core temperature, and sweat will be better distributed across the body to optimize cooling. Sodium concentrations within sweat will decrease in order to help offset electrolyte imbalances that occur during heavy sodium loss. Glycogen usage significantly increases when exercising in the heat. After acclimation, glycogen usage will not be as high as prior to acclimation. This will spare glycogen stores, which are limited and can negatively impact performance when diminished.

In order to appropriately acclimate to training in the heat, you should start slowly and train during cooler parts of the day. Do not attempt to acclimate by training during the hottest part of the day or by conducting high-volume or high-intensity bouts in the heat. Instead, start increasing volume and intensity after the two-week acclimation period.

INDEX

ABOUT THE AUTHOR

Will Peveler is a noted physiologist with a teaching and research focus on the physiological and biomechanical factors that influence sport performance and is professor of exercise science at Liberty University. Dr. Peveler has been riding and racing since 1994 and has coached cycling collegiately. He is the author of the Train Like a Pro book series, *The Complete Book of Road Cycling*, and *Racing and Triathlon Training Fundamentals*.

9 781538 139561

FROM PROTEST TO POLICY

FROM PROTEST TO POLICY
Beyond the Freeze to Common Security

PAM SOLO

BALLINGER PUBLISHING COMPANY
Cambridge, Massachusetts
A Subsidiary of Harper & Row, Publishers, Inc.

International Standard Book Number: 0-88730-112-6

Library of Congress Catalog Card Number: 88-6206

Printed in the United States of America

Library of Congress Cataloging-in-Publication Data

Solo, Pam.
  From protest to policy.

  Includes index.
  1. Nuclear arms control—United States. 2. Anti-nuclear movement—United States. 3. United States—National security. I. Title.
JX1974.7.S515 1988   327.1'74'0973   88-6206
ISBN 0-88730-112-6

To the Solos—
Paul, Rita, Mary Beth, Kathy, Davey, Barb,
and the ones they love

CONTENTS

FOREWORD

In a macabre way, we can thank Hiroshima and Nagasaki for thus far preventing World War III. But the fear of nuclear war may not last forever. Accidents happen. Lunatics rule. Passions burst. A nuclear war could erupt, despite our best efforts to avoid it.

The first widespread peace movements emerged after the devastations of World War I, the war to end all wars. Then came World War II and Hiroshima and Nagasaki, which finally forced people to get serious about peace. As Robert Graves asked,

> What, then, was war? No mere discord of flags
> But an infection of the common sky.

From the fiery close of World War II, decades passed and dozens of religious, territorial, and political disputes lunged into wars. A few, like Korea and Vietnam, swelled into superpower faceoffs.

By the 1970s, the religious and secular communities that make up the peace movement renewed their resolve. Whether prompted by Vietnam or by the nuclear threat, this revitalization was long overdue. Peace is not simply the absence of war. Peace is more difficult to sustain because its goals are more nebulous. Peace requires the organization and implementation of policy.

Protest, on the other hand, is easy. Protest is more like war. Protest borrows the exhortive rhetoric, the tactics (mobilizations and marches), and the paraphernalia (arm bands, buttons, and flags) of military campaigns. A peace march and a military parade have much in common.

Pam Solo's book, *From Protest to Policy* uses the Freeze Movement, in which she played a key role, to chronicle the tension between mounting protests and making policy, between exhorting and educating, and between grass-roots organizing and governing. This is a fascinating and important story.

—**Representative Pat Schroeder**

PREFACE

The Freeze movement was not born in the mind of one individual or even in the minds of several individuals. It was given life through the interaction of many serious people looking for a way to act meaningfully on their values and their desire for peace.

The history of the Freeze movement is a history of one community after another developing local leadership and a corps of volunteers who became resident experts on the arms race. The story of the Freeze that can never be adequately told would be the story of heroic commitment by thousands of individuals of time and talent. Scientist, church leader, professional woman, working mother, civil rights activist, feminist, father, peace activist, environmentalist, lawyers, doctor, stockbroker—each had a personal history with the bomb. Incalculable hours were spent organizing, researching, writing, meeting, educating, petitioning, and doing electoral and legislative work.

Alan Kay in Boston put the first money into the Freeze idea. He was followed by so many others who knew that tangible resources have to be put behind our values. There were few who paid personal costs as high as those of the activists who traveled the country and the world arguing for and educating about the Freeze. Most are known only inside the movement. It is probably safe to say, however, that the Freeze could not have happened without the intellect and personal commitment of Randall Forsberg. She traveled and spoke—

teaching as few know how—about the arms race. She gave people information. More importantly, she gave them a feeling of power. It was Randy Forsberg and her colleagues in the Boston Study Group who took the idea of a freeze and researched it in detail. She wrote it up, and the handful of national peace organizers turned her proposal into an organizing tool. With it, they captured the attention of antinuclear activists throughout the country. It was all of these factors—the intelligence and vast knowledge of Randy Forsberg, the good timing and savvy organizing of the initiating group, the willingness of some to travel and organize for the better part of eight years, the widespread yearning for a political consensus, the desire to make a difference, and the spirit of cooperation and collaboration—that made the Freeze movement happen.

The Nuclear Weapons Freeze Campaign became, in just three years (1980–1983), one of the largest grass-roots social change movements in the history of the country. Almost as quickly as it came, however, it seemed to fade from the political landscape.

> After great pain, a formal feeling comes—
> The Nerves sit ceremonious, like Tombs—
> The stiff Heart questions . . .

> Emily Dickinson

This line from Emily Dickinson captures my own feelings since the 1984 elections, the turning point for the Freeze movement. Many of us in the movement felt its potential slipping through our fingers. We could not hold on to it, much less translate its massive public support into real political power that could force the enactment of a mutual U.S.-Soviet halt to the production, testing, and deployment of nuclear weapons.

The core questions I ask in this book are: Can the Freeze, or any citizens' movement, gain the power to move from protest to policy? Is national security decisionmaking susceptible to public opinion? What kind of organization must the movement have to ensure that it gains the momentum, visibility, and political power to translate public concern into policy?

More specifically, did the Freeze have an impact on national security definitions and decisionmaking? Was the impact great or small? When was it strongest, and why? When was it weakest, and what accounted for its weaknesses?

As one of the movement's founders and organizers, I have devoted many hours of reflection to understanding what happened socially and politically to the movement.

Despite our years of work in building one of the largest movements in the history of the country, we have not yet changed policy. At least, not in the ways we had intended. As the 1984 elections approached, it seemed clear that we would not be able to muster the political power to move from protest to policy. The movement's co-optation and erosion came from both without and within, as the story that follows will explain. But the internal crisis of the peace movement became evident to me in March 1983, as I walked through the cobblestoned streets of Potsdam in East Germany.

I was in East Germany as part of an AFSC delegation investigating the impact on its people and politics of American and Soviet deployments of intermediate-range missiles. I stayed with a young woman who is part of the peace movement in East Germany, such as it is in a police state. Through Christiana's eyes, I saw the world from the East. I felt her longing for freedom and democracy, but this desire did not compete with her commitment to socialism. Nevertheless, I felt her rebelliousness against the Soviet Union's domination and her anger at her own government's apparently absolute control over her personal choices.

Looking at night from Potsdam toward the West, we could see the flickering lights in the homes, stores, and office buildings of West Berlin. "I cannot go to the West. My grandmother goes each year because she is retired. I have an aunt and cousins in Australia. My mother traveled there last year because her sister was sick. It was very hard for me and for my father. My father had to see her travel alone to a strange place. For me . . . my mother was going somewhere I cannot know. I cannot share it with her."

We asked each other questions about everyday life where we lived. She asked me, could people share apartments in the United States? What did the western United States look like? Where had I been able to travel? But mostly we talked about politics and our respective views of the worlds we had inherited. I asked about the camps, the Holocaust, and whether she talked to her parents about it. "This is our greatest question to our parents," she said. "Where were you? How could you let this happen in our country?" In East Germany the youth are asking their elders the hard questions.

I was deeply challenged by this twenty-eight-year-old woman and by the other religious and young people in East Germany working for peace. Listening to their conversations and watching their faces as they talked about the risks and the costs they would pay for the sake of freedom and democracy. I saw immediately that they were not making rhetorical or self-congratulatory comments. And yet they talked, knowing that the state reacts swiftly and forcefully to suppress any action it does not sanction.

The circumstances in which East Germans live force them to a certain depth of reflection and consciousness of choice. Yet the danger is part of life, just like making music together, sharing friendships, or raising happy children. They feel a solidarity with the people of Chile and Central America, who are constantly on their minds—even minimizing their own danger in comparison.

But the comparison of their lives to ours was startling. I felt that these young people understood better than we do what it was going to demand of us all to stop the arms race. They knew that the struggle is not free of risks and costs, and that in taking those risks they are taking individual responsibility. I was more frightened than ever about the fragility of our freedoms in the United States in the face of increased militarism. The need to safeguard and extend freedoms to others seems more than obvious, but my experience in East Germany showed me another urgent need: greater political, intellectual, and moral depth in our own movement.

Christiana's question to her parents and her grandparents—"Where were you, how could you let this happen?"—reverberated through my head as I walked the sidewalks of Denver. There are too many similarities between our own times and the 1930s. Ours is a time filled with hate, increasing acceptance of violence as the norm, and categorizations of whole groups of people as expendable. A national security policy built on the threat to use nuclear weapons of mass destruction has become an organized, bureaucratized, and legalized holocaust system that is not morally different from the Nazi system.

We need a massive citizens' movement to counter the militarization of our society. That movement will be made up of ordinary people prepared to take individual responsibility. Are we up to the challenge?

ACKNOWLEDGMENTS

My thanks go first to Deborah Mapes. It is difficult to overstate the importance of Deb's work and contributions. She spent hours of tedious research and editorial work on the manuscript. Deb retraced the assault on the Freeze movement by the organized Right Wing and drafted these initial sections. I am grateful for her investment of time, energy, and intelligence as well as for her companionship and friendship.

I am grateful to the Bunting Institute at Radcliffe College and President Matina Horner and the support of Radcliffe throughout this project. Others who gave support and to whom I owe thanks are Wade Greene, Paul Aicher, and the Peace Development Fund. Special thanks also to the Institute for Peace and International Security for the exchange of ideas, for feedback on the manuscript, and for providing a base for continuing to organize while writing the book.

Writing a book is a team project. I'd like to thank those who have given generously of their ideas, time, and encouragement: Everett Mendelsohn; Mary Anderson; Michael Jendrzejczyk, who was my partner in this work for a decade; Paul Walker; Ted Sasson, who read and discussed the ideas with intelligence and enthusiasm; Naomi Chazan; Steve Van Evera; Jane Sharp; Andrea Avayzian; Gail Pressberg; Melinda Fine; and my Bunting Institute Work Group, Ava Baron, Luellya Hillis-Colinvaux, Eileen Julian, and Sandy Zagarell.

I am grateful to the people at Ballinger Publishing, particularly Carolyn Casagrande and Carol Franco.

I want to thank those people who have challenged me by their own efforts at social change: Isabel Letelier; Elise Boulding; Dorothy Day; Judy Danielson; Helen Caldicott; Christiana Hoch; Patricia Schroeder; the Sisters of Loretto, particularly Cecily Jones; Marian McAvoy; and Mary Luke Tobin.

Lastly, the great irony of working to end the threat of nuclear war is that the constant knowledge of it can rob one of a sense of life itself. Fighting this detachment from life is a personal part of a very political struggle. My gratitude goes to those who keep me open to life in the face of so much death, especially my family; my Denver "family," Marian McAvoy, Kathleen Mullen, Vicky Reeves; and Rochelle Friedman.

1 SECURITY PAST AND PRESENT
Which Way to the Twenty-First Century?

A mass movement like the Freeze did not just appear from nowhere, nor was it sparked by the extremism of the Reagan administration alone. Years of grass-roots education and organizing by groups and individuals aiming to build a new, local, and democratic power base from which to influence national policy spawned the Freeze movement. That base has grown in size, in sophistication, and in determination to move from the periphery to the center of national security decisionmaking.

While policy remains essentially unchanged, and is even somewhat more belligerent, the domestic and international politics of national security decisionmaking have been fundamentally altered. In 1975, most Americans did not even know that nuclear weapons were researched, tested, manufactured, and deployed in their backyards. Millions of Americans now assume that they have the right to enter the decisionmaking process when it involves the "national interest." Increasingly, the American people expect results from political leaders. The secret cult of nuclear weapons has begun to fall apart.

In this regard, the Freeze has been a significant success. A growing number of people are ready to reject the arms control elites as the high priests of the national security state, move beyond the narrow focus on arms control, and get on with redefining national security in the nuclear age.

Much of the national peace movement, however, is still caught between the liberal arms controllers' belief that negotiations can

1

limit the arms race as well as maintain superpower relations and the belief of conservatives that the foreign policy goal is U.S. superiority and a rollback of the Soviets. Arms control and what Robert Karl Manhoff calls the "cognitive regime of the cold war" are the ties that bind liberals and conservatives together in political consensus.[1] These ties must be broken and a new political language must be developed if any progress toward disarmament and real security is to be made.

This imperative has been dramatically underscored by the government's response to the Freeze movement. Reagan's accommodations to the Freeze reaffirmed for the current policymakers the utility of negotiations in "managing" European and American public opinion. Governments will always try to co-opt public sentiment when it reaches a certain intensity by using negotiation to propose cosmetic changes. If peace activists stay within the narrow arms control framework and avoid the tougher but essential task of redefining the terms of the security debate, both the movement and public sentiment will inevitably be co-opted. The focus of debate too often shifts to questions of which weapons systems to support and which to oppose. Obviously, this has a frustrating and demoralizing impact on grass roots activists.

Those people around the country who are nevertheless ready to move into a much tougher political debate need to know that this debate is linked to a political program and a winning political strategy. Clearly, national security policy can only be changed step by step. Incremental or transitional measures such as a freeze or a comprehensive test ban are feasible goals; the public can rally around them and hold decisionmakers accountable.

Everett Mendelsohn says, "We all agree that policy changes incrementally. The question is, where are we incrementally headed."[2] The analysis presented within these pages argues that the strengths and weaknesses of the first wave of the Freeze movement can become the foundation upon which a second, more powerful wave of peace activism can be built.

THE FIRST COLD WAR

You must know very well that in my view we should be working for a "historical compromise" between the superpowers and the blocs with the goal of withdrawing United States forces and bases from both Europe and Asia and withdrawing Soviet forces and bases from Central Europe, East Europe and Afghanistan etc? That should be the goal of our common work and anything else is merely episodes on the way. If we cannot persuade President Reagan to respond to the extended test moratorium offered by the Soviet Union, then we are certainly not going to get a freeze out of the Reagan Administration. I will regard with benevolence a revival of freeze pressure upon an administration subsequent to Reagan, but I do feel the United States peace movement should be raising its sights to more radical and more ambitious goals, such as the roots of the Cold War itself, since I think that paradoxically, by taking the easy route of the lowest common denominator, the necessary criticism of the United States militarism has been blunted.[3]

This position of British historian E. P. Thompson summarizes what I think are the central lessons and challenges for the future of the American peace movement. The experience of the Freeze movement supports the conclusion that peace advocates will continue to fail or fall short of their goals unless they radically alter the terms of the debate and challenge the deep structures of militarism. Progress in disarmament will never be made until the fossilized tenets of cold war doctrine have been replaced with practical principles that face the world as it is but refuse to accept the permanence of violence.

These new principles will need to break through the mind-numbing rules that dictate current approaches to international negotiations. Most importantly, the government, corporate, and academic bureaucracies that President Eisenhower warned us about will have to be either converted or coerced by nonviolent means into using these new principles. It is these bureaucracies that unquestioningly determine a future that can only result in a never-ending arms race and perpetual cycle of confrontation and violence.[4] World War III will not be ignited by accident, though some mishap such as an Iraqi missile accidently hitting a U.S. frigate in the Persian Gulf could have set in motion the responses for war. Nuclear war by accident is plausible, but we must accept more responsibility for it. World War III will happen because we endlessly plan for it in our minds. Our social, economic, and governmental institutions are based on it. British peace researcher Mary Kaldor calls this predisposition the "war of the imagination," and it does not depend for its prosperity on any actual use of weapons.[5]

Peace movements before the Freeze also tended to focus on weapons as the central problem to war and peace. They have based arguments and political programs on the assumption that modern technology had made war as a solution to conflict obsolete.

But weapons do more than serve as a symbolic exchange of power and dominance in the superpower competition. Though the technological imperative is important, the arms race is also driven by cold war confrontation. We learn only half the lessons of history if we ignore the political, moral, economic, and social forces set in motion by the transformation of the international order into a war system. It is worth reviewing that history before suggesting a new perspective on the cold war, militarism, and arms control.

Just before the First World War, Ivan Bloch, a Polish industrialist, wrote what he hoped would be a definitive study demonstrating that war had become

> [a] practical impossibility and that the only alternative [to war] was the development of mechanisms for international arbitration. . . . Even in the leading circles of Europe hardly anyone will deny that it will be possible to bring our means of annihilation to such a degree of perfection that war must become completely impossible. But the question is: have we not already reached such a stage of development in military apparatus, does that sum total of conditions not already exist under which we must eliminate war, since it has not only become a shattering experience, but also politically fruitless.[6]

Bloch's studies assembled a mountain of data suggesting that the "development of weaponry since the Franco-Prussian war dictated that any future war would entail the unprecedented slaughter of combatants."[7]

An estimated 19,619,000 people died in the First World War.[8] Still, Bloch's lesson on technology was not learned. The horrors of World War I, with its unprecedented number of deaths and its new weapons, did not prevent the Second World War. After the war, a vigorous peace movement emerged for a time, with students, clergy, and women forming its core.[9] But it did not develop a political program capable of capturing and giving direction to the isolationist mood of the American public and Congress. Peace organizations were temporarily able to build antiwar sentiment out of this isolationism, but it would prove to be shaky ground on which to build a durable peace movement.

Pacifist organizations were at their peak during these years, until 1937. The resurgence of European militarism and the election of Hitler jolted the U.S. peace movement.

Ironically, and tragically, the renunciation of war by Americans coincided with Mussolini's seizure of power in Italy, the Nazi triumph in Germany, and the growth of Japanese militarism. . . . Successive layers of the peace movement broke away in anguished response. Moreover, those with an ethical revulsion to war could not fail to reserve a special shudder for the peculiar horrors of fascism. The destruction of individual liberty, the glorification of hatred, and, perhaps the ugliest of all, a series of anti-Semitic attacks that raised the ancient pogrom to the status of a state religion, sickened the American peace activists, and led many to conclude that war represented the lesser of two evils.[10]

Albert Einstein and Reinhold Niebuhr were two of the first and most notable to break away from the peace movement. Einstein thought that a "new attitude" toward peace was needed because "the existence of two great powers with definitely aggressive tendencies makes an immediate realization of the movement toward disarmament . . . impracticable. The friends of peace must concentrate their efforts rather on achieving an alliance of the military forces of the countries which have remained democratic."[11] In 1939, Einstein joined Leo Szilard in proposing to President Franklin Roosevelt that an atomic bomb project be set up; they feared that the Germans were already approaching success on an atomic weapons project. Their proposal was eventually adopted in 1941.[12] Both Szilard and Einstein would later lead the effort to control the weapons they had helped to develop.

Meanwhile, demonstrations by the peace movement against Hitler began in the spring of 1933. American public opinion being predominantly isolationist, however, the demonstrations encountered fierce opposition to providing refuge for European Jews. Pacifists reacted to events in Europe by working to save Hitler's victims, even though less than 8 percent of Americans were willing to welcome those victims into the United States.[13] Anti-interventionist forces—led by an organization called America First—capitalized on this reluctance by using racism and anti-Semitism to bolster right-wing arguments against entering World War II.[14]

To deal with the dilemma posed by the right wing trading on isolationism, the peace movement tried to claim "isolation" only from a policy of war, not from world affairs. Franklin Roosevelt—like the New Right after Vietnam and Ronald Reagan after the Iranian hostage crisis—read public opinion and appealed to its isolationism and fear by arguing that we must stay out of war but be prepared for it.

The peace movement of the thirties was eventually pressed to the margins of the political discourse. It had not been able to effectively react to Axis aggression and brutality, nor to the international political realities of the Second World War. When the United States entered the war, any criticism of war became un-American. The peace movement was all but dead except for the religious pacifists supported by organizations like AFSC.

In the Second World War, the so-called rules of war were radically changed. The role of targeted civilian populations became more central to military strategies, and technologies, bureaucracies, and society adapted to the higher level of acceptable governmental violence. The massive deaths of combatants in the First World War were far overshadowed by the Nazis' methodical extermination of millions of Jews and other Europeans, and then by the American use of nuclear weapons against the cities of Hiroshima and Nagasaki.

The world itself was radically altered by the war. With most of the European states seriously weakened in its aftermath, the prewar international system was in collapse, leaving only two countries, the United States and the Soviet Union, to prevail as the dominant world powers. So it was, with the end of the war in sight, that Stalin, Churchill, and Roosevelt met in Yalta to determine the shape of postwar Europe. Within a few months, however, Roosevelt died, and Churchill was turned out of office by Britain's voters and replaced by Clement Atlee. Stalin was left to deal with Roosevelt's successor, Harry Truman, who was inexperienced in foreign affairs.[15] Germany had surrendered by April of 1945, and even though Japan's surrender was imminent, Truman made the decision to bomb Hiroshima on 6 August 1945. Three days later, the United States bombed Nagasaki. Historian Martin Sherwin argues that the use of the bomb against Japan was the first salvo in the East-West conflict, Truman having intended to send a message to Stalin as much as to bring the Japanese to surrender.[16]

Cold war politics started very early on in the postwar period, stimulated in part by the politics of the bomb itself. The British and the Americans had been conducting atomic projects in great secrecy, without informing the Soviet Union, then our ally. The Soviets' work on the bomb had begun in similar secrecy in 1942, two years after the United States and Great Britain had formed the Manhattan Project.[17] The United States tested the first bomb on 16 July 1945. Days after the test and only weeks before its use on Japan Truman is reported to have told Stalin that the United States "had a new weapon of unusual destructive force." Truman later wrote that Stalin replied that he was "glad to hear of it and hoped we would make good use of it against the Japanese."[18] Truman and Churchill were convinced that Stalin had not grasped what the president was referring to. They were mistaken; by the time of the Potsdam Conference in the summer of 1945, the Soviet Union had a full-scale bomb project under way, which Stalin had not revealed to Truman and Churchill. Soviet military analyst David Holloway speculates that "had Stalin been told about the bomb, his postwar attitude might not have been any different. Western secrecy contributed to Soviet suspicion and spurred the Soviet Union to develop its own bomb."[19] But mutual suspicion and secrecy sunk even deeper roots.

The late 1940s and early 1950s brought Soviet advances in missile technology and warhead developments. On 29 August 1949, the Soviet Union tested its first nuclear weapon. Washington knew of the Soviets' atomic weapons program, but it had not expected the Soviets to have the bomb until 1950. This early Soviet success shocked government leaders and led to Truman's decision to accelerate the American program on thermonuclear weapons.

The cold war and the arms race had been set in motion. "The Grand Alliance gave way to a global antagonism between two hostile coalitions, one led by the United States and the other by the Soviet Union. . . . One of them, the United States, had been little involved in the old system; the other, the Union of Soviet Socialist Republics, had been mostly excluded from it in the years between the two world wars. . . . They shared little except distrust."[20]

Postwar competition, secrecy, national ideologies, suspicion, and mutual ignorance compounded the dilemma for U.S. policymakers.

The two related questions that have always confronted those in the West who have to shape policies toward the Soviet Union[:] What is the connection between Marxist-Leninist ideology and Soviet foreign policy? . . . Does a totalitarian practice at home necessarily produce a foreign policy that is totalitarian in intent, committed to overturning the international system and to endless expansion in pursuit of world dominance? The policies of Adolf Hitler seemed to confirm that a powerful relationship did exist between such domestic practice and international behavior.[21]

In answer to these questions, the National Security Council, in a report commonly known as NSC-68, laid out the essentials of postwar U.S. foreign policy: "The Soviet Union, unlike previous aspirants to hegemony, is animated by a new fanatic faith, antithetical to our own, and seeks to impose its absolute authority over the rest of the world. Conflict has become endemic." While George Kennan, ambassador to the Soviet Union, had argued for a policy aimed toward containment of the Soviet Union, NSC-68 transformed containment into a doctrine of military competition and confrontation with the Soviets:

> As for the policy of "containment," it is one which seeks by all means short of war to 1) block further expansion of Soviet power, 2) expose the falsities of Soviet pretensions, 3) induce a retraction of the Kremlin's control and influence and 4) in general, so foster the seeds of destruction within the Soviet system that the Kremlin is brought at least to the point of modifying its behavior to conform to generally accepted international standards. . . . It was and continues to be cardinal in this policy that we possess superior overall power in ourselves or in dependable combination with other likeminded nations. . . . Without superior aggregate military strength, in being readily mobilizable, a policy of "containment"—which is in effect a policy of calculated and gradual coercion—is no more than a policy of bluff.[22]

Historian John Gaddis has called NSC-68—which was declassified and made public only in the late 1970s—a document that is as important to the shape of U.S. policy as the Constitution.[23] This report called for a tripling of the 1950s military budget and an expansion of air, sea, and land forces, both conventional and nuclear. NSC-68's recommendations for a militarized containment rollback policy led to what Daniel Yergin calls the "national security state"— a government within a government.

"NEGOTIATIONS AS USUAL"

It is simply not enough to look at the technologies and at attempts to control them without also looking at the political, economic, and social foundations upon which war and governmental violence are now firmly established as human institutions. Furthermore, for the peace movement to move from moral protest to moral *and* political force, I believe it must also connect its opposition to war to the historical, psychological, and moral roots of governmental mass murder inaugurated during the Second World War. The peace movement, like the larger society, has not faced the other lesson about the roots of modern warfare and the arms race: the lasting influence of the death camps themselves. War and human civilization were changed by *both* the genocidal policies of the Third Reich and the American use of nuclear weapons against Japan.

Today the central moral assumption of military strategists and policymakers—those who approve military doctrines and budgets—is the same assumption made in more primitive forms of slavery: some groups of human beings are expendable. The economic and political objectives usually invoked in the "national interest" to justify acts of war and violence incur domestic costs that are deemed acceptable. But the burden of these military costs is disproportionately shared by working people and the growing number of poor people. We can accept the presence of increasing numbers of homeless in our cities. We can support authoritarian governments in order to oppose totalitarian ones. To counter terrorism, we can support terrorist acts. We can train guerrilla fighters to overthrow regimes we disagree with, in the name of freedom and democracy. We can destroy the village in order to save it.

Richard Rubenstein explores this erosion of the worth of the person and the link between slavery and war in his book, *The Cunning of History.* According to Rubenstein, German society institutionalized a set of moral and political assumptions that made everything that happened at Auschwitz "legal." "We ignore this linkage, and the existence of the sleeping virus in the bloodstream of civilization, at risk of our future."[24]

Weapons of mass destruction are a symbol of the war system now sanctioned by government and integrated into our way of thinking through the reiteration of cold war beliefs. Like the presence of death camps in German society, the omnipresence of nuclear weapons in our society represents the political relationships, legal assumptions, and bureaucratic momentum behind the arms race. The acceptability of mass casualties from nuclear war and from small-scale conventional wars is at the heart of the war system that now consumes vast amounts of our nation's resources and human talent. Over 25 percent of American scientists are said to be working directly or indirectly on the development of weapons of mass destruction. In the United States, over 70 percent of all research and development funds in the federal budget are spent on military R&D. This leaves under 30 percent for every other operation of government, such as regulating and legislating in the areas of environmental protection, transportation, education, health, and social services. In addition to the use of public resources for military purposes, the expanding role of military research at universities reinforces the growing militarization of our society.[25]

The institutions which develop the technologies and the targeting strategies for warfare are held together by a belief that not only are some lives worth more than others but that all lives—from the entire population of the United States to the rest of the earth's inhabitants—are, under some circumstances, expendable and worth the risk of nuclear war. Our governments have strategies to enforce this belief, including psychological warfare, routine targeting of civilians, and the threat of launching unlimited nuclear warfare against the "enemy," inevitably involving the entire globe as a consequence. We must examine the realities of racial hatred within our own society and the ways in which we are mobilized to support our government's foreign policy when it declares the enemy to be the embodiment of evil—as with the Soviet Union—or distrustful, greedy, and bloodthirsty terrorists, as it portrays the Arabs. The psychology of the enemy and the role it plays in animating a threat system is critical. By setting up an enemy, the expendability of human beings is justified; social and governmental institutions are transformed and put in the service of planning for war, or "defense."

We and the Soviets have enslaved ourselves and the rest of the world to this threat, which is codified in cold war doctrine: the belief system that rules our thinking about the U.S. global role and the actions dictated by that role. "Security" is ensured by engendering fear not only in the enemy but in one's own population, to sustain its support. The cold war requires that both the United States and the Soviet Union have an enemy. Intimidation and unpredictability provide continuity and power to those who control the weapons. A "credible deterrent" convinces the enemy that you have the intention, determination, and ability—as well as the support of your population—to strike with impunity if your political objectives require you to do so.

The political objectives change as alliances shift and "vital interests" evolve. Protecting these vital interests provides the latitude that both Eastern and Western bureaucrats need as an excuse to mobilize the threat system against each other, or against each other's surrogates in the Third World. This threat system must eventually be dismantled. It is rooted in methodical, premeditated governmental violence. This threat system is a total system, which we might also call militarism: a way of thinking about the world and one's place in the world that is characterized by the promotion of aggressive, belligerent, and violent acts, with the intention of dominating and controlling international affairs. Militarism requires the domestic bureaucratization of these beliefs, through what President Eisenhower termed the "military industrial complex," and an enemy presenting a constant threat from both without and within. This cold war regime dictates political thought and imagination—by controlling the direction of domestic policy and transforming most foreign policy into a matter of military alliances and military intervention.[26]

Arms control negotiations—begun as a means of breaking out of the deadlock of East-West confrontation—have become a mechanism for managing the progress of the cold war, by elaborately, systematically, and mutually ratifying military advances on both sides. It seems that negotiations were never seen by cold war strategists—such as Paul Nitze, author of NSC-68—as a way to stop advances in weapons.

At the inception of the cold war, NSC-68 codified the purpose of negotiations:

> What, then, is the role of negotiation? . . . The public in the United States and in other free countries will require, as a condition to firm policies and adequate programs directed to the frustration of the Kremlin design, that the free world be continuously prepared to negotiate agreements with the Soviet Union on equitable terms. . . . The terms must be fair in the view of popular opinion in the free world. . . . A sound negotiating position is, therefore, an essential element in the ideological conflict. . . . For some time after a decision to build up strength, any offer of, or attempt at, negotiation of a general settlement could be only a tactic. Nevertheless . . . it may be desirable to pursue this tactic both to gain public support for the program and to minimize the immediate risks of war. . . . Negotiation is not a possible separate course of action but rather a means of gaining support for a program of building strength, of recording, where necessary and desirable, progress in the cold war.[27]

Arms control negotiations since that time have remained constrained by this original ideological purpose. Today politicians and arms control experts may argue that arms control is a vehicle for reducing levels of arms and working toward general and complete disarmament, but the process has become—if not so intended from the beginning—another hostage to the cold war. The rules of counting weapons, their elaborate systems of classification, the public posturing, and the private bickering over meaningless minutiae by both the United States and the Soviet Union have turned arms control negotiations into an unnecessarily tedious process. The tedium masks the net effect of negotiations: to serve as a superpower forum for scoring points against each other and, in collusion, for quieting their own citizens or allies and sustaining domestic support for military spending.

The arms control process, as currently conducted, merely legitimizes military buildups, defers real disarmament, and, more often than not, generates increased political competition instead of reducing it. The prospect that traditional negotiations will become the forum for progress toward disarmament is slim at best. Negotiations will lead toward disarmament only with sustained public pressure and a demand that the political relationships be changed in the process.

The peace movement faces this fundamental challenge: how to force the United States and the Soviet Union—the two parties with the dominant roles and most of the weapons—into taking action, while avoiding the trap of "negotiations as usual." One of the greatest hopes for real arms reductions lies in a serious round of independent reciprocal initiatives by the superpowers.[28] One side would initiate an action and call upon the other side to respond, with both sides committed to the promulgation of the step into a treaty within *months* of establishing the step as a mutual initiative. President Kennedy, in response to public pressure and concern over radiation effects, took such an initiative by unilaterally stopping atmospheric warhead tests and calling on the Soviets to respond. This led within weeks to signing the Limited Test Ban Treaty. But the United States missed another such opportunity when President Reagan refused to respond to the Soviets' unilateral moratorium on underground tests in 1985–1986. This could have led to a comprehensive test ban treaty and encouraged further steps toward the goal of disarmament.

The cold war was formed by the postwar world and has shaped policy since 1950. The militarization of containment policy remains the dominant political framework for defining what is acceptable in public policy debates.[29] But we are on the threshold of the twenty-first century. It is no longer 1945, and the world out there—the Soviet Union and the growing nonaligned movement in the Third World—can no longer be managed by cold war doctrine. This fossilized thinking remains largely unchallenged in the United States, even while the European peace movements have begun to develop a vision and a politics for a "new Europe."

THE NEW SECURITY DEBATE

The peace movement needs to get moving. If it is to initiate changes, generate new ideas, and function as a mediating force between the fossil of cold war doctrine and the brutality of militarism on the one hand, and a future of genuine security without nuclear arms on the other, it will need to change itself.

Both Democratic and Republican leaders have failed to construct a foreign policy that accounts for the increasing dangers of the arms race and the complexities of pragmatic relations with the Soviet Union and the nonaligned movement. As Italian peace movement leader Luciana Castellini remarked, "In political parties, the tendency is to think that what is rational already exists, so it becomes impossible to even conceive of a different world. The present is colonizing the future."[30]

Political parties will not generate new ideas; nor can we count on the imaginations of political or academic elites. The Freeze movement gave arms control new popularity on Capitol Hill, but that popularity has more to do with domestic politics and competition for votes than it does with a willingness to consider serious policy alternatives. Because cold war doctrine is the dominant ideology and acceptable framework for political discourse between liberals and conservatives, the margin of difference between the two parties is located between right-of-center and far right political perspectives. The political debate on Capitol Hill must remain within the boundaries of what is viewed as respectable thinking. "Respectable thinking" considers only what is acceptable to the Pentagon and powerful defense contractors. Traditional arms control provides a way for politicians to tinker at the edges of the kinds of changes needed, thus avoiding real policy changes. (One need only recall how support for a freeze was used to leverage support for the MX missile and the introduction of the Midgetman missile.)

Liberal Democratic use of arms control for domestic political gain is as dangerous as far right opposition to arms negotiations, because it feeds the public illusion that something is being done. The story of the political support for the Freeze by Democratic presidential hopefuls and the Democratic party only underscores the need for greater autonomy and sophistication in the peace movement. Unless the movement's leaders are visible and active voices in the public discourse, alliances with Democratic liberals who do not share the far-reaching goals of the movement turn the national debate on security policy into a political football. The current Republican and Democratic debate certainly will not introduce alternative security policies for democratic discussion.

The peace movement must combine a new political independence with its newly acquired sophistication in working with politicians. By understanding power dynamics and then entering the political arena with greater intellectual and moral clarity, the peace movement can better understand the reward systems that politicians respond to and can be wiser about when, how, and whether to compromise and confront.

The peace movement can generate the new security debate within which alternative policy could be made. The network of local peace groups—either autonomous or affiliated with a wide variety of national organizations—is hungry for resources and new programs and is also eager to generate that new debate. Groups throughout the country have been meeting to try to formulate a new direction for the movement, following the losses of 1984. Working groups on common security, the formation of movement study groups, think tanks, training sessions on strategy building, and attendance at national education conferences by local activists—all underscore the grass-roots strength of the peace movement. For example, in February 1987 over 300 activists from 40 states and over 100 organizations gathered in Cambridge, Massachusetts, to attend a national conference, "Generating the New Security Debate: Challenges and Strategies for the Peace Movement," sponsored by the Institute for Peace and International Security (IPIS). The merger of SANE: Committee for a Sane Nuclear Policy (SANE) and the Freeze is also a signal that the peace movement recognizes the need for reorganization and political leadership. But organizational strategy does not substitute for political strategy.

Policy will not change in ways the peace movement wants it to until the movement itself proposes and simultaneously works toward a long-range political program and immediate policy options. Holding such an education and action program in dynamic tension is essential and possible. Without this approach, the movement's local groups will continue to find themselves running from issue to issue, and national impact will remain marginal at best.

The peace movement knows best what it is against. Also knowing what it stands *for* is central to the task of developing a more effective peace movement; developing a clearer moral framework is one way it can move from protest to policy.

This new framework could define the preferred method for achieving the movement's aims as those actions that resolve conflicts with less and less resort to violence. This renewed movement would be motivated by the conviction that we are seduced by violence and have developed a habit of war. The threshold for acceptable violence has been lowered since the Second World War by the military interventions of both superpowers, as well as by the proliferation of sophisticated conventional and nuclear weapons to nations around the world.

The movement could adopt this rejection of violence on practical, intellectual, and moral grounds. These days, the self-righteousness of both religious and political fundamentalists makes some people reject the use of the word "moral." It has become a cover for right-wing activists promoting actions by the government that would dictate our private and personal choices and behavior. I am suggesting, however, that the movement advocate a morality we can all share; that is, one that guides public life and rejects the legitimacy of violence.

> Violence is essentially wordless, and it can begin only where thought and rational communication have broken down. Any society which is geared for violent action is by that very fact systematically unreasonable and inarticulate. Thought is not encouraged, and the exchange of ideas is eschewed as filled with all manner of risk. Words are kept at a minimum, at least as far as their variety and content are concerned, though they may pour over the armed multitude in cataracts: they are simply organized and inarticulate noise destined to arrest thought and release violence, inhibiting all desire to communicate with the enemy in any other way than by destructive impact.[31]

While pacifists have long rejected violence, what is new in Thomas Merton's formulation is the recognition of how the political utility of war and violence evolves and what it leads to. This radical idea is based on the realization that there are severe limits to the military "solution" to complex regional and local conflicts in this nuclear age. For example, military strength could not prevent the taking of U.S. hostages in Iran. Ironically, the only use the Reagan administration could find for its military arsenal in fighting for the release of the hostages was to sell those arms to Iran. Selling arms to Iran provided the covert funds to arm the Contras in Nicaragua. Foreign policy was privatized and the Constitution was subverted, in the name of freedom and democracy. Meanwhile, the world became less secure, not more so, and regional conflicts in the Middle East and Central America intensified. Military solutions seem even more unpromising as superpower involvement in the Persian Gulf grows.

The new public morality that could guide foreign policy-making requires first the development and then the international institutionalization of mechanisms for dismantling governmental violence. The use of military force to attain foreign policy goals would be delegitimized and replaced by peacemaking policies. Just as the human rights covenants codify and define human rights, the peace movement could advocate "security rights" rooted in the principled goal of ridding the international system of violence.

Resolving conflicts with less and less violence over time is an effort that can be defined and its progress measured. The measurement of foreign policy proposals and decisions would be: *Do they reduce the levels of violence and increase freedom and development?* Any governmental action that escalates or encourages violence, particularly against civilians, would be opposed vigorously. Any governmental action that promotes political settlement of differences, reduces the likelihood of violence, and promotes freedom and self-determination would be just as vigorously supported by this new movement. It could develop an inventory of violence-inducing behaviors by governments; ways of measuring those behaviors; and ways of naming and rating the governments that promote violence as well as those governments that promote political dialogue and peaceful settlement of conflicts.

Bombings, assassinations, transfers of offensive weapons, transfers of nuclear capabilities, and conventional arms sales to regions of conflict are all violence-promoting actions by governments. What we need to acknowledge is that this violence-promoting behavior not only leads to deaths in conventional wars, counterrevolutionary wars, and so-called low-intensity conflicts, but also fuels other forms of violence: hunger, disease, illiteracy, and so on. Conflicts within and between states often develop from the conditions of poverty accompanying social and political oppression. When human beings are vulnerable to disease, malnutrition, starvation, and illiteracy, violence is being done, and the seeds of war and social conflict grow.

There is a simple, practical, yet profound relationship between violence and human vulnerability. Thus, another indicator of "not-violent" governmental policy would be how it increases the quality of life, and how it reduces human vulnerability.[32] The deeper connections between the goals of development and disarmament must be illuminated. These ties already demonstrate the trend toward more and more transfers of human and financial resources into militarily defined security. By linking governmental violence to human vulnerability, the priority of persons—human life—will return as the animating center of peace action.

A new wave of peace activism oriented this way will gain moral authority, public support, and political power. Such a movement will conduct short-term campaigns, but will also keep growing only if it enlists the support of people for their lifetimes. A permanent public mobilization must be part of the dream. Just as John Muir and others saw into the future when they sought to preserve natural beauty and the wilderness for generations to come, the peace movement can preserve—even in a culture fixated on instant results and immediate gratification—a sense of the future. While governments and bureaucrats cannot seem to plan for the future beyond the next five years, the peace movement must demand action now and promote a public morality that moves beyond mere survival and toward an internalized belief that we do "borrow the future from our children" by the actions we take today.

To achieve the goals of preserving life on the planet, averting nuclear war, and reducing the loss of lives in conventional wars—through citizen peace initiatives (such as Witness for Peace) and governmental action (such as the Contadora and Five Continents Peace Initiative)—the movement should also promote healthy psychological and physical development at home. Some in the Scandinavian peace movement have suggested making the quality of life for children the measurement of a successful security policy. We could consider some similar standard, as developed and advocated by groups like the Children's Defense Fund.

Of course, all of this requires that we develop and act on such an agenda through the major institutions of our society. Churches as well as civic and social organizations could initiate awareness of these political and moral equations by calling for our security rights and demanding that they be translated into the rule of law, nationally and internationally. Governments and politicians will give the people what the people want only when the people demand it.

There are lingering and long-lived effects from the first phase of the Freeze movement that can become the foundation for the next era of peace activism. Hardheaded evaluation and acceptance of the past's limitations and failures can not only help us avoid repeating mistakes, but can even encourage us to build on them in the peace work ahead of us.

THE FREEZE CAMPAIGN:
A FOUNDATION TO BUILD ON

The Freeze movement burst onto the political scene in 1980, just as Ronald Reagan assumed the presidency. While Reagan and many of his top appointees were talking soon thereafter about fighting and winning nuclear war in Europe and about the need to gain nuclear superiority over the Soviets, a gathering storm of opposition was building throughout the United States and the NATO countries.

The Freeze movement began as a way of breaking the deadlock that the traditional process of arms control had on U.S.-Soviet relations and on disarmament. The Freeze proposal hoped to sidestep the trap of negotiations, challenge the theory of bargaining chips, and prevent the rise of a new cold war between the United States and the Soviet Union.

Initiated as it was when both the United States and the Soviet Union acknowledged "essential equivalence" in their respective nuclear forces, the Freeze proposal was an idea whose time had come. Parity was about to be eroded by new deployments of weapons designed for a preemptive first strike. The technological developments represented by the Soviet SS-20 and SS-22 and the U.S. MX, Pershing II and cruise missiles reinforced perceptions on each side that the other was preparing for a new round of the arms race.

The bellicose language and almost naive bravado of the Reagan administration detonated public concern and response. But the Freeze movement was not just a reaction to the extreme rhetoric and overtly dangerous policies of the Reagan administration. It was a social movement intentionally and methodically organized by long-time peace organizations and activists.

Those who organized the movement wanted to create a permanent public mobilization to freeze the nuclear arms race in place—as a first step toward disarmament and toward confronting the increased militarization of foreign policy, made so apparent during the Vietnam War. The freeze proposal called on the United States and the Soviet Union to "initiate an immediate, verifiable, mutual halt to the production, testing, and deployment of new nuclear weapons and their delivery systems." The goal of the movement was to make a freeze on nuclear weapons government policy. The Freeze proposal was not meant to be merely a symbolic statement against the threat of nuclear war, or yet another peace movement slogan. The movement intended to get a freeze through either presidential action or congressional mandate in the form of funding cutoffs.

The movement hoped to use a variety of grass-roots organizing strategies to push the president and Congress to enact a freeze. The primary strategies were public education and action leading to direct pressure on the president, legislative action in Congress, and grass-roots involvement in the electoral process. Initially, the campaign had a five-year time frame for achieving its goal. While this deadline infused its network and day-to-day work with a sense of urgency and purpose, the campaign tried as well to provide its rapidly expanding grass-roots organization with a sense of orderliness and methodical planning.

The diverse national and local groups that made up the Freeze movement of 1980–1986 can continue to function as a protest movement. They can keep dissent possible, and they can make it impossible—or at least more difficult—for the government to do what it is inclined to do when it has no visible opposition. The peace movement has traditionally been a protest movement. Since at least as long ago as the Second World War, this has been the primary role of organized peace opinion in the United States.

This role has been vital in protecting and preserving basic civil liberties and in limiting military adventurism during the Kennedy, Johnson, Nixon, Carter, and Reagan presidencies. It is well documented that presidents have considered using nuclear weapons from the Korean War through the Vietnam War. But protest movements contributed to presidential decisions to not initiate, or threaten, nuclear attack. Organized and effective protest is no small accomplishment.

The Freeze movement, however, aspired to make government policy out of its proposal for a mutual halt to new nuclear weapons. The Freeze should be measured against that goal of being a political movement capable of shaping policy.

The equivalent of a coup took place in 1980 when Reagan's election knocked the Democratic party out of the political ring. For the first two years—if not for his entire presidency—Ronald Reagan functioned without an opposition party. The Democrats either rushed toward the right or remained cautious about taking on a "popular" president.

Despite the bipartisan agreement on cold war politics maintained through the Carter years, Reagan's election brought on the collapse of liberal and centrist positions, creating a vacuum that the Freeze movement was ready to fill, at least for the first two years of the Reagan administration. The Freeze, however, was being pulled in two opposite directions; it was sympathetic to one and needed the other to reach its goal of freezing the arms race.

The first was that mass of groups and individuals desperate for political leadership. They found little or no hope in the Democratic party. Liberals had been defeated in November of 1980 not only by right-wing political organizing but by the acquiescence of liberals to the right-wing political agenda and rhetoric. Jimmy Carter had caved in, and Senate liberals such as Frank Church had followed suit. Politics abhors a vacuum, and the Democrats had left a very large one.

Support also came from those pulling the freeze in the other direction with their narrower political agenda. Prominent arms control experts and former government officials (many having been formally denied access to the administration) were looking for a base from which to challenge and reenter the political debate. The endorsement and participation of public officials like Paul Warnke and William

Colby added credibility and visibility to the movement. The Freeze movement, in turn, could be supported by those who had been shut out of the inner workings of the State Department and the Pentagon to confront their nemeses in the national security establishment and in the Reagan administration.[33]

Support for the Freeze campaign was rounded out by groups fighting to save social programs and environmental safety standards. These organizations gravitated toward the Freeze movement because it was one of the only avenues for progressive politics and because they could support its commonsense proposal.

The Freeze caught the press, Congress, and the administration off-guard. What had seemed to be a national mandate for Reaganism was dramatically challenged by the Freeze movement alone, which, as a protest movement had an astounding impact. It forced accommodations from congressional and executive decisionmakers and from national security elites. While policy remains essentially unchanged, it has been far from unchallenged. The logic of the arms race and the forces propelling it were deeply shaken by the Freeze movement. The Freeze can rightfully claim many accomplishments, from educating the public to forcing members of Congress to become conversant with weapons systems and military doctrines so that they can strongly challenge the administration on arms control policy. The Freeze changed the issues and the language used by politicians to discuss them.

Because of the Freeze movement, Ronald Reagan had to move toward the center on arms control policy. The man who had spent his political career opposing every major arms control agreement, and who was dogmatically opposed to dealing with the Soviets, became pragmatic. Within two years, President Reagan was converted. He pledged his commitment to arms control and "nuclear weapons reductions." Chastened by public opinion, Reagan learned to mute his bellicose statements about the Soviets and nuclear war so as to give at least the appearance of negotiating arms reductions with the Soviets.

And here is the ironic twist for the Freeze. When Reagan moved toward the center and "got religion" on arms control policy, accommodating to the realities dictated by public opinion polls, he deflated the Freeze movement and disarmed his political foes in Congress and in the 1984 presidential race. Public opinion was further tranquilized by the president when he denounced the immorality of nuclear deterrence and offered his vision of a world rid of the threat of nuclear war, in his "Star Wars" speech of 23 March 1983:

> What if free people could live secure in the knowledge that their security did not rest upon the threat of instant U.S. retaliation to deter a Soviet attack, that we could intercept and destroy strategic ballistic missiles before they reached our own soil or that of our allies?

The President answered that question with "a vision of the future which offers hope. It is that we embark on a program to counter the awesome Soviet missile threat with measures that are defensive." He continued by announcing

> a comprehensive and intensive effort to define a long-term research and development program to begin to achieve our ultimate goal of eliminating the threat posed by strategic nuclear missiles . . . and free the world from the threat of nuclear war.

Masterfully, the president appealed to the American public's fear of the Soviets, fear of nuclear war, love affair with technology, and its newly confirmed belief that deterrence will fail over time. Congressional debate was disciplined and further stifled as the president used the "promise" of Geneva and the need for bargaining chips at the negotiation table to derail congressional initiatives on arms control.

The very same movement that shocked the administration, the Democrats, and the media in 1982, was diverted, diffused, and disillusioned by 1984. The Freeze struggled to prevail on four fronts. First, it had to avoid being reduced to the staging ground from which Democratic presidential hopefuls could badger Reagan, which could only lead to the Freeze being further sloganized and trivialized by friends and foes alike on Capitol Hill. Secondly, it needed to respond directly to the arms control initiatives of the president as well as to his escalating red-baiting tactics. The third front required a response to the army of right-wing opponents and its attacks. This network was coordinated to include the president and major political allies such as Senator Jeremiah Denton and Congressman Larry McDonald. The fourth challenge was keeping the grass-roots campaign growing, finding tactics to keep it mobilized and visible, and developing political leadership so that Freeze policy proposals could be distinguished from those of the president and Congress.

As it took on these four fronts, the movement narrowed its agenda, which in turn constrained its educational program and confined its politics. The Freeze opted to hold onto its early visibility and the respectability brought by the support of political and arms control elites. Woven throughout its efforts to deal with these challenges was the movement's inability—if not conscious choice—to refrain from raising political issues. It chose to address the freeze on technical grounds, that is, on terms acceptable to and defined by the administration, congressional allies, and right-wing opponents. It strayed from its own original goal of breaking out of arms control "negotiations as usual" and challenging the new militarism.

According to James Skelly of the Institute on Global Conflict and Cooperation:

> The great strength of the freeze was its initial breakout from the dominant discourse. . . . The energy behind the early freeze movement was a testimony to the fact that it had liberated large numbers of people from their imprisonment in the regime of truth constructed around nuclear weapons. It allowed people who had previously been part of the culture of silence around nuclear weapons to speak, and as such threatened to reinvent a political discourse around foreign and military policy. . . . President Reagan, sensing in his own way that the freeze was an attempt to break out of the discourse, tried to suggest both that he was constrained by the discourse and that the freeze was not enough of a break with it by saying that the freeze "isn't good enough, because it doesn't go far enough." . . . That which had originally contributed to the recapture of political voice by citizens on the issue of nuclear weapons, now began to make them increasingly silent.[34]

The words, the arguments, the way the movement shaped and defined the public discourse—these were critical to the Freeze's ability to gain political power. The movement was engaged in a "war of ideas,"[35] and early on it began to erode one of its most potent stratagems: its break with the dominant discourse of arms control and the cold war.

The educational work of the campaign was no longer a vibrant movement-building tool but a caboose pulled along behind the engine of pragmatic politics, which were increasingly dictated by the vagaries and vulgarities of Washington politics. The education program of the movement was simultaneously far-flung and narrow. Fact sheets on the details of treaty verification and on the history of intervention rolled off the presses. Each one demonstrated an isolated depth of information and the research abilities of Freeze staff and volunteers. But no political program or vision of an alternative security system in the nuclear age gave them coherence or meaning.

The politicians needed us, and (we thought) we needed them. The pressure to narrow the agenda, limit the arguments, and remain "respectable" seemed compelling at the time: How else were we to build a grass-roots power base and get a foothold within the power structure?

These seemed like worthwhile, short-term compromises because the freeze was primarily a strategy—a genuine first step in building a movement with the political and social power to define national security and change policy. The shared assumption of movement leaders was that a win on the nuclear weapons freeze would create a "political vortex" and other steps would then follow naturally. The naivete of this assumption is one of the critical areas to be explored in the following pages.

Still, it didn't take long for many of us to see that the Freeze was a mile wide and an inch deep. The core organizers soon realized that we were in a political cul-de-sac. We were lacking a way to deepen the movement's own understanding of the problems on which it was working. As a consequence, the movement was also unable to keep educating the public and policymakers. More importantly, the narrowing of its agenda deeply influenced the movement's ability to define the problem and set the terms of the debate. The grounds on which it could debate the nuclear arms race became more and more limited; its increasingly technical arguments were determined by the "lowest common denominator" rather than by politics.

As it lost sight of political strategy, the Freeze became an end in itself. The larger analysis—the more far-reaching political program the Freeze was meant to initiate—became secondary. A Freeze "fundamentalism" dominated key political opportunities, thus preventing the campaign from asserting its leadership or using its power effectively. The only agreement was on the Freeze proposal itself; later, shakier agreement was maintained on various mutations of the original proposal. Suspended altogether were decisions about the movement's position on deterrence and on the abolition of nuclear weapons, without which firm decisions could not be made on the direction of its educational progam or the steps that would follow the enactment of the freeze.

Furthermore, the Freeze movement found itself unable to focus political opposition on the cruise and Pershing II missiles (the very weapons it meant to stop), much less on the MX missile. Some critical organizing was derailed or postponed because congressional supporters feared the charge of unilateralism (mainly a public relations problem I will argue here) as well as the possibility of igniting the deeper debate about NATO and extended deterrence.

By keeping political issues on the sidelines, the Freeze was also transformed into an arms control movement—not a peace and disarmament movement—and its attention became riveted on technical debates that damaged its popular base. As the debate became more technical, the American public increasingly tended to leave it to the experts. The less political direction the movement gave to its elite supporters, the more minimalist its agenda became, which simultaneously sent those supporters the signal that they could set the movement's political program. Just as Congress sought the least common denominator as its operational style, so did the movement. Having filled the political vacuum in 1980–1983, the Freeze subsequently traded in its leadership role for that of a special interest lobby.

Herein lies the organizing challenge, and the intellectual, moral, and political challenge, for the movement's organizers and strategists: *can we inspire a social movement capable of generating sustained public support for a new vision of U.S. global responsibilities, with a specific political program and policy objectives to which we can hold decisionmakers accountable?*

It is important to look at the Freeze as a social movement that grew out of the activism and political learning of the 1960s and 1970s. These social and political roots are important to bear in mind as we attempt to evaluate the Freeze's political impact and assess its future, because the movements of the future are embedded in our past and even now are gestating in our recent past.

To move from protest to policy, a movement must also have an intellectual and moral framework for acting and thinking; otherwise, it will fail. That framework must be explicit in the life of the movement. It is not static; an intellectual and moral grounding gives the movement vitality and cohesion.

As I look more closely at the Freeze movement and draw lessons that are instructive for moving from protest to policy, my analysis will be based on four related, but distinct, components of movement building:

1. *Identify and name the problem as well as the social, political, and economic forces at work.*

2. *Raise public awareness and mobilize natural and potential allies.*

3. *Translate that public awareness into a power base to be used on behalf of movement goals and political objectives; anticipate adversaries; identify and evaluate unexpected opponents.*

4. *Build the institutional capacity to operate on all these levels at once.*

Animated by its beliefs and values, and informed by its commitment to knowledge and understanding, a movement hopes to act historically, not just in the immediacy of constantly changing political realities. But the clearer the movement is about its social-change model and about both its long-range and near-term political program and goals, as it works with elites and retains its independence it is more likely to successfully navigate the very complicated waters of power politics.

2 NAMING THE PROBLEM
Crisis or Opportunity?

The first step to building an effective movement is to understand the nature and history of the problem to be worked on, to name that problem, and then to develop, among organizers as well as the public, ever more complex understandings of the problem.

A vital problem that the core organizers of the peace movement need to begin with is assessing the roles various forces play in shaping national security policy. Social, economic, civic, and political forces have different histories. Each exerts a different influence on security decisionmaking. Analyzing these influences provides the context within which a movement chooses a realistic political strategy and measures its own power. Similarly, by naming and differentiating among the adversaries—attempting to anticipate their arguments, resources, and interests—a movement's political and educational strategies can be further refined and targeted. Through accurately identifying the various players on the field, a movement can more methodically enlist the support of natural allies, recruit other potential supporters, minimize the opposition, and possibly convert opponents.

Power is constantly shifting, and movement organizers must make nuanced judgments from the changing and ever more sophisticated information at hand. Commitment to an action-reflection-research process enables a movement to change its own definition of the problem as this new information and experience accumulate.

By anticipating power dynamics, a movement can shape these dynamics, not just respond to them. These dynamics include historical alliances, the impact of cultural values, and the economic or social power that different groups have over the problem. The continuing identification and assessment of the role and power of social and political forces helps to build an intellectually rigorous and politically sophisticated movement.

Another major task of a movement is to keep control of the agenda; that is, to maintain and expand its role in setting the terms of the debate. A movement must fight for the legitimacy of its ideas. Research and reflection are ongoing mechanisms by which movement organizers can anticipate and forecast the shape of the public discourse they intend to inaugurate through action and education strategies.

A routine movement activity is sorting and evaluating the short-term and long-term impacts of its actions. What effect did the action have on policymakers? What effect on the public? How have alliances and power relationships shifted or changed as a result? How does the problem look from the perspective of other people and groups? How should we integrate this new information as we plan for further actions? These are questions that organizers need to ask if they are to continue clarifying the problem, crafting strategy, and moving closer to policy changes. A movement must remember that its goal should be changing policy and solving problems, not just witnessing against a wrong. Its commitment to developing its own base of information will not only empower a movement to more effectively shape the political discourse but will also ensure that its program and representatives are taken with growing seriousness by security decisionmakers and elites.

PEACE MOVEMENT ORGANIZING
IN THE SEVENTIES

The Freeze movement had its genesis in the environmental movement and in the antiwar activism of the late sixties and early seventies. These movements drew the attention of academics, futurists, and politicians to the interdependency of international, ecological, and economic systems. New understandings developed about the delicate balance of the ecosystem; the damage being done by man-made pollutants, which respect no national borders; energy shortages and limited resources; the deepening division between rich and poor nations; and the impact of increasing militarization on accelerating conflicts in the Third World. The seventies saw a heightened awareness of U.S.-Soviet competition for influence and power, dramatically underscored by the Vietnam War. A sense of urgency permeated elite circles of both conservatives and liberals when the United States experienced defeat in Indochina.

Peace and environmental activists entered a new era of organizing. They attempted to focus popular attention on a new vision of the U.S. global role in energy, foreign, and military policy. Environmentalists focused on appropriate technology and nonpolluting renewable energy resources, on shifting away from vast consumption of world resources and toward a sustainable, "small is beautiful" stewardship of the earth. Environmentalism evolved from a conservation ethic into a sophisticated movement that initiated specific environmental protection measures and influenced policymaking. A responsive constituency in the peace movement took up environmentalism's idea of the "right sharing of the world's resources." At the grassroots level, a massive, community-based campaign against nuclear power plants and waste storage sites was spawned. In the midst of the burgeoning environmental movement, peace activists were beginning to focus their efforts on the extreme edge of militarism: the military-industrial-academic complex and the threat of nuclear war.

Campaign to Stop the B-1 Bomber

The American Friends Service Committee (AFSC) initiated the campaign to stop the B-1 bomber—later joined by Clergy and Laity Concerned (CALC)—as the Vietnam War was winding down. Both groups had come to the conclusion that a "permanent war economy" had been established and that corporate influence over national security policy needed to be exposed and opposed.[1] An AFSC Subcommittee, National Action and Research on the Military-Industrial Complex (NARMIC), had documented the revolving door between the Pentagon and private corporations, which were doing research, development, and active lobbying through political action committees (PACs). NARMIC uncovered an informal set of structures and relationships between the public and private sectors and revealed the disproportionate influence that defense contractors have over national security policy. Individuals had built their entire careers going back and forth between government and corporate life, acting as guardian angels for their favorite and most profitable weapons system. The "national interest" was becoming the same as the corporate interest.

AFSC and CALC were concerned that the drive toward technological innovation and greater sophistication in weapons of mass destruction, combined with a permanent war economy, meant an indefinite future for our country of arms races and interventionary foreign policy. Their efforts to stop the B-1 bomber were joined by local organizers around the country and a powerful national political campaign resulted.

During the campaign's early development, there was lively discussion and debate about the campaign's lack of alternatives to the permanent war economy. Before too long, however, organizers found a way to make national military spending a local issue. The "conversion" strategy addressed the difficult economic problems of jobs and the impact on workers at plants with military contracts. By 1977, the momentum of the B-1 bomber campaign led to President Carter's cancellation of this new weapons system.

Rocky Flats Campaign

But not every community was home to a major B-1 contractor, although many had other weapons contractors in their backyards. A few community-based peace groups decided to take the basic politics of the B-1 campaign and apply them in their own communities. Chiefly in Colorado and California, activists began an entirely new strain of peace organizing that would give birth to a nationwide network of campaigns focusing on local nuclear weapons facilities.

In 1974 the staff of the Colorado AFSC formed the Rocky Flats Action Group (RFAG), whose purpose was to draw state and national attention to the country's only plutonium trigger factory, located just outside of Denver, Colorado. RFAG developed a unique marriage between environmental and peace activism. Colorado was fertile ground for this new form of organizing because the Atomic Energy Commission (AEC) had scheduled 40,000 nuclear weapons detonations in the Rocky Mountains for the purpose of stimulating the flow of natural gas. Called Project Plowshares, the AEC plan made it plain to the Colorado activists that there were very fundamental connections between the military and commercial nuclear industries.

After significant pressure from RFAG, Colorado Governor Richard Lamm and Congressman Tim Wirth appointed a citizens committee to monitor this top-secret nuclear weapons facility, the first such committee in the country. The committee's success as an advocate of public health and safety was significant. Its basic recommendation was that plutonium operations at the plant be phased out and the workforce and usable facilities converted to non-nuclear use. In conjunction with RFAG, the committee forced a new level of Energy Department openness, legitimized community concerns, and helped to educate the public and local officials about the presence and dangers of nuclear weapons production in our backyard.

RFAG blended environmentalism's popular appeal and focus on changing policy with peace activism's community-organizing skills and campaigning experience. In Colorado it was a winning combination, producing a political orientation summed up in the campaign's main slogan, Rocky Flats: Local Hazard/Global Threat. In the meantime, the Lawrence Livermore Laboratory in Livermore, California was the focus of Bay Area groups, led by the War Resisters League (WRL) and the AFSC San Francisco office. By 1978, the Labs Conversion Project had further exposed the scientific and academic link to the arms race, sparking a debate in the California university system and around the country about that connection.[2]

Some peace organizations, including WRL, AFSC, CALC, and the Women's International League for Peace and Freedom (WILPF), began meeting to form a national coalition to bring coordination and coherence to this new, grass-roots, antinuclear movement. In 1977 they formed the Mobilization for Survival (MOBE), whose slogans encapsulated its aims: Zero Nuclear Weapons, No Nuclear Power, and Fund Human Needs.

The forming of MOBE was not a welcome initiative, however, to many environmental organizations, who mistrusted the peace groups and felt that the success of campaigns focused on commercial nuclear power would only be set back by any link to nuclear weapons. Fearing that political issues would cloud their work, environmentalists were most anxious that the problem of the Soviet Union not be brought up. Ferocious struggles broke out.

For a while, a myth had persisted that the two nuclear industries were technically, institutionally, and politically separate. But the facts about the governmental and corporate links between the commercial and military technologies began to be researched and were eventually exposed by local activists. Those working at the community level had seemed to have little problem making the connection. In spite of the national organizers' disagreements, many peace and environmental activists had already formed working relationships and were producing documentation on these institutional links as well as on the impact of radiation on humans, whether released from a commercial power plant or from a plutonium trigger plant run by the Department of Energy.

A political accommodation was finally reached among the national staffs of peace and environmental groups. But local activists did not want the initiative to be taken over by East Coast-based peace organizers, whom they felt did not fully appreciate the new politics being hatched in the process of taking on the arms race in one's own hometown. So local activists proposed to the MOBE steering committee that national demonstrations be called: one at a commercial nuclear power plant in Barnwell, South Carolina and the other at the Rocky Flats nuclear weapons facility.[3] This solution satisfied local and national organizers, environmentalists, and peace leaders. On 29-30 April 1978, thousands of demonstrators turned out in South Carolina and Colorado to dramatize and confront the nuclear age. Civil disobedience at both facilities further escalated the political debate about the future of nuclear technologies.

The demonstration at Rocky Flats was followed by daylong training and workshops on how to build a campaign against the nuclear weapons plant in your backyard. Workshops covered: the health and biological effects of low-level radiation; how to use the environmental impact statement (EIS) procedure to get information and assert a community's right to know; the structural relationship between private corporate contractors and the Department of Energy, for whom contractors manage weapons facilities; the weapons complex itself; economic conversion planning; transportation of radioactive materials; and nuclear waste. The demonstration helped to stimulate organizing throughout the country. In response to the flood of inquiries from around the country, the Colorado AFSC and the national office of the Fellowship of Reconciliation (FOR) formed a joint project to build a nationwide network of cooperating campaigns. The Nuclear Weapons Facilities Task Force (NWFTF) was formed, with Steve Ladd (from the California Labs Conversion Project) as chair.

NWFTF was facilitated by Michael Jendrzejczyk for FOR and by myself for AFSC. Each of the approximately sixty campaigns around the country was either autonomous or linked to one of the national peace groups, with each local group participating in this strategy-building network. The ad hoc nature of NWFTF circumvented turf battles and bureaucratic inertia, while keeping the focus on local organizing. The national group confined itself to facilitating actions and cooperative strategies, which were agreed upon at the annual meetings.[4]

Strategies emphasized local hazards as well as the global threat of nuclear weapons production, testing, and deployment. (For example, campaigns used the EIS process and numerous other environment-oriented strategies to expose the immediate and long-term impacts of the nuclear trap.) The goal was to give people an entry point in their own communities for understanding that the arms race is not something "out there" but an everyday reality with profound impact on our lives. Campaigns began everywhere—from Hanford, Washington to Amarillo, Texas, from the Draper Labs at MIT in Cambridge, Massachusetts to Los Alamos, New Mexico, the state where it all began. These local campaigns generated heightened political consciousness and a tidal wave of public concern.

Through NWFTF, AFSC and FOR published *Makers of the Nuclear Holocaust.* For the first time, information about the vast network of plants, federal agencies, and corporate contractors was made public.[5]

NWFTF was important not only because it developed an important grass-roots network upon which the Freeze was later built, but because it was intentionally focused on organizing and political action, not on the internal organizational issues and sometimes bureaucratic tendencies of the peace movement. But as soon as the 1978 demonstrations were over, many of these dynamics began to take root in the national organizations. For example, MOBE member groups began competing for funds and credit with the very vehicle they had created to build that kind of support for the coalition.[6]

The demonstrations and organizing had been politically successful, catching the attention of the press, elected officials, and the funding community. The MOBE staff wanted to continue the coalition. But member groups felt it had served its short-term purpose, which was to get the strategy wheels in motion and then let the local groups work under their own steam. The member groups withdrew to build their own programs. Rather than closing its doors, the MOBE became another peace organization. But there was, in fact, nothing to naturally keep MOBE together—no political program, no set of demands. Its broad slogans—Zero Nuclear Weapons, No Nuclear Power, and Fund Human Needs—did not provide a substantive political program or plan of action.

The organizational evolution of MOBE was similar to that of SANE and the Freeze. Both SANE (formed in 1957 to organize for a test ban treaty) and the Freeze were formed as vehicles for the various peace groups and individuals to coordinate and focus their resources on effective political action. Each eventually became a separate organization unable to sustain the original function of coordinating program work among independent affiliated organizations.[7]

But even with the growing competition for leadership and access to funders, antinuclear organizing grew and the creativity seemed endless. The movement was well prepared for a quick response to one of the disasters it had warned about: the near meltdown of a nuclear power plant.

Three Mile Island

The accident at the nuclear power plant at Three Mile Island (TMI) in Pennsylvania accelerated concern about the immediate and long-range impact of nuclear technology. Ironically, it riveted attention as well on the larger impact of using nuclear weapons. The political and tactical division among organizers between the two orientations dissolved with the near meltdown on 28 March 1979. The antinuclear movement gained credibility and momentum as the country listened closely to newscasters comparing the potential radiation release from the plant to the fallout at Hiroshima. The "theoretical" accident was happening, and the threat to the health and lives of people in Harrisburg, Pennsylvania, became an organizing impetus for millions whose imaginations could no longer escape the nuclear terror. Campaigns against weapons facilities and nuclear power plants spread even more rapidly in the wake of the accident. These campains were giving voice to the deep and commonly held feelings of fear and dread in the nuclear age.

After TMI, the flesh and blood reality of the nuclear age came knocking on the doors of official Washington. The nuclear arms race took on a human face as its victims told their stories before a panel of community leaders in 1980 at the first national Citizens' Hearings for Radiation Victims, held in Washington, D.C. The hearings, initiated by the Environmental Policy Institute, AFSC, and FOR, brought together workers from weapons and commercial facilities. The victims of the nuclear age were not only the people of Hiroshima and Nagasaki still suffering radiation effects decades later. The trail of victims from exposure to low levels of radiation had been blazed throughout the country over the decades of the nuclear age: Navajo uranium workers; inhabitants of the Marshall Islands; workers in weapons facilities; the 250,000 atomic veterans who marched into mushroom clouds under military orders;[8] the thousands of "down-winders" exposed to radiation from Nevada testing for whom cancer and leukemia have become a way of life in southern Utah. As invisible as the radiation, these people represented one of the nagging questions about security in the nuclear age. What were we doing to ourselves, to our land, to our water—all in the name of security?

The idea for the citizens' hearings emerged from Senator Edward Kennedy's 1979 travelling hearings, when victims first told their stories in Salt Lake City. Kennedy's hearings were the first forum to give legitimacy to the assertion that lives had already been taken by nuclear weapons production and testing. Former Secretary of the Interior Stuart Udall's lawsuits on behalf of radiation victims in southern Utah, and the revelations of Eisenhower's admonition to the AEC that they "keep the American public confused," all added to the urgency and anger that people were feeling.[9]

The citizens' hearings sparked government response and helped to enlist the medical community's involvement in the antinuclear movement. The hearings supplemented the ongoing policy organizing on Capitol Hill under the tireless leadership of Bob Alvarez of the Environmental Policy Institute and Kitty Tucker, a Washington attorney active on radiation victims' cases, including the Karen Silkwood case.[10] In addition to lobbying, Alvarez and Tucker steered others toward the appropriate officials, agencies, and commissions to press for both compensation for radiation victims and protective guidelines for radiation exposure in workplaces and communities.

Alvarez and his assistants had a shrewd understanding of Washington politics. Their ability to work with local groups and with the critical scientific community became a central resource for those of us hoping to protect our communities from the immediate dangers of weapons production and testing and working to raise the stakes so that the more fundamental policy of nuclear deterrence could be debated. Not until it was debated in the town squares would it be discussed in the halls of Congress. A long-term strategy was in the making.

A key reason for the early success of the antinuclear movement was its grounding in solid research, which informed the questions it raised about human health and safety—questions the federal government and health professionals had either suppressed or neglected. After the Three Mile Island accident, large-membership environmental groups—such as Friends of the Earth and the Sierra Club—took up the issue of nuclear weapons in a wholehearted and enormously effective manner. The collaboration between peace and environmental activism on the nuclear issue was launched, and a new peace movement had been hatched. Education, nonviolent direct action, and legislative efforts were all now focused on the multidimensional trap of the nuclear age.

Scientists, religious leaders, and professionals such as physicians and lawyers were getting organized, strengthening the social network necessary to launch a national movement around a unified goal. Dr. Helen Caldicott rejuvenated Physicians for Social Responsibility (PSR) in 1979.[11] Scientists had passed resolutions at the annual meetings of the American Association for the Advancement of Science (AAAS), calling for special sessions on the arms race, health effects of low-level radiation, and international relations; they also established an AAAS working committee on arms control and disarmament.[12] *Science* magazine began to publish articles on these issues.

Churches had become increasingly involved in the peace movement after the Vietnam War. The Interfaith Center for Corporate Responsibility (ICCR) had been founded to work with Catholic religious orders and the major Protestant churches on socially responsible investments. Through ICCR, shareholder resolutions were filed with most of the major military and nuclear weapons contractors, including Rockwell, Monsanto, General Electric, and Westinghouse. ICCR coordinated these resolutions by working closely with local campaigns and with the religious groups holding stock in these companies. While no company withdrew from nuclear weapons production, the educational benefit within the religious groups, at the shareholders' meetings, and in the business community was more than worth the effort.[13]

At the local level, members of the religious community were often centrally involved in nuclear weapons facilities campaigns. Their involvement deepened as the nuclear debate filtered up to national and international church bodies, whose attention to the issue of the arms race was further stimulated by the dialogue between scientists and church leaders. For example, the MIT chaplaincy and NWFTF initiated an independent discussion center at that university on the occasion of the 1979 World Council of Churches (WCC) meeting to raise the issues of the arms race. Mike Jendrzejczyk and I worked with MIT chaplain Scott Paradise and professors Jonathan King, Joseph Weizenbaum, George Wald, Bernard Feld, Philip Morrison, and Everett Mendelsohn to organize a coffeehouse and discussion center for WCC delegates from around the world. As a result, WCC passed a resolution on the arms race and initiated hearings on the arms race, which happened in Amsterdam in November 1981. WCC went even further and made the arms race a major theme at its international meeting in Vancouver, Canada, in 1986.[14] The National Council of Churches (NCC) was similarly organized to put the issue of the arms race higher on its agenda.

POLITICAL SCENE IN THE LATE SEVENTIES: ASSAULT BY THE RIGHT WING

Right-wing forces had dominated the foreign policy picture since the emergence of the cold war in the late 1940s. The late 1970s found the right wing mobilizing again to deal with what it considered to be a weakening of American military strength.

In 1975, Eugene V. Rostow, Paul Nitze, Lane Kirkland of the AFL-CIO, and others began to talk about the idea of rejuvenating the Committee on the Present Danger, which had been established in the 1950s.[15] They consulted with James R. Schlesinger (then secretary of defense), who offered strong encouragement for their efforts. In November 1976, the formation of the revived Committee on the Present Danger was publicly announced; its purpose was "to alert American policy makers and opinion leaders and the public at large to the ominous Soviet military buildup and its implications, and to the unfavorable trends in the U.S.-Soviet military balance."[16]

While the committee declared itself to be independent from the government, many of its original 141 members had previously held top administration posts—including Theodore C. Achilles (formerly a counselor for the State Department), Karl R. Bendetsen (former under secretary of the Army), William J. Casey (former chairman of the Securities and Exchange Commission and a former under secretary of state), and William E. Colby (former CIA director). In fact, when Reagan came into office in 1980, many other members would be forced to resign from the committee before accepting positions in the Reagan administration.

In 1978, the American Security Council (ASC) formed the Coalition for Peace through Strength to lobby against the SALT II treaty and ultimately spent $8 million to defeat the treaty.[17] According to ASC, they reached 100 million Americans through the showing of their anti-SALT television "documentary," *The SALT Syndrome.*

President Jimmy Carter's administration was under siege by this New Right, which took every opportunity to criticize Carter's responses to international events. The Soviet invasion of Afghanistan, the overthrow of the Nicaraguan Somoza government, and the taking of American hostages in Teheran, each of these events deepened the Democratic party's internal foreign policy crises and strengthened the right-wing position in domestic politics. The New Right accused Carter of a failure of moral and political will as he publicly acknowledged that there were limits to the use of military force in the conduct of foreign policy.[18]

Americans were still confused about the lessons of the Vietnam War, hesitant to commit the lives of their children to war but fearful and angry about the vulnerability they felt. Anti-intervention sentiment seems always to involve the contradictory desire to stay out of war but to remain in control of international developments. The right wing read this confusion, disillusionment, and ambivalence in public sentiment and moved to fill the vacuum left by a floundering president and a rudderless Democratic party. Conservatives successfully portrayed Carter as the embodiment of the Vietnam Syndrome—the failure of moral and political will that infected the American public after Vietnam and eroded public support for U.S. military intervention abroad. In right-wing terms, America was getting pushed around, and Carter's weak response indicated a failure of nerve and a failure of leadership.

The MX Missile

Having cancelled the B-1 bomber as a result of public opposition, President Carter was under enormous pressure to propose a weapons system he could endorse. The cancellation of the B-1 was a peace movement "success," but with its cancellation came the introduction of other weapons systems long on the drawing boards, including the MX missile, the Stealth bomber, and cruise missiles. Carter's choice was the MX, which would satisfy the Pentagon and right-wing pressure groups, while providing Carter with the political space to get the SALT II treaty ratified by the Senate.

His administration proposed to put the MX on racetracks, first in farm-rich Nebraska and then in Utah and Nevada. A coalition of farmers joined with Nebraskans for Peace to stop the deployment of the MX. They successfully persuaded the Air Force not to base the system in Nebraska. Carter's scheme then moved west, and so did the protest.

The MX provided even more grist for the antinuclear activism spreading through the country. Its racetrack basing mode, its cost, and its first-strike ability were exposed by Nevada and Utah community groups. For Utahans, the MX added insult to injury. Not only had they been exposed for decades to radiation from aboveground nuclear weapons tests, but now they would be targeted for a Soviet preemptive first strike in the event that the MX was deployed. SANE staff organizers Marilyn McNab and Mike Mawby travelled to Nevada, Utah, and other potential MX sites to organize grass-roots efforts to reject President Carter's plan to shuttle the MX underground through Utah and Nevada. Local NWFTF activists joined with the groups in each area and formed the Coalition Against the MX—a coalition of disarmament, arms control, environmental, ranch, Native American, and religious groups. Paul Walker and Gordon Thompson of the Union of Concerned Scientists (UCS) contributed to these efforts through their research and publications.[19] They also arranged a midwest speaker tour to help local groups confront the Air Force. The Carter administration's proposed MX plans even mobilized conservative Mormon leaders. In an unprecedented action, the Mormon leaders issued a statement not only opposing the MX but calling for ratification of the SALT II treaty and for movement by the superpowers toward disarmament. In addition to the entire hierarchy of the Mormon church, all four senators from Utah and Nevada opposed the MX plan.

Developing at the same time as the Coalition Against the MX was the Coalition for a Comprehensive Test Ban. Former workers from the Nevada Test Site joined the downwinders to form the grass-roots base of this coalition. The Nevada Test Site workers had already sued the Department of Energy over the radiation effects they were suffering. This coalition was joined by AFSC and FOR, through NWFTF, as well as by the Committee for National Security and the Environmental Policy Institute. Janet Gordon, Preston Truman, Las Vegas Franciscans led by Father Louis Vitale, and other local activists were key organizers in this effort. The central leadership for this group came from the communities most affected, although groups such as Greenpeace also joined the coalition and participated in demonstrations at the Nevada Test Site.

In December 1980, the coalition held a national conference in Salt Lake City to discuss organizing for a comprehensive test ban. After the conference, the coalition continued to work to heighten awareness about testing through local organizing and through postcard mailings to the White House whenever tests were scheduled.

The Committee on the Present Danger

But right-wing pressure was unrelenting and highly organized. Conservative PACs and the Committee on the Present Danger used every accommodation from the president and the Democrats to escalate their pressure and demands. Those who had formed the first Committee on the Present Danger in the fifties and had sold the cold war to the American public were once again on the move and intended to regain power over U.S. foreign and military policy. Their goal was to rearm America and restore the public's belief in the merits of military force in U.S. foreign policy. Halting SALT II was their litmus test for progress toward launching the second cold war.

They also formed new PACs to defeat liberal foreign policy champions like Senators George McGovern and Frank Church. The National Conservative Political Action Committee (NCPAC), Richard Viguerie, Terry Dolan, and others dominated political reporting with their aggressive and highly visible commentaries. The New Right's claims that America had gone soft, had lost its nerve as a world leader, and was being "pushed around" internationally seemed to be reinforced each day the Iranian hostage crisis dragged on.

Carter bent to the right-wing political pressures, and so did other Democratic leaders. In the fall of 1979, Senator Church, liberal chair of the Senate Foreign Relations Committee and a key target of

NCPAC and other right-wing groups, released old information about Soviet troops in Cuba; it was an attempt to paint a hard-line image of himself for his Idaho voters. For days the story played prominently in the news, but faded when it was revealed that these were not new troops, that the CIA and the White House had known of their presence since the Cuban Missile Crisis. Church's desperate maneuver played into the hands of his right-wing opponents.[20]

Thus, hopes for SALT II were further eroded in the Senate. Church lost his Senate seat months later. Senator George McGovern lost his as well. The Capitol Hill cloakrooms were filled with rattled members of Congress who feared they would be the next target of the New Right. The capitulation of so many Democratic liberals to right-wing pressures may demonstate either the power of the Right or the lack of clarity and commitment to a post-Vietnam alternative foreign policy, or both. That there were not organized and forceful progressive voices articulating the lessons of Vietnam in the political arena must also be faced by those who decry the right wing and condemn actions such as Senator Church's.

New Deployments in Europe

The political situation in Europe was equally volatile. The Social Democratic (SPD) and Labour parties lost elections in West Germany and Great Britain. NATO allies were considering a U.S. proposal (initiated in response to Chancellor Helmut Schmidt's concern over America's commitment to extended deterrence) to deploy 572 new medium-range missiles on European soil. The United States asserted that Pershing II and ground-launched cruise missiles would counter Soviet conventional strength; offset Soviet deployments of SS-20s and SS-22s; further couple the nuclear and military futures of the United States and its European allies; preserve bargaining chips for negotiations; offset the perception that the West was falling behind the Soviets in nuclear forces; and enable Allied forces to catch up numerically to Soviet intermediate-range forces. Whatever the political or military problem, the cruise and Pershing II missiles would be the cure-all.

In December 1979, the NATO allies took the so-called dual-track decision, which was to proceed with deploying the cruise and Pershing II missiles in Holland, Italy, Belgium, Great Britain, and

West Germany *and* to simultaneously pursue negotiations in Geneva. This decision reflected Europe's ambivalence about America as a guarantor of its security as well as its fear of the Soviet Union. The Europeans do not want to be militarily abandoned by the United States, but they also fear that the United States will get carried away by its confrontation with the Soviet Union and thus harm European interests. NATO allies wanted to believe in the American nuclear umbrella. They also wanted to ensure that the Americans would continue talking with the Soviets.[21]

Negotiations could, perhaps, keep détente alive. Whatever the political or military utility of these new weapons, real or perceived, they helped to spark a new peace movement throughout Europe. Knowing full well what military doctrines these weapons and their technical innovations represented, European activists pointed out the politically destabilizing and first-strike capabilities of the cruise and Pershing II missiles and began to mobilize public opposition throughout the Continent and Great Britain.

Back in the United States, right-wing efforts to sway public opinion about U.S. foreign and military policy under Carter and the Democrats was aided by the Iranian hostage crisis, followed by the Soviet invasion of Afghanistan in December 1979. The right wing's arguments against SALT II were both technical and political. Their claims that the United States was behind in numbers were matched by their assertions of aggressive Soviet behavior and intentions. The invasion reinforced and seemed to prove the claims being made most prominently by the Committee on the Present Danger.

On 3 January 1980, Carter withdrew the SALT II treaty, which was finally going on the Senate's agenda for ratification after seven long years of negotiation. The treaty had become hostage to the Afghanistan invasion and to domestic political battles over the direction of U.S. foreign policy.

PEACE MOVEMENT SEEKS A UNIFYING PROPOSAL

In every respect, the situation looked bleak for the peace movement: the political ascendancy of the right wing and its cold war politics; increasing international tensions and the dissolution of détente between the superpowers; the unraveling of support for the SALT II agreement in the Senate; the growing militarization of relationships with Third World countries by both superpowers; the increased possibility of direct confrontation between the United States and the Soviet Union; the rising threshold of acceptable violence in the Third World; and the proposed deployment of a new generation of first-strike weapons.

Even with the strong and growing antinuclear movement, organizers accurately judged their own marginality to the larger political struggle. In numerous consultations and meetings, assessments were made of the New Right's political agenda, its strength, and how it might be countered.

Many groups wanted the peace movement to put its resources behind fighting for the SALT II treaty, to draw the line against the Right in that arena by using the momentum of the antinuclear movement and the network built during the B-1 campaign. In general, however, peace groups did not have a consistent response to SALT II. Some groups opposed it for being arms control as usual. Others supported it because losing SALT II would have enormous domestic ramifications. Still others supported it not only for this reason but because the treaty at least established the principle of parity on which more far-reaching disarmament proposals could be built.[22]

Indeed, the Carter administration was so desperate for SALT II support that it organized an ad hoc committee to lobby the peace groups. Although national organizations were encouraged to take a position on the treaty, Robert Leavitt reports that the Carter administration

> strongly discouraged arms control and disarmament activists and groups from pushing SALT II at the grassroots level, fearing identification of the treaty with such activists and organizations. (Ironically, some within the Administration, apparently unaware of this official discouragement, grew angry at the peace movement for failing to support their treaty.)[23]

But the groups could not agree to make SALT II the priority. The inadequacies of the treaty and of arms control negotiations had caused many groups to give it only nominal support, or even to oppose it. Those supporting the treaty found they could not translate that advocacy into a program that could inspire grass-roots involvement.

There was an unspoken consensus by the spring of 1979 that a coordinated movement and a policy proposal with some teeth to it were both needed. Key national and local activists in AFSC, FOR,

CALC, and the network of local campaigns cooperating through NWFTF were searching for just such a proposal and were ready for a new level of cooperation. AFSC, CALC, and the Washington, D.C. Sojourners community had all been calling for a nuclear moratorium. But the moratorium idea being promoted by AFSC, CALC, and Sojourners seemed too broad and imprecise to become a winning policy proposal. It lacked the pragmatism that could ignite and inspire those who wanted to take action, who wanted more than a symbolic statement.

What seemed like a popular demand, a nuclear moratorium, needed depth and detail if it was to be taken seriously by politicians and the press. What activists instinctively were moving toward—the idea of a halt—slowly took shape as various experts tested the idea in scholarly journals and in political settings.

Sojourners lobbied one of their board members, Senator Mark Hatfield, to introduce legislation. In June 1979, he proposed as an amendment to SALT II a mutual U.S.-Soviet freeze on strategic nuclear weapons deployment; of course, this amendment suffered the same fate as SALT II. The freeze idea was originally outlined by Richard Barnet just a short time before, in the Spring 1979 issue of *Foreign Affairs*; he defined it further in his July testimony before the Senate Foreign Relations Committee.[24]

AFSC Goes to the Soviet Union

Meanwhile, Terry Provence of AFSC had not only been promoting a moratorium idea but had organized an AFSC delegation to the Soviet Union in 1979. Everett Mendelsohn of Harvard led the trip, joined by Terry Provence, Dr. Helen Caldicott, Reverend William Sloane Coffin, Wendy Mogey, Marta Daniels, Dr. Bill Harris, Arthur Macy Cox, and myself. Cox was a Soviet specialist and military analyst and was formerly with the CIA. He rejuvenated the freeze idea during this trip and pushed the Soviets to respond to his proposal for a mutual freeze with or without the ratification of the SALT II treaty. Cox argued to them that the United States and the Soviet Union had agreed to the essential equivalence between their nuclear forces. This parity opened the way for a bilateral halt and could radically alter the politics of negotiations by transforming the Geneva talks into more than just a setting for the management of the arms race. With a mutual halt in the production, testing, and deployment of nuclear weapons and delivery systems, the negotiations might reach a formula for reducing the 50,000 nuclear weapons stockpiled by the two superpowers.

With the skills of a consummate diplomat, Mendelsohn delicately and forcefully guided discussions on the Cox version of a freeze, taking the idea through the U.S.S.R. Institute for the USA and Canada, up to the Foreign Ministry, where the delegation met with the Soviet SALT II negotiators. The AFSC delegation came home prepared to push the freeze idea further.

Discussions of the freeze idea were also proceeding in the Boston Study Group, whose members were military analysts and scientists, including Philip Morrison, Phylis Morrison, Paul Walker, Randy Forsberg, and George Sommaripa.[25] Sommaripa and Forsberg were also exploring the freeze concept, and Forsberg later drafted the "Call to Halt the Arms Race," which was the most formal and detailed articulation of the freeze proposal. It called on the United States and the Soviet Union to agree to an immediate, verifiable comprehensive halt to the production, testing, and deployment of new nuclear weapons and their delivery systems.

The Soviets' interest needed to be tested, their seriousness challenged. The only possible test would be their reaction to the U.S. government proposing a mutual halt. It was therefore worth the effort to lobby our government to propose a freeze. The idea of a bilateral halt, at a time when both superpowers acknowledged parity and public awareness was high, could be successfully argued with policymakers and would be simple, understandable, and accessible to the public.

Organizing Around Freeze Idea Begins

With news of the AFSC discussions with the Soviets, Forsberg's "Call to Halt" gained keener attention from core activists in the national organizations. An organizing group made up of Mike Jendrzejczyk, Terry Provence, Carol Jensen, Wendy Mogey, Patsy Leake, Randy Forsberg, and myself began meeting in late 1979 to develop a national campaign around the freeze. On 14–16 October 1979, the Riverside Church in New York attracted more than 1,000 people to its convocation to reverse the arms race. At the MOBE annual national convention in December 1979, Randy Forsberg presented the freeze idea to the 600 participants. Currie Burris of CALC said that this speech stimulated "a moment of redefinition" for the various people gathered.[26]

Those of us acting as the core organizers contacted members of various groups—including some grass-roots organizers from New England, Colorado, and New York—and arranged a 8 February 1980 consultation in Nyack, New York, "Alternatives to the New National Security Consensus."[27] The groups who gathered at this meeting hosted by FOR discussed many military, economic, foreign policy, and nuclear issues. The group suggested numerous proposals that would address these issues, including eight specific strategy ideas. The freeze was only one of these strategies, which included, for example, sending delegations to Washington and Moscow to present alternative policy proposals and organizing street demonstrations and teach-ins at the Democratic National Convention.

Participants had "a strong feeling that we must seize the current situation as an opportunity to articulate an alternative vision of American interests."[28] If the lessons of Vietnam could be sustained and integrated into changes in U.S. foreign and military policy, the peace movement would have to initiate and nurture that learning. Those lessons could best be debated, understood, and acted upon if the national security policies of our country could be decoded and demythologized by citizens. The potential for a new period of public education and action seemed ripe, in spite of the rise of right wing influence. Just as drafting young boys into the military had brought the war in Vietnam to America's dinner tables, so might the draft of all of us as unknowing, unapproving "soldiers" in a nuclear war bring security policy into our living rooms.

As the ad hoc strategy group continued to meet throughout 1980, the freeze idea emerged as the unifying goal for which the peace movement had been searching. The peace groups embraced the freeze because they saw its potential as a policy proposal and as a grass-roots organizing vehicle. The movement was looking for something small enough to accomplish but big enough to lead to other policy changes. Forsberg had argued for the freeze as a first step in "confining the military to defense as a route to disarmament." This made sense to the peace groups in the context of the SALT II debate. Such an argument also refined the peace groups' call for a nuclear moratorium, which could begin a process of more far-reaching changes in U.S.-Soviet relations and the arms race.

At a second meeting on 27 February 1980, various groups (AFSC, CALC, FOR, and the Institute for Defense and Disarmament Studies [IDDS]) decided to print and distribute "The Call to Halt the Arms Race." The Ad Hoc Task Force for a Nuclear Weapons Freeze was formed to spread the freeze idea. The group met throughout the spring to discuss strategy for building the campaign. In April we distributed 5,000 copies of "The Call to Halt," which now had endorsements by a number of academics and peace activists.

In this first phase of organizing, we began to seek endorsements of politicians, scientists, arms controllers, and other prominent leaders. Prominent endorsements gave the freeze proposal visibility and credibility and were part of an intentional public awareness strategy. This strategy was particularly important because of the Freeze movement's goal of changing national security policy, which traditionally had been made behind closed doors. Much of the public was not conversant with the terms of U.S. security policy. As people began to examine the freeze proposal, it would be more credible to them with the endorsements of prestigious scientists, arms control experts, and politicians, as well as respected community leaders such as clergy and directors of professional organizations. It would, of course, be important for people later to become knowledgeable about national security so that they could form their own judgments on candidates and policy proposals.

The early freeze organizers had difficulty getting support from one constituency, the liberal arms control community. Randy Forsberg had sought comments and endorsements from people like Herbert Scoville of the Arms Control Association (ACA), Jeremy Stone of the Federation of American Scientists (FAS), and Admiral Eugene LaRocque of the Center for Defense Information (CDI). They all declined to support the freeze during its early stages for a variety of reasons, including its broadness, its comprehensiveness, and the perceived problems of verification. Jerome Grossman of the Council for a Livable World explained how many lobbyists working in Washington felt about the freeze:

> People had a lot of doubts about it. When it was first presented to the Council, I mean, who was Randy Forsberg, and what was so great about the idea anyway? The Council had carved out a role, an expert role, and the freeze

seemed to have a lot of holes in it, a lot of unanswered questions. So the Council was loathe to pick it up. . . . It's very important for us to maintain our credibility, to be known as very sober people who aren't swept away, are not emotional peaceniks.[29]

But some associated with these organizations—including Grossman, George Rathjens, and the famed chemist George Kistiakowsky of the Council for a Livable World—were among the first signers, as individuals.

Eventually, our active recruitment in the arms control community brought in some of the nation's most prominent figures. Within months, Scoville, Stone, and LaRocque supported and became centrally involved with the freeze. Among the many other endorsers were William Colby; Averell Harriman, former under secretary of state and ambassador to both Great Britain and the Soviet Union; Henry Cabot Lodge, former ambassador to the United Nations; Paul Warnke, former director of the Arms Control and Disarmament Agency and the chief SALT negotiator; and Jerome Wiesner, past president of MIT and science advisor to President Kennedy. Vice Admiral Ralph Weymouth of the U.S. Navy joined Eugene LaRocque as one of the retired military officials endorsing the freeze. Scientists included Bernard Feld and Philip Morrison of MIT and Frank von Hippel of Princeton. The freeze was brought into formal religious circles by Harvey Cox, a Harvard Divinity School professor and disarmament spokesman.

By the summer of 1980, CALC and FOR had formally endorsed the freeze at their annual national conferences, and AFSC's national board had also endorsed the idea. These endorsements were significant because they provided the Freeze movement with a "large and solid base of experienced local activists and organizers, who had . . . developed extensive ties within their [local] communities."[30] Several other groups made the freeze an organizing priority: IDDS, WILPF, Sojourners, the Riverside Church, World Peacemakers, Pax Christi, and the disarmament working group of the Coalition for a New Foreign and Military Policy. The freeze idea caught on quickly with its natural supporters, most of whom were loosely connected as a result of antinuclear and antiwar organizing in the sixties and seventies. The antinuclear movement, in particular, had woven a web of personal and political contacts, both locally and nationally, among religious people, peace activists, and environmentalists.

In May 1980, the New York AFSC's disarmament program, the New Manhattan Project, began to organize both Democratic and Republican delegates to the national conventions that summer. The freeze proposal, Minority Report No. 21, was submitted to the floor of the Democratic convention by John Kenneth Galbraith. The proposal made it to a voice vote—over the protests of the New Jersey delegation—but lost. It did gain 40 percent of the delegates' support, however, which was a substantial victory considering that President Carter personally lobbied against it. The convention efforts also helped to build a congressionally based, grass-roots network of activists in the metropolitan New York area.

Throughout the summer of 1980, Randy Forsberg and George Sommaripa developed a strategy proposal for a freeze campaign. This proposal included a discussion of the larger national security issues, the freeze campaign as a first step toward public discussion of these issues, and specifics about the campaign they envisioned. In September they presented this to about thirty local and national peace activists meeting in New York. While some members of the group felt ready to plunge ahead, most felt that a larger conference with many local organizers from various peace groups was needed to launch a freeze campaign, since people who were going to be a part of the movement should define what would be done and how to do it. Planning began for this national conference.

Local Organizing for Referenda

Simultaneously, peace activists in western Massachusetts were organizing referendum campaigns around the freeze proposal. In 1979, Randy Kehler, Frances Crowe, and other colleagues at the Deerfield Traprock Peace Center—which was trying to organize the local community around nonviolence and global disarmament—had heard of the freeze idea from Jim Wallis of the Sojourners community. They decided to put a nonbinding referendum question on the November 1980 ballot. The referendum called on the president to propose to the Soviets a mutual freeze on nuclear weapons; it also called for the money saved to be put toward increased funding of human needs. The referendum was an overwhelming success: voters in fifty-nine of sixty-two towns in three state senatorial districts of western Massachusetts passed the referendum by an overall margin of 59 percent.

Ninety-four thousand people voted for the freeze proposal, and 65,000 against it.

But on the same date, 4 November 1980, powerful Democrats lost big when the darling of the New Right shocked everyone by actually winning. And he won big. The Reagan revolution had begun.

In western Massachusetts, Ronald Reagan won by the same margin as the freeze did. This should have served as a red flag to freeze organizers, in western Massachusetts and elsewhere. Reagan certainly did not come into office supporting a freeze. If the same voters who wanted a freeze also wanted Reagan, there would need to be some serious public education. Organizers throughout the country were heartened by the Massachusetts victory, but the schizophrenia in the Massachusetts vote would persist in public opinion throughout most of Reagan's presidency.

Reagan was sworn into office and within months began to talk about fighting and winning nuclear war. This reckless talk divided the Reagan administration from mainstream public opinion. When millions demonstrated against nuclear weapons throughout Europe in the fall of 1981, the echo from the streets of Bonn, Rome, London, Paris, and Amsterdam reverberated throughout America. As Elizabeth Drew said, "The movement took off because a number of people did careful groundwork, and because the Reagan Administration gave it traction."[31] For the "Teflon president," as Representative Patricia Schroeder named him, Reagan's arms policies became his one sticking point during his first term.

3 TO THE VILLAGE SQUARE
Education and Recruitment

> *The facts of nuclear energy should be taken to the village*
> *square and from there the decision made about its future.*
>
> —Albert Einstein

Having identified the nature of the problem, its history, and the social, political, and economic forces involved, a movement must go on to the second step of designing a public education program and recruiting its allies.

For a movement to develop a mass base that has the potential to develop political power without being co-opted, its educational strategy must be an integral and lively part of its program. A protest movement is likely to only present alternative information. Information is important, but only education derived from that information will prepare a mass base for the long-term struggle of moving from protest to power.

To do this, a social change movement must develop the political literacy of those it would educate. This educational strategy understands that learning new ways of problem-solving leads to political involvement of the mass base. In Paulo Freire's words, this means moving beyond the "banking concept" of education.[1] Even though "literacy"—the ability to read—may be more widespread in the United States than in developing countries, our schooling does not foster the ability to think analytically. As Freire sees it, information

51

is "deposited" in the learner's mind. Many people seem to have closed their accounts upon leaving school. Any interest in world affairs has been overshadowed by the clutter and stress of daily life, and participation in politics is decreasing. More people watch the television comedy "Family Ties" than voted in the 1986 elections. Given the permeation of our culture by immediate results, "fast-forward," and "instant replay," a movement must promote political literacy with a dynamic education strategy that recognizes the peculiarities of our culture and language and does not overlook the continuing impact of television on our political life as a nation.

A movement should not simply make its own "deposit" in the public awareness. On the contrary, a movement's educational work should not only deliver alternative information and knowledge but empower more and more people to understand and take action on those issues that deeply affect their lives. Such education attempts to identify the values underlying not only the political discourse but the ways we think. It offers alternative concepts, language, and public values—a new public morality—out of which alternative security principles and policies can be formulated.

The peace movement must pay great attention to the relationship between culture and politics, remaining deeply aware and critical of the popular perceptions that guide policy. This means examining the language, concepts, fears, values, and images used by spokespeople for the Pentagon, the State Department, and the White House as they attempt to sell a particular policy to the American public. By paying particular attention to the themes and presentations of key spokespeople, movement leaders can anticipate public response and determine more precisely how to shape the movement's statements.

Some of the key foreign policy themes of the Reagan administration—prosperity, fighting terrorism, the Strategic Defense Initiative (SDI) as a way to move beyond nuclear weapons, fear of the Soviets, and a call that America become first among nations and the leader of the free world—have been tested through survey and market research. They are winning themes strategically presented, and they appeal to the strengths and weaknesses in the American psyche. They are used to sell a conservative formulation of American foreign policy. The conservative movement is adept at packaging and testing its themes, but they are not all packaging. These themes also work because they are linked to the political structures and ideology of powerful and deeply entrenched conservative organizations that have made themselves into the dominant force in U.S. foreign and military policy.

A movement can give people information that will empower them to see the contradictions between the words and actions of politicians. The educational goal is to motivate people not only to read the newspaper, but also to decipher the significances, nuances, and real meanings behind the words they find there. In the short run, a movement offers a new way of thinking and talking about foreign and military policy and helps people imagine that change is possible. The next step after learning that change is possible is demanding that it happen and organizing politically behind those demands.

A movement's challenge becomes more complex as it tries to expand its base of support. It must continue to develop the core constituency, which is gaining greater sophistication and needs meaningful action and learning opportunities. At the same time, a movement must attend to the job of creating entry points for more new people. It must simultaneously strive toward greater sophistication and greater accessibility.

Articulating the problem is a common entry point. Participation in the antinuclear movement began for many with the naming of radiation and health issues. Immediate action opportunities at the local level, like those offered by the Freeze, serve as another kind of entry point. But each act and every level of learning should carry with it the seeds for more far-reaching understanding and action. Each act should be small enough to accomplish, but big enough to make a difference.

Participation should lead to each individual's investment in finding solutions. The psychological, financial, and working commitment of many individuals creates mass cohesion and stamina—the basis for political power. In turn, the visibility of the organization's strength and growing political power deepens individual participation and commitment.

The third step in movement-building is to translate public awareness into a power base. While an informed citizenry is crucial to achieving changes in the national security state, change will not spontaneously trickle up from an outraged and active citizenry. There are powerful and institutionalized forces and ways of thinking that dominate the debate and the decisionmaking. These forces will not be easily moved. Therefore, any social change movement must have plans for achieving greater degrees of power on behalf of its goals.

It must try out a variety of tactics but, in general, it must demonstrate its willingness to use its growing power by raising the cost of inaction by decisionmakers. By pressing them to negotiate toward realistic solutions to the problem, a movement is moving into the circle of decisionmakers, and the power balances are beginning to shift.

Building a power base requires clear and repeated articulation of political demands. As that articulation grows louder and more insistent, politicians, other decisionmakers, and the media will start to see those in the movement as part of the circle of "actors" with whom they must deal. As a movement thus asserts its power in the political arena, it can press decisionmakers toward decisions *other* than those they would have made without the movement's influence.

In raising the cost of inaction by decisionmakers, a movement must decide when and how to escalate the pressure behind its demands. It needs its own "voice," that is, independent representatives recognized by the public, the media, and the political world. A movement's leaders need to not only decide on appropriate tactics but develop a sense of political timing so that they know when it is best to apply different tactics. Most importantly, a movement's leaders must have both moral and political clarity to guide them and the movement as a whole in taking responsible political risks on behalf of their goals. Some such risks are likely to entail nonviolent action tactics, including information and education efforts, civil disobedience, boycotts, strikes, pickets, electoral and legislative work, legal demonstrations—and any other nonviolent tactic that creates a social drama around the issue.

Building this power base, through political pressure, organized actions, and effective leadership is neither a random nor an entirely controllable process. Strategists within a campaign must constantly sort out those elements that are in its control, those elements out of its present control but within its reach, and those elements out of control and out of reach. Such assessment is crucial to decisions about what strategies to focus on, how to respond to events, and how to best mobilize a movement's limited resources.

LOCAL ORGANIZING AND NATIONAL STRATEGY

As word spread about early successes, more local groups around the country took the initiative to organize for the freeze. In Vermont and New Hampshire, organizers who were mostly local AFSC staff organized to put the freeze on town meeting agendas. Community governments that usually dealt with taxes, land use, leash laws, and streetlights were asked for the first time to pass judgment on a foreign policy issue. The response in these communities was telegraphed throughout the country.

Even while a national freeze conference was still in the planning stage, commitment to the freeze grew among key organizers and within the peace groups as they considered the first strategy proposals written by George Sommaripa and Randall Forsberg, which were amazingly detailed and comprehensive. They articulated their view of how national security policy is made and how it could be changed:

> For the President and Congress to act together to stop nuclear-weapon production does not require a negotiated treaty ratified by two-thirds of the Senate. A treaty is needed to formally bind the United States through successive Congresses and Presidents. But a President, upheld by only one-third of either House or Senate, can simply veto all authorizations and appropriations incompatible with a freeze. Similarly, either the House or the Senate, by a simple majority, can cease authorizing or appropriating funds for nuclear-weapon development, procurement, testing and modification. Thus, the U.S. side of a freeze could be achieved without the treaty negotiation and ratification process *if* the American people convince the Congress and the President to support the freeze and to propose it to the U.S.S.R.[2]

Most of these assumptions about the formal decisionmaking process remained operative throughout the Freeze campaign.

Forsberg and Sommaripa tried to anticipate some of the other forces shaping national security policy. Reason and logic alone could not provide the political power needed by a citizen's movement to become one of those forces:

> The forces of inertia, of confused ideologists, and of organized groups with a personal stake in the arms race . . . have too strong an influence on Congress and the Executive to be overcome directly, purely by logical argument. To

overcome these forces, we must convince a substantial portion of the American public that a freeze is feasible and verifiable, as well as desirable; and that they must make this demand known to their elected officials in the Federal government. . . . The more Senators and Representatives we convince, the more plausible and convincing our case to the general public; and the more people we convince, the easier it will be to persuade members of Congress to support the freeze, district by district and state by state.

The solution to translating growing public awareness into political power lay in widening the public support base, paying particular attention to elites in the business and academic communities:

The universities have been conspicuously absent from attempts to disengage the U.S. from its military emphasis during most of the last 35 years. . . . We need to show conservative American businessmen that big government, centralization and heavy taxation are direct outcomes of support for the military. . . . As unions face the prospect of high unemployment and declining social services, interest should rise in reasonable, safe proposals for reductions in military spending that would be offset by conversion to more labor-intensive civilian production and improvement in the quality of education, health, child care, public transportation, and affordable energy housing.

The Sommaripa and Forsberg paper described the roles of foreign governments, the international peace movements, and the United Nations in achieving the freeze:

. . . The British, French and Germans are vying to have nuclear weapons, imported or domestic, on their own territory. This official attitude seems to be held by small elites who, in turn, are influenced by a small number of articulate Americans. We should be no less able to systematically arouse pro-freeze support in European countries. Canada's Trudeau, speaking at the U.N. Special Session on Disarmament in 1978, has already advocated a strategy of "suffocating" the nuclear arms race, by stopping nuclear weapon tests, missile flight tests and fissionable material production. Stopping the nuclear arms race is also advocated by Sweden, Japan, Mexico, probably advocated by Austria's Chancellor Bruno Kreisky, and possibly by Yugoslavia. An attempt should be made to link current, grassroots opposition to new U.S. nuclear weapons for Europe in Britain (including a Labour Party plank), the Netherlands and West Germany to the broader freeze concept. . . . While the U.N. has all the disadvantages of official bureaucracy and caution combined with the lack of power typical of private groups, it does provide such arrays of nationalities within convenient reach as to merit the search for courageous, articulate sponsors of the moratorium.[3]

The paper went into detail about technical debates that would emerge about the proposal:

The concept of the nuclear-weapon freeze outlined in the *Call* is built on years of public, unclassified research, writing and debates. . . . At present, our opinion is that actual U.S. and Soviet military production facilities for weapon-grade material and warheads are known and that a freeze on production in these facilities can be verified by national means. . . . It does seem likely, however, that production of small numbers of warheads from existing stocks of weapon-grade material in other, clandestine facilities, not presently in use, might proceed without detection by existing national means. Nevertheless, in the case of the United States and the Soviet Union, such production would be trivial when set against (1) the tens of thousands of warheads already in the inventories of both sides, (2) the unknown exact quantity of existing warheads and weapon-grade material, and (3) the well-known and highly verifiable numbers of long-range missiles and aircraft in both countries. . . . It is a conscious choice of the bilateral freeze effort to concentrate on the civilization-busting inventories of our own country and the Soviet Union, rather than the city- or country-busting potentials of the smaller powers. In the context of the existing numbers of U.S. and Soviet warheads, and the freeze on delivery vehicles and testing, the production of a few more warheads clandestinely would be militarily insignificant and purposeless and politically highly risky.[4]

It was ambitious, comprehensive, and more methodical than anything the peace movement had produced since the end of the Vietnam War. What is most notable about the Sommaripa and Forsberg document, and the draft strategy papers leading up to the first national conference, is the degree to which the freeze proposal was intended to significantly change both the political environment and U.S. foreign and military policy. Sommaripa and Forsberg included a thirty-page outline on why priority should be given to a bilateral nuclear freeze as the first step toward global disarmament and a world without war.[5] It was a step that could circumvent the trap of arms control and negotiations as usual *and* initiate the reversing of militarism.

FIRST NATIONAL NUCLEAR WEAPONS FREEZE CONFERENCE

The early organizers could not have chosen a better time for launching the national conference. The political mood among activists was ripe. On 10–12 March 1981, 300 people from thirty-three states attended the First National Nuclear Weapons Freeze Conference at Georgetown University in Washington, D.C.

Setting Goals and Strategy

A strategy planning committee had drafted a strategy paper, based on the work of Forsberg and Sommaripa, that would be reviewed and debated by conference participants.[6] Much of what they had written about the long-range political context, movement building, and political power was left out of the draft. Still, the Georgetown strategy paper described in somewhat broader terms the nature of the problem and the goals of the Freeze movement:

1. Reduce tension between the United States and the Soviet Union
2. Halt development of first-strike weapons
3. Halt production of nonverifiable cruise missiles
4. Maintain nuclear parity between the United States and the Soviet Union
5. Set the stage for real reductions in nuclear weapons
6. Improve the prospects for stopping the spread of nuclear weapons to other countries
7. Strengthen the economy
8. Increase national and international security

It briefly analyzed the political problem each goal addressed and how a freeze would alleviate each of these problems.

The strategy paper mapped out a three-to-five year strategy for achieving a comprehensive, bilateral freeze. It envisioned four phases to the campaign: (1) demonstrating the potential of the freeze; (2) building broad and visible public support; (3) focusing that support on policymakers and creating a major national debate; and (4) winning the debate and making the freeze a national policy objective.

Small groups analyzed the paper and provided input to a strategy synthesis group. This group produced a report to the conference as a whole. The conference affirmed the substance of the strategy synthesis report and forwarded it to the national committee, with the direction that it would oversee the rewriting of the strategy paper.

While the report gave general guidelines about tactics, schedules, resources, and relationships with the media, it failed to discuss the larger political context and the movement's vision of a freeze as a first step toward its goals. Although the conference discussed the eight goals in the original strategy paper, it could not come to agreement on them. The conference agreed on the freeze as an immediate policy goal, but did not define it in two key ways: how to implement a freeze, and what would follow a successful freeze.

Those who came to Georgetown saw different futures after a freeze. Debates were heated. Some groups felt that the freeze strategy was already too narrow and that they could not adopt it as their first priority. One of these groups was MOBE. While MOBE was an early sponsor and supporter of a freeze—and continued to support it in general—this group didn't take it on as a priority. Bruce Cronin of MOBE said, "The main reason was that the freeze was focusing on the weapons, talking about nuclear madness, saying that these weapons have to be stopped. Our feeling was that it was much more involved; we thought it was more important to look at the policies, the context in which the weapons are developed."[7] Also with an eye on the future, long-time peace and labor activist Sid Lens argued long and vehemently against inserting the word "verifiable" in the proposal. He maintained that this word would later be used against the Freeze movement by those who argue against all treaties because of technical issues of verification, and that the movement would be diverted into these technical debates.

The conference was unprepared to make the enormous number and range of political and organizational decisions confronting it. The agenda was packed, and no one had given much thought to how the campaign would be structured after the conference, much less to issues of political strategy for the long run. Partly because of this lack of preparation, the process of narrowing the movement's analysis and vision, as well as its political strategy, began very early on. But this was also due in part to the formation of the Freeze campaign as a coalition. Coalition politics work best when the goals are narrow and the term of the coalition is finite. As organizers at the Georgetown conference sought the least common denominator acceptable to the largest number of people, the long-term vision and politics of the Freeze became secondary.

A major fault line within the campaign emerged at the Georgetown conference: between those who saw the freeze as an arms control step separable from changes in international political relationships and those who felt changes in those relationships were essential.

The peace movement has often experienced this split, and it continued to plague the campaign as it unsuccessfully attempted each year to reach consensus on long-range goals and determine what its most effective near-term strategies would be. The split could have been handled more effectively if the core organizers had reached greater clarity from the beginning about what would come after a freeze.

But there was early disagreement among the leaders themselves. Even some of those involved in the first meetings that led up to the founding conference forgot the political roots and original vision of the Freeze. The campaign's first national coordinator, Randy Kehler (who served from 1981 to spring 1985), saw a freeze as the end to the nuclear arms race and felt that other issues were tangential. In Kehler's view, the Freeze was about itself and was never intended to serve any other political agenda:

> The Freeze was never presented as a cutting edge to a whole larger vehicle to get at militarism fundamentally. I knew a lot of people believed that had to be done. I believed that. . . . But from the very first meeting I attended as a newcomer, which was that September 1980 meeting, that's not how the Freeze was presented. . . . I don't think in any of our literature we even mentioned the word "militarism." Militarism to me is a whole way of thinking that has to do with how you solve conflicts through armed force.[8]

Kehler and others felt that a purely antinuclear stance might provoke political debate and changes, but that these were not issues the campaign itself should address as its central priority or program. Others advocated that a freeze was not only a first step toward dismantling nuclear weapons but could also be used to demand changes and measure progress in U.S.-Soviet relations, the future of both Eastern and Western Europe, and the superpowers' use of conventional force in the conduct of foreign policy. They argued that this "nuclear weapons only" focus of the campaign kept it from addressing any issues related to U.S.-Soviet relations, the trade-off between nuclear disarmament and conventional buildup, and the myth of Soviet conventional superiority and Third World intervention.

All these differences could have led to healthy political debate and more refined positions within the campaign. Instead, as the discussions widened to include more and more people and the movement literature was developed by more and more activists, these central issues were moved even further to the campaign's periphery.

Politically, however, these issues occupied center stage. Congressional debate and arguments posed against a freeze by academics, conservative opponents, and the press raised all of these critical questions. The Freeze was unprepared to debate them, much less take positions on them, even though it eventually became clear that solutions to the arms race require changes in the political relationship between the superpowers and among the superpowers, their allies, and the Third World.

Whether or not all Freeze activists knew about the political roots of a freeze, and embraced them or not, is now beside the point. Even with the movement's limitations, however, Kehler argues quite rightly that without the Freeze there would not be the debate about the merits of arms control, the future of U.S.-Soviet relations, and security in the nuclear age that is now taking place in the peace movement and among arms controllers. The Freeze movement achieved minimal learning at the popular level, but helped to intensify the national debate among defense and military analysts.

Structuring a Coalition

The task of the Freeze movement was huge; to confront national security policies and the bureaucratic forces behind them would require an unprecedented sophistication and organization. Any political campaign experiences tensions provoked by both external challenges and internal pressures. Figuring out how it can respond to these pressures and keep moving forward demands political acumen and organizational clarity.

The Freeze was trying to change the way peace organizing was done at the same time that it took on the national security establishment. This was no small task given that the peace movement, centered on the East Coast since the First World War, was working from a very traditional model of lobbying in Washington. The Freeze was attempting to develop an organizing model that moved beyond traditional Washington lobbying politics and, at the same time, beyond the marginalized image and tactics of the sixties' antiwar counterculture. The Freeze hoped to implement a politics that could reach mainstream opinion, institutionalize the peace movement in local community life, and bring pressure on Washington through these local power bases.

It was a tall order, but the Freeze was intentionally designed to be a new peace movement—locally based and democratic in both principle and practice. Instead of relying on isolated, individual supporters to periodically write letters to Congress or come together for demonstrations called by national groups, the new peace movement would build local peace organizations with political power, eventually representing a permanent peace constituency throughout the country. That political victory would stimulate the implementation of the long-term political program of the movement, while increasing the staying power of the movement. Rooting peace action in the life of local communities was a political strategy that required a commitment to a democratic organizational style. Democratic decisionmaking would ensure that strategies and programs stayed rooted in communities, building the local power bases that could change national politics.

To this end, Freeze founders believed that the citizenry could be informed and aroused, thereby awakening a morally passive government and gaining the political power to confront the forces perpetuating the arms race and militarism. The Freeze movement's ferocious commitment to democratizing the national security debate made it potentially one of the most powerful movements in U.S. history. The doctrines and institutions that drive the arms race were to be questioned "in the village square." The Freeze established a new assumption in American political life: that the people could have a voice in determining what is in their national interest. Taking for ourselves the option of defining our own security, in the face of some forty years of cold war confrontation and nuclear weapons buildup, was a radical change, and it was initiated by the Freeze movement.

While the Freeze's commitment to democratic procedure represented the organizing and cultural preferences of those initiating the movement, it was also an instinctive response to militarism. The secrecy, the cult of expertise, and the bureaucratization of military-mindedness cut people off from decisions that effect their lives so profoundly. This realization solidified the Freeze's commitment to democracy as both a goal and a way of conducting its business.

It was originally envisioned that national peace groups and national organizations representing churches, labor, women, and civil rights—in addition to the various local networks of all these organizations—would be the members of that cooperating body called the Freeze. Additionally, masses of individual citizens who were previously uninvolved would become very active with the Freeze. It took many people gathering together to organize the town meetings and the city and state referenda. After the referenda votes, these local organizers would form more permanent community Freeze groups. With this network of national and local groups, a new cooperation could be built and with it a growing power base. The new coalition had to be diverse, presenting a new image and a different and unpredictable social base for the peace movement—one vastly expanded from either the antiwar or antinuclear movements.

In the beginning, the Freeze movement was just such a coalition— a network of organizations brought together to build program and strategy and divide the labor. It recognized that the limited resources of individual organizations could achieve greater results if some new collaborative model could be invented, one that allowed for organizational diversity and pluralism but also unified and coordinated for the purpose of gaining political power.

While the power to hold decisionmakers accountable works best when voters are watching their own representatives and local officials, national policy is actually made far away in Washington. Isolated local efforts without a unifying program and strategy could be meaningful in the short run, but without national political impact in the long run. This new peace movement needed national coordination to maintain cohesion and exert the power it was developing by its local presence. It needed a national presence as well.

There were few models from which to draw a design for the structure of this new peace movement. It was not easy to reject the traditional lobbying model of Washington groups and curb the tendency of peace organizations to marginalize themselves in language and style. The changes in style, organizing approach, and image that the Freeze hoped to make required the invention of new models; those who knew the old ways of doing things had to be asked to give them up.

To ensure that the Freeze would not fall into the old models, the decision was made to set up an office as a clearinghouse instead of as a top-heavy organization. A site in the middle of the country was chosen as both a symbolic political statement and as a way of keeping the Freeze from getting caught up in the old behaviors and ways of thinking so dominant in Washington politics. A clearinghouse would also ensure that a wide variety of national organizations would remain involved and commit resources to the routine work of the campaign. St. Louis, Missouri was eventually chosen by the national committee in July 1981, although the Institute for Defense and Disarmament Studies (IDDS) continued to serve as the interim center until December 1981, when the National Clearinghouse opened. Consistent with the original plan that the Clearinghouse be a coordinating center, the national conference outlined its responsibilities:

1. Monitor Freeze activities, endorsements, and resources
2. Maintain address lists
3. Respond to information requests and do networking
4. Publish a national Freeze newsletter
5. Maintain files on task force and coordinating committees
6. Assist task forces

Delegates to the first conference mandated that the final authority for review of Freeze strategy would be given to the national conference, which would meet and review strategy annually. This was the arena where local organizers could voice opinions on the national direction of the campaign. At the first conference, all persons attending could vote. After that, while anyone could attend the conference, votes were limited to one per congressional district and one per national organization participating. Local groups could also help to shape strategy through their participation in state networks.

In between national conferences, however, the national committee was responsible for decisionmaking. The national committee was mandated to meet twice a year—or more often if necessary—and make the major, ongoing decisions of the campaign, including the hiring, firing, and supervision of the Clearinghouse staff. It also had the authority to appoint an executive committee—and determine the constituency and number of its members—to oversee decisions between national committee meetings.

In the early stages, the national committee reflected the coalition nature of the campaign. Its forty-five members represented: each task force (one person); each regional caucus (one person); major constituency groups; and contributing organizations ("any group that has contributed and will continue to contribute to move forward the work of the Freeze").[9] A majority of the representatives were from the national organizations actively supporting the Freeze. Because the Freeze was originally a *coalition*—not an *organization*— it was appropriate that the organizations making up this coalition be represented in the decisionmaking bodies. In 1982 there were about twenty-five national organizations represented on the national committee. (The number fluctuated with the development of the campaign.)

The first conference set up eight task forces to do the work of the campaign.[10] While the national conference outlined the overall strategy and goals, it was up to the individual task forces to define the specifics of implementation. They reported their progress back to the national committee. Consistent with the coalition nature of the Freeze, the task forces assembled for particular short-term projects and disbanded when the projects were done. Any interested person could volunteer for a task force, and chairs were also named on a volunteer basis. A large percentage of task force members were local representatives.

From the early meetings of the ad hoc strategy group that planned the first national conference, there had already been some infighting among the national peace groups—about where the coordinating center would be, how interim decisions would be made, who had authority to make them. These disputes had preoccupied the original organizing group, breaking down trust and bringing up organizational turf issues. While the initial disputes were eventually resolved, similar disputes occurred throughout the campaign's early years. In particular, the question of decisionmaking authority and who would have it continuously plagued the campaign.

Hours of meetings were devoted to deciding the location of the Clearinghouse instead of to refining the details of a structure that would build local groups, keep national organizations involved, and reach the mainstream of American society. As much as it dragged out, the Clearinghouse debate was easier than clarifying the details of how the Freeze would put its organizational strategy into operation.

Some of the organizational strategy questions, however, had real relevance to questions of political strategy. Where the campaign would be based symbolized a profound political statement and an intentionally different organizing strategy. This would be a new peace movement—grass roots-based and democratic because that was the *only* way to change policy.

SUMMER 1981: PUBLIC AWARENESS GROWS

The network of churches, grass-roots organizers, and local activists quickly responded to the idea of a "halt to the production, testing, and deployment of nuclear weapons," as well as to the new level of collaboration and cooperation of the national groups. The flurry of activity in 1981 soon proved that the Freeze idea was one around which a wide coalition, rooted in grass-roots, antinuclear sentiment, could be built.

The Freeze began identifying more of those it thought could be counted on for support: the established peace and antinuclear groups, both local and national; churches; medical, scientific, and legal professionals who had begun to form their own organizations; and liberal Democrats. Not so certain but potential supporters seemed to be unions, moderate Republicans, organized minority and women's groups, arms control experts, and foreign governments. Freeze organizers learned early on that the European peace movements enthusiastically supported a U.S. peace movement that managed to develop at all during Reagan's tenure.

In its early stages, the Freeze was a dazzling success at raising public awareness and at setting the terms of the debate. The political culture was permeated by a swarm of Freeze organizers. Churches, schools, universities, families, community and civic organizations, town meetings, city councils—all were asked to endorse the "Call to Halt the Arms Race." The judgment of some was more technically informed and sophisticated, but for all the people who voted, sat on church boards, or worked on committees for the hundreds of endorsing organizations, nuclear weapons policy became *their* problem. In these acts, their moral and political judgment and their values were mobilized. What had been a debate among national security elites in government, academic, and corporate circles was now up for discussion in every setting an organizer could imagine. The shroud of secrecy had been pulled back, and the assumption that national security policy had been made rationally was fundamentally challenged. "Arms control as usual" was challenged. The seeds for democratizing national security decisionmaking had been planted.

The diversity of organizations both endorsing and actively promoting the freeze was remarkable. By September 1983, 156 national and international organizations had endorsed the Freeze, including the U.S. Conference of Mayors, the Young Women's Christian Association, the American Nurses Association, Friends of the Earth, the American Association of University Women, and the National Conference of Black Lawyers. Many of these groups became actively involved by establishing peace and justice committees or by making some other commitment to promote the Freeze or other disarmament efforts.

Organizers realized from the start how important it would be to get the support of unions. Major efforts in this area yielded good results; the Freeze had the endorsement of nineteen major unions, including the American Federation of State, Council, and Municipal Employees, the United Farm Workers of America, the Coalition of Black Trade Unionists, and the American Federation of Teachers. The endorsement and active role of William Winpisinger of the International Association of Machinists and the efforts of Freeze staff member Gene Carroll, who worked with the unions, were central to this success.

Professional organizations developed, many of them with the central goal of achieving a freeze. While Physicians for Social Responsibility (PSR) had been founded in 1961, it was dormant through the late sixties and early seventies. Around the time of the Three Mile Island accident, it was revived through the efforts of Helen Caldicott and other Boston physicians, in conjunction with the Council for a Livable World. PSR organized nationwide symposia on the environmental and medical effects of nuclear explosions. Through "bombing runs," the physicians made the nuclear threat real to local communities by analyzing the effects of a one-megaton bomb on the community being addressed. The PSR symposia, like the NWFTF campaigns of the 1970s, generated awareness and action around what was happening in people's backyards. Not only did they recruit local physicians but they also fueled the organizing on local weapons plants and on the government's proposed civil defense plans.

The physicians' movement helped to legitimize the popular fear of nuclear war; it also helped to build the Freeze momentum because it encouraged people to look for a way to deal with new information and with their fear. Supporting the Freeze proposal was the practical and realistic way for many people to take action.

From its 1979 membership of a few hundred doctors, PSR grew to a membership of 20,000, with 125 local chapters by 1982; membership and the number of chapters doubled between 1981 and 1982. According to Christopher Jones, resource coordinator, as of 1987, PSR's dues-paying membership is 30,000, with 155 chapters nationwide and about 20,000 other supporters.

Soon, other professionals began to organize around the Freeze. The chaplaincy at Harvard University organized a "waging peace" conference that included occupation-specific workshops. Many occupational groups formed at this time supported the primary goal of a bilateral freeze. Among them were the Computer Professionals for

Social Responsibility, Artists for Survival, Nurses' Alliance for the Prevention of Nuclear War, High Technology Professionals for Peace, Lawyers' Alliance for Nuclear Arms Control, and Communicators for Nuclear Disarmament. Furthermore, the business community was reached, owing in large part to the efforts of Alan Kay, Stanley Weiss, Don Carlson, and Harold Willens (author of *The Trimtab Factor*), instrumental in forming Business Executives for Nuclear Security. All of these new professional groups brought in a segment of the middle class that had traditionally been uninvolved in the peace movement.

The Freeze also had support in the worlds of art and entertainment. Musicians Stevie Wonder, James Taylor, and Joan Baez, along with actresses Jill Clayburgh and Patti Davis (President Reagan's daughter), endorsed the Freeze. Groups such as Artists for Survival and Musicians Against Nuclear Arms (MANA) emerged. Graphic artists lent their talents to doing Freeze publicity, and other concerned artists began to arrange exhibitions on the themes of disarmament and peace. Numerous films were produced.

The educational world picked up on the Freeze. Young children, high school youth, college students, and educators all got involved. In November 1981, the Union of Concerned Scientists (UCS) sponsored teach-ins on the arms race; over 450 college campuses nationwide participated. To follow up on the success of the teach-ins, UCS launched a new organization, United Campuses to Prevent Nuclear War (UCAM-United Campuses). UCAM has a network of contacts at colleges and universities that, when founded in 1982, focused on organizing new student groups. Also, in November 1981, Hampshire College in Amherst, Massachusetts, sponsored a conference to train students in how to organize around the Freeze; over one hundred students from across the country participated.

Then high school students and their teachers launched the Student/Teacher Organization to Prevent Nuclear War (STOP). They funded a student Freeze campaign project, which organized a student Freeze lobby on Washington, D.C. Following the successful House vote on the freeze (4 May 1983), 150 students delivered 15,000 petition signatures to the Senate—which was supposed to be voting on the freeze within a few months—and they lobbied swing senators. The high school students also organized a press conference that got national and international coverage; even reporters from the Soviet news agency TASS covered the event.

Younger children got involved through organizations like the Children's Campaign for Nuclear Disarmament. They wrote thousands of letters to President Reagan, urging him to reverse the arms race. Mothers and grandmothers got involved as they became aware that the threat of nuclear war haunted their children's chances of making it to adulthood.

Educators for Social Responsibility (ESR) was formed to develop curricula and train teachers about nuclear issues at all classroom levels.[11] Although many peace studies programs existed at colleges and universities prior to the emergence of the Freeze movement, many more were now formed, and numerous individual courses on the nuclear arms race were newly offered.[12] Educators endorsing the Freeze included Richard Falk of Princeton, Notre Dame's president Theodore Hesburgh, and Roger Fischer and John Kenneth Galbraith of Harvard.

While many of the most established peace groups were religiously based and had their roots in the nineteenth and early twentieth centuries (AFSC, CALC, and FOR), the Freeze movement brought the arms race to the attention of new religious constituencies, including 144 Catholic bishops, the United Presbyterian Church, the American Lutheran Church, and the Union of American Hebrew Congregations. The endorsement of the Unitarian-Universalist Association represented 173,000 members. The Freeze got quite a boost when it received the endorsement of the National Council of Churches and the World Council of Churches. Pope John Paul II was an endorser, and numerous bishops and clergy took active roles in promoting the Freeze and disarmament. Women's religious orders led the way in the Catholic church. For example, the Sisters of Loretto were one of the first groups to endorse the Freeze, pledging to gather signatures around the country. Other orders followed their lead. On 14–16 October 1979, the Riverside Church held a convocation to reverse the arms race; it was attended by more than 1,000 people. And on 28–31 May 1982, there were 3,000 church services for peace, planned to coincide with the opening of the U.N. Second Special Session on Disarmament.

The Freeze movement became the vehicle for U.S. citizens to deepen their political understanding. The local debates and the sense of having some effect on the everyday political debate during the early 1980s invigorated and informed the development of the movement.

FALL 1981: REAGAN CHAMPIONS NUCLEAR WARFIGHTING STRATEGIES

The White House responded to the Freeze rather mildly at first, while continuing and even escalating its bellicose rhetoric about the Soviets. As some administration officials were criticizing the Freeze, the president was, ironically, helping to catalyze it. Just as the State Department and other official spokespeople for the administration were arguing that the president had an arms control plan and shared the public's concern over nuclear war, a presidential press statement would detonate a new round of bad news for the White House. In March 1982, for instance, Reagan's comment on the question of limited nuclear war was: "I could see where you could have the exchange of tactical weapons against troops in the field without it bringing either one of the major powers to pushing the button."

Reagan spoke openly of fighting and winning a nuclear war in Europe and of his determination to deploy cruise and Pershing II missiles in Italy, Belgium, Great Britain, West Germany, and the Netherlands. In testimony before the Senate Foreign Relations Committee in November 1981, Alexander Haig backed up the president by speaking of contingency plans in the NATO doctrine for firing a nuclear "warning shot" in the midst of a conventional war in Europe.

The European peace movement—seeded during the later Carter years by the development of the neutron bomb and the announcement of the cruise and Pershing II missile—grew rapidly in response to the nuclear saber rattling of Reagan and his appointees. As early as October 1981, the administration had helped to provoke massive demonstrations by millions of people in Bonn, London, Amsterdam, and all across Europe. The Reagan administration, with an almost naive bravado, had deepened public concern on both sides of the Atlantic.

Nuclear war fighting strategy was being promoted by administration officials at national press conferences, in speeches, and before Congress. While Carter's Presidential Directive 59 (PD-59) was seen as the first official statement that nuclear war could be fought and survived, it did not contain any specific proposals for implementation. In the fall of 1981, the Reagan administration drew up a document to supersede PD-59. As reported by the *Los Angeles Times*, it "specifically requires the Pentagon to draw up a plan for turning the policy declaration into military reality." That policy declaration was that

> ... in the nuclear war-fighters' view, which Reagan's National Security Council appears to accept, a nuclear war might be fought over a period of several months with selective strikes at primarily military targets. At the end, they believe, one side could emerge victorious, with enough of its resources and population intact to begin over. . . . *They specified that 20 million U.S. fatalities would represent an acceptable cost.*[13] (Emphasis added)

The administration was soon promoting the new warfighting strategy at all available opportunities. Deputy Defense Secretary Frank Carlucci: "I think we need to have a counterforce capability. Over and above that, I think we need to have a warfighting capability." Defense Secretary Caspar Weinberger: "If you have developed the ability to take out their missiles, you have achieved a degree of deterrence." Navy Secretary John Lehman: "You have to have a war-winning capability if you are to succeed." James P. Wade: "We don't want to fight a nuclear war, or a conventional one either, but we must be prepared to do so, if such a battle is to be deterred, as we must also be prepared to carry the battle to our adversary's homeland. We must not fear war."[14]

One of the most poignant and revealing exchanges during the hearings for Eugene Rostow's nomination to the directorship of the Arms Control and Disarmament Agency occurred between Senator Pell and Rostow:

> PELL: My question is, in a full nuclear exchange would a country survive?
>
> ROSTOW: The human race is very resilient, Senator Pell.

Rostow was approved for the directorship.

Probably the most infamous comment was made by T. K. Jones, the deputy under secretary of defense for strategic and nuclear forces: "Everybody's going to make it if there are enough shovels to go around. . . . Dig a hole, cover it with a couple of doors and then throw three feet of dirt on top. It's the dirt that does it."[15] Jones's comment forecasted the "civil defense" planning that was to come later.

FREEZE LEGISLATION INTRODUCED
IN HOUSE OF REPRESENTATIVES

By February 1982, as the second National Nuclear Weapons Freeze Conference convened in Denver, it was increasingly apparent to the press and to some Democratic politicians that the Freeze was becoming a genuine grass-roots movement with potential political power. Leading political figures in Colorado, including Representatives Patricia Schroeder and Timothy Wirth, were invited to address the conference. Even before the Denver conference was over, phone calls to and from Senator Edward Kennedy—as well as initiatives from Congressman Edward Markey's office—catapulted the Freeze campaign into the national limelight through the introduction of legislation.

Congressman Markey sent a staff member, Peter Franchot, to the conference. Formerly on the staff of UCS and an antinuclear activist, Franchot "immediately took to the Freeze. He had done enough public interest work to become a fair judge of grass roots campaigns and how they could catch fire—and of how a politician could ride the crest of a movement's wave, if he or she were willing to take a few chances.[16]

"The Freeze is going to sweep this country. . . . I can feel it in my bones, and there's no reason why we shouldn't be in the middle of it," said Franchot.[17] Markey and Congressman Jonathan Bingham (D-NY) each had freeze legislation floating around Congress in the months prior to the Denver conference. This was much sooner than the campaign had intended. By introducing freeze legislation in early February 1982, Markey and his staff positioned themselves on top of the crest of the wave.

Douglas Waller, another Markey aide, sought support for Markey's resolution from Senator Gary Hart. What better fit, he thought, than the senior senator from Colorado announcing his cosponsorship of freeze legislation on the eve of the movement's biggest national gathering, taking place in Denver? But Hart's spokesperson, Larry Smith, declined for the senator after raising questions about whether the proposed freeze would allow for certain modernizations in delivery systems and for reliability testing. Smith said that Hart would be developing his own arms control proposal, which he eventually introduced as STOP (Strategic Talks on Prevention) in response to Reagan's START program (Strategic Arms Reduction Talks.)[18] Although he had not yet announced, Hart was also by this time looking toward the 1984 presidential race.

But neither Bingham nor Markey's legislation pleased some of us in the campaign, for reasons of timing as well as content. Bingham's resolution left out any consideration of nuclear weapons production; Markey's called on the president to propose a halt in the context of negotiations. Both were resolutions without legislative "teeth"; they put the movement in a supplicant's position vis-à-vis the president.

And indeed, both resolutions were viewed by Congress itself as "symbolic." According to Waller, Markey seemed torn from the very beginning between treating the freeze as a symbolic representation of public concern and treating it as a serious policy proposal. Waller told Markey, "All we are talking here about is a symbolic measure. . . . Let's explain that the freeze is the first step toward reductions and let's not worry about details at this point. . . . We're concerned in this resolution with making a statement."[19] Waller was passing along the advice given to him by numerous others around Capitol Hill, including Bob Sherman, an aide at that time to Congressman Thomas Downey. Sherman said, "You'll have verification problems with parts of it."[20] In fact, many in congressional circles perceived verification as a major stumbling block to achieving a freeze. They would continue to focus on verification issues throughout the proposal's life in Congress. The Freeze movement would get overly involved in these concerns, responding to them as real obstacles rather than technical excuses to stall progress. Verification issues ended up influencing the campaign's decision to call for a quick freeze rather than a comprehensive freeze in 1984. According to David Doerge, a defense analyst with Members of Congress for Peace Through Law, "It's our job here to study the ramifications of these new weapons systems, to decide whether or not to build them and to put into some practical sense what those people out there are telling us. And what they're saying is that it's time to stop. Up here, we have to do more than just say stop. We have to figure out how to stop."[21]

In spite of the glamour and attention this very hot public issue would bring the congressional supporters, Markey and his staff (and later Kennedy's office) also recognized that introducing freeze legislation would provoke a real political debate for which they needed to be prepared. The congressional supporters felt that they would be the mediators between the Freeze activists, who were serious, and the legislation's opponents, who were equally serious about challenging the freeze proposal on both substantive and symbolic grounds. Allies in Congress realized that the administration and the right wing would bring serious resources to bear against the Freeze movement. Congressional supporters needed to quickly get educated on some of the technical questions of a freeze. This was an area that found most staff out of their depth.

In addition to the problems of timing and content, the movement knew it did not yet have a grass-roots base established around the country that was strong enough to win the freeze. The movement had a schedule; at this stage, the plan was to be still building the grass-roots base.

> Once we have a substantial base of support we can focus it on policy-makers and work on making the Freeze a national policy objective. . . . But let us be careful about moving too rapidly into these other phases before we have a sufficiently large and broad base of support. While the issue is filled with urgency, we can do more harm than good by a premature attempt to win at the national level.

At this stage the Freeze might have had the power to stall the move into a legislative strategy, on the grounds of both premature timing and undeveloped content. Markey and Bingham's efforts, however, were eclipsed after the Denver Freeze conference when a much more visible and powerful congressional player now also recognized the political potential of the Freeze movement.

Senator Edward Kennedy's presidential campaign was already well under way. Kennedy phoned Forsberg and Kehler soon after the Denver conference ended, proposing to introduce freeze legislation in the Senate cosponsored with his Republican colleague, Senator Mark Hatfield from Oregon. Senator Hatfield was no newcomer to the idea of a freeze. In 1979 he had introduced the moratorium legislation as an amendment to ratification of the SALT II treaty. Kennedy had begun to explore the freeze idea in response to hearing his Massachusetts constituents' often repeated concerns about nuclear war. Chris Paine, a young arms control expert working for Jeremy Stone at the Federation of American Scientists (FAS), was asked by Kennedy's office to put together a freeze resolution and to serve as Kennedy's liaison with the Freeze campaign.

Looking back, both Randy Kehler and Randy Forsberg agree that there were many problems with the Senate legislation. At the time, Kehler was unaware of the implications of changing the language of the legislation:

> To me they were just words. . . . I said, how many people are going to look at the fine print here. The fact is, the general public is going to see this as a Freeze bill. And it's going to have Kennedy's and Hatfield's name on it and a lot of others. And I didn't realize that in fact those words would take on real meaning, and that they would shift the whole definition in the way that the Freeze was talked about by all the elites . . . and that it would be hard for us then to get away from the definition that those words implied.[22]

Kehler, therefore, relied heavily on Forsberg and Chris Paine to determine whether language changes would seriously affect the legislation. "I can only assume they knew the implications of the words, but they didn't know the political implications any better than I did. . . . There's a real difference between the implication of the words and the political implication."[23]

Forsberg agreed that the legislation was stripped of real meaning; she had particular problems with large chunks of the legislation being stripped away in order to deal with the verification issue.

> The retired head of the Interagency Verification Review Team from the CIA, Howard Stertz, wrote a piece in *International Security* on verification of the freeze. What he used as a definition of the Freeze was the Kennedy/Markey resolution. And he said, "If the freeze had been a call for a comprehensive freeze, it might have been verifiable." . . . and as far as one can tell, he never read the Call to Halt the Nuclear Arms Race; all he read was the resolution. But he says 'That's not what has been put before us, what's been put before us by Congress is a freeze with many loopholes to let everybody's favorite weapons system through.

But she attributes the problems at that time mainly to confusion at the top leadership level of the movement: "People in the Washington office were not clear about what they were for and against and supporting and opposing and negotiating."[24]

Because the Freeze was imprecise in its view of how a freeze should be enacted, and because it was inexperienced in congressional politics and legislative operations, it bowed to the legislators' judgment that Congress should only advise the president and not claim any authority over the arms control process. Later, Freeze strategists would press supporters on the Hill to change that relationship to the president by using their congressional budget authority. In fact, as early as September 1982 the Freeze's strategy task force had suggested that Congress be lobbied to cut off funds unless and until the president proposed a freeze. But when the time came, the Freeze did not yet have the political power to offer or press for such alternatives in its first negotiations with politicians.

This dilemma was a constant one for the Freeze. The collaboration with Kennedy, Markey, and other congressional liberals led to the narrowing of the Freeze campaign's political demands not only because of inevitable negotiations over legislative language but because the media increasingly turned to politicians and not to the movement itself for explanations of Freeze goals. As movement organizers and politicians both worked to turn the Freeze into a political force, their conflicting agendas and radically different views about a freeze as viable policy proposal came to the surface. But without the support of Kennedy and all the prominent liberal support he brought with him, the Freeze no doubt would have taken much longer to build. The question was not whether to seek the cooperation of major political figures, but how and when the movement could allow itself to be used by political supporters so as to transform that support into meaningful action. A movement can hope for the support of politicians who find themselves in principled agreement with the movement's message. But such support will only be given if it does not create trouble in their Districts or with powerful constituents.

FREEZE LEGISLATION INTRODUCED IN SENATE

The legislation went forward. On 10 March 1982, the Kennedy-Hatfield resolution (S. J. Res. 163) was introduced into the Senate with seventeen cosponsors. In the House, Markey, Conte, and Bingham introduced freeze legislation (H. J. Res. 434) with 122 cosponsors. Soon the political benefits of supporting the Freeze became apparent to more and more political figures as the grass roots demonstrated its support in one congressional district after another: Freeze referenda were organized and passed; town meetings voted for a freeze; and city councils registered in favor of a halt to the arms race.

Within days of the introduction of the Kennedy-Hatfield resolution, the Freeze was getting the attention of the White House:

The Reagan Administration is beginning to pay some attention to the protest movement against the nuclear arms race, but it is not really dealing with the anxiety and philosophy behind this outcry. It is paying attention, reluctantly, for political reasons. The Republican leaders in Congress are telling the Administration that they cannot pass the Pentagon budget during the present economic crisis against the rising opposition to Mr. Reagan's military budget, with its emphasis on new nuclear weapons.[25]

The administration's early responses reiterated the arguments that an imbalance in nuclear forces gave the Soviets the advantage, particularly in Europe; that the U.S. goal was to redress this imbalance; that bargaining chips were needed in Geneva; and that there were many technical questions about the verifiability of a freeze. Reagan went on to argue that congressional initiatives would undermine his hand in negotiations; that a freeze would make the Soviets see nuclear war as advantageous to their position; and that a freeze would be less likely to mitigate the threat of nuclear war than Reagan's preferred position of negotiating for weapons reductions.[26]

These arguments were contradictory, but effective against a fledgling movement and its Senate and House supporters, most of whom were using the freeze as a symbolic statement against the administration's arms control proposals. They were even less prepared than the movement was to substantively address the arguments in the administration's counterattack.

Promises of negotiations had been successfully used in the past to halt peace movement momentum. This again became a major tactic in the Reagan administration's attempts to stifle the Freeze and its proposal, which, according to a 11 March 1982 State Department statement, would "freeze the United States into a position of military disadvantage and dangerous vulnerability" and deprive the administration "of a credible chance to negotiate a good strategic arms reduction agreement." The State Department promised that alternative proposals for opening the American position in a new round of negotiations on long-range atomic weapons would soon be brought to President Reagan for his approval. At the same time, State reiterated the administration's concern that the Freeze proposal "could add to the sentiment against nuclear weapons already present in Western Europe."

The battle lines were beginning to be drawn. While many members of Congress signed onto the freeze resolutions, others introduced their own arms control legislation. Some did this to distinguish themselves from the Freeze pack; others did so to join the administration in outright opposition to the Freeze movement. The administration and Republicans in Congress were under pressure to "take some action soon to persuade the public that the Administration is serious about arms control."[27]

By 28 March a compromise had been worked out between a bipartisan congressional coalition and the White House. Senators Henry Jackson and John Warner were joined by six Democratic and Republican colleagues in sponsoring a resolution calling for a "mutual and verifiable nuclear forces freeze at equal and sharply reduced levels." Kennedy and Hatfield pointed out that "the presence of the word *freeze* in the Jackson-Warner Resolution is a rhetorical trick," and indeed, this resolution was designed to confuse and undercut the Kennedy-Hatfield resolution by calling for a freeze *after* reductions, which allowed for the addition of major new weapons systems in the meantime. The need for modernizing the U.S. nuclear force was a keystone of the administration's arguments, and the Jackson-Warner resolution maintained that priority.

After a fifteen-minute meeting with Warner and Jackson on 30 March, Reagan endorsed their freeze legislation. On the same date, Warner and Jackson introduced the legislation in the Senate, and William Carner, a New York representative, introduced the same resolution in the House. Senator Warner announced that his new resolution was "consistent with the President's objectives"; it would allow the president to go ahead and deploy new strategic bombers and submarines before a Soviet-American agreement on arms reduction had been reached.

This freeze after reductions was supported by representatives in both houses of Congress, from both sides of the aisle—*as well as by many who supported the Kennedy-Hatfield resolution.*[28] Elizabeth Drew observed that

> some Senators signed the Jackson Warner resolution because they didn't understand it. . . . Some signed because they were anxious to have their names attached to something that called for a freeze. Some signed both the Jackson-Warner and the Kennedy-Hatfield resolutions because they wanted to sign everything in sight that had the word "freeze" in it and because they wanted, as they say in Washington, to "buy political protection."[29]

This attempt to co-opt the word "freeze" from the movement met with a sharp reaction from Kennedy and Hatfield. Kennedy called the Jackson-Warner resolution a "blank check for the Reagan Administration to continue the nuclear arms race" and labeled it "dangerously deceptive because it pays lip service to the concept of a freeze, while actually pushing the nation into yet another spiral of the arms race."

By the late winter of 1982, arms control was one of the most popular subjects on the Hill, and legislation cascaded onto the House and Senate floors. Everyone, particularly presidential hopefuls, wanted to distinguish themselves on this issue. Having declined the role of Senate sponsor of the Freeze legislation, Gary Hart introduced his rather vague STOP legislation. His proposal was intended to encourage the United States and the Soviet Union to engage in talks that would go "significantly beyond the questions of force levels and redirect our attention on the more fundamental problems of prevention of war." Representative Albert Gore also introduced legislation, which called for a moratorium of four to five years on *selected* weapons systems. It would allow each superpower to develop and test two new systems, but not to deploy them. Gore's legislation was totally at variance with the Freeze movement's critique of arms control and with its fundamental aims. His idea was simply to use "freezing" the most "dangerous" U.S. and Soviet weapons systems as a strategy in negotiations.

The Gore proposal foreshadowed a concept later introduced by Senators Sam Nunn and William Cohen called "build-down." Their build-down proposal called for the dismantling of older weapons as they were replaced by newer systems. Masquerading as part of the Freeze movement, both Gore's proposal and the build-down created loopholes you could drive a whole new weapons system through. And that was their purpose: to allow "modernization." The Speaker of the House, Tip O'Neill, also decided to play it safe. Noting that the House had started similar discussions on 14 October 1969, about the Vietnam War, he declared, "That was the start of the day when the war began to wind down." With equal confidence in the ability of Congress to halt the arms race, O'Neill endorsed both the Kennedy-Hatfield and Gore resolutions.

Pressure on the United States from the NATO allies was also growing as the West European peace movements became more powerful. Reagan was scheduled to tour Europe in June 1982, and the Allies warned him that there would be demonstrations against the cruise and Pershing II missiles. Bending to the intensifying pressure, Reagan was forced not only to support the Jackson-Warner legislation but to announce plans for strategic arms reduction talks with the Soviets. But from the beginning, the talks were seen by the Administration as a way to deflate public concern.

As the debate in Congress intensified, differences within an already weak Democratic party began to surface. Representative Les Aspin warned, "We could have the arms controllers and the freeze proponents beating up on each other, instead of Ronald Reagan." In spite of Aspin's concerns, the freeze and arms control debate was indeed used against Reagan by the Democrats. In fact, the administration retaliated in late April 1982 by attacking the Democrats' use of arms control. Vice President George Bush welcomed "the emergence of the nuclear freeze issue in the national political debate," with the caveat that the debate should be nonpartisan. "This issue is far too important to the U.S.—to the entire world—for partisan demagoguery." Even as it attacked the Democrats, the administration was suddenly eager to identify with the motives and goals of the Freeze campaign.[30]

The administration was not just responding defensively; it was launching a counteroffensive against the movement and the Democrats. White House officials announced that they had devised a new way to control intermediate-range nuclear missiles: the so-called zero option. This would entail the elimination of already deployed Soviet intermediate-range nuclear forces in exchange for the United States foregoing future deployments. As reported in the *New York Times*:

> Officials said President Reagan indicated that he wanted to deliver a dramatic speech on the subject probably before leaving for Europe in June, and that he wanted negotiations with Moscow to begin by the end of June. . . . The Administration's main concern, according to the officials, is to go on record quickly with a simple and comprehensible plan to show that the Reagan team is for peace, thus taking some of the steam out of the nuclear freeze movements in Europe and the United States.[31]

By the late spring of 1982, the battle lines were fully drawn.

4 SUSTAINING THE MOVEMENT
Chills and Thrills in 1982

At the same time that the first three steps of movement building occur, an institutional ability to operate on all levels at once must be built. The movement's organization provides continuity and the context for the ongoing process of research and analysis; that is, the organizers can thus communicate with each other and participate in formulating the goals of the organization. They can also more effectively coordinate the popularization of the organization's message through education and action strategies. The organization can then represent the accumulating power of the larger movement to both the media and politicians.

The challenge of setting up decisionmaking structures and methods of communication and participation can generate participatory, democratic organizations that foster creativity and involvement as well as stimulate activity. On the other hand, the challenge of this task can lead to bureaucratization, which fosters the marginalization of the movement. Such an organization turned inward is susceptible to co-optation and internal competition.

Since the Vietnam War, the peace movement has come to favor consensus decisionmaking, though its organizations are often run by traditional parliamentary procedure. Because the movement inspires and attracts many volunteers, it must, by its very nature, make decisions that are as close to consensus as possible. Volunteers are not "required" to work for something they do not believe in; movements are supposed to be something one participates in out of beliefs and principles. This is a practical matter. The imperative to reach consensus also comes, however, from a desire among many in the movement to create institutions that run counter to the hierarchical, intimidating, and alienating organizations and governments at the local, state, and national levels. These movement values are laudable. But "participation" can become prized as a value in and of itself. Consequently, in peace movement culture, the commitment to democracy has sometimes been more a way of opting out of the larger society than a means through which many can find a way of taking power and shaping that society.

The Freeze movement was faced with such a turning inward, particularly as it began to lose visibility and control of its own agenda. The burnout of experienced organizers and committed volunteers, in addition to an anti-leadership bias that fueled competition among individuals, also fostered the proliferation of committees, consultations, and long-distance conference calls in lieu of making timelier decisions. As power issues became more complex—both within the organization and in its work with the political world and the press— the movement emphasized its internal decisionmaking process even more vehemently. It was as though the inability to shape events outside the movement, fears of dealing with those in power, fears of assuming a place within that power structure, and finally, the lost opportunity to assume that place—all led to process being raised to the level of a belief system and becoming a primary purpose of the organization.

There were these internal dynamics that contributed to the movement's loss of political potential during the key years of 1982–1984. But there were external obstacles as well. Both need to be examined as we continue to examine the Freeze—a powerful protest movement that could not institutionalize its momentum into political power or translate its proposal into government policy.

GRASS-ROOTS CAMPAIGN MUSHROOMS

From April through December 1982, the Freeze movement had its first opportunities to assert its leadership, direct the public discourse away from traditional arms control (to an extent consistent with its own politics), make public demands on its supporters in Congress to take stronger and more decisive action, and, most importantly, intensify its pressure on the White House.

As the debate was heating up in Congress, the grass-roots campaigns were mushrooming throughout the country. Vermonters voted at town meetings to support a mutual freeze on nuclear weapons by the United States and the Soviet Union. The issue was voted on in more than two-thirds of Vermont's cities and towns and overwhelmingly won voter approval, passing in 155 of them, while being rejected in only 22.

Similarly, freeze resolutions were introduced in the state legislatures of Maryland, Ohio, Minnesota, Vermont, Kansas, Washington, Maine, Massachusetts, Oregon, Connecticut, New York, and Wisconsin. The Freeze's grass-roots strategy was working.

City councils, town meetings, state and local government agencies, all became involved in "making" nuclear weapons policy. But even as the movement was asking them to endorse the Freeze proposal, the federal government, through the Federal Emergency Management Agency (FEMA), was calling upon local governments to make civil defense plans for the unthinkable. The mass evacuation plans of FEMA provided another context within which community organizers could confront the nuclear war system.

The California Freeze movement reinforced the potential power of the movement when Californians for a Bilateral Nuclear Weapons Freeze Initiative filed 750,000 signatures to put the Freeze proposal on the California ballot in November 1982. The campaign in California, which represents 10 percent of the national electorate, was probably the single most important one for the movement from a political perspective.

Major religious support for the Freeze proposal had already developed; it was soon reinforced by the Catholic bishops' statement. By late April, almost half of the 280 active bishops in the United States had endorsed a proposal for a freeze on nuclear weapons. (Eventually, a total of 144 Catholic bishops endorsed the Freeze proposal.)

In 1980, the physicians' movement had been internationalized when Bernard Lown founded International Physicians for the Prevention of Nuclear War (IPPNW). (In 1986 they would receive the Nobel Peace Prize.) This global network of doctors emphasized exchanges with Soviet counterparts. On 7 April 1982, IPPNW called for a freeze. Ten days later, the National Academy of Sciences publicly called "on American and world leaders . . . to intensify with a sense of urgency, their efforts to reduce the risk of nuclear war and the spread of nuclear weapons."[1]

Unprecedented numbers of people not only endorsed the Freeze but became actively involved. In addition to the numerous occupation-based groups that were formed, the Freeze attracted quite a large force of volunteers working in local and state Freeze offices. In March 1982, the Freeze campaign counted 20,000 volunteers working in 149 offices in 47 states.

Furthermore, support for a freeze cut across geographic lines. There was some level of Freeze activity in 326 congressional districts—in other words, 75 percent of the total number of 436 congressional districts.

> Voters passed the Freeze proposition in the industrial states of Massachusetts, Rhode Island, New Jersey, and Michigan; in the western states of California and Oregon; in the northern plains states of North Dakota and Montana; in at least one major sun-belt area, Dade County (Miami), Florida; in rural areas such as Izard County, Arkansas; in the mid-western cities of Kearney, Nebraska, and Columbia, Missouri; and in large metropolitan areas such as Philadelphia, Chicago, and Denver.[2]

Support for a freeze also cut across political lines, winning solidly in Republican areas such as Suffolk County, New York and Springfield, Missouri. This grass-roots endorsement translated into bipartisan support.

The Freeze generated enough popular support among U.S. citizens to reach an 81 percent favorable rating in national polls by April 1982.[3] In the first half of 1982, 2.3 million signatures were collected on freeze petitions and presented to the U.S. and Soviet United Nations missions in June.

The media was forced by the weight of public interest and concern into the stream of education and involvement. Media attention started locally, covering the referenda, but eventually the national media picked up the freeze issue. In March 1982, there were at least twenty-five articles in the *New York Times* on a nuclear weapons freeze. Defense correspondents started to get more educated. The publication of books by *Time* magazine defense correspondent Strobe Talbott and by the *Boston Globe*'s Fred Kaplan were just the tip of the iceberg; bookstores across the country were adding entire sections on nuclear war. The writing and research in this field skyrocketed.[4] Several journalists on the national security "beat" attended the Freeze national conferences. Other journalists added peace and disarmament issues to their agendas. Some Washington, D.C. peace groups held weekly seminars on peace issues and invited national media representatives.

In addition to covering the movement itself, the issue of the arms race was elevated to greater priority by editorial boards and publishers throughout the country. A *New York Times* editorial was warm to the Freeze movement because it put healthy pressure on a recalcitrant president:

> Mr. Reagan won applause last fall when he finally promised to revive the SALT talks, renamed START. But START hasn't started and probably can't before June. . . . Reagan seems determined to look tough, whatever the political price. He knows what 500,000 freeze signatures mean in California. Yet his Administration's response to all the alarm is typified by Secretary Haig's denunciation of the freeze proposal as "devastating." Mr. Haig may be right about the technical merits. But so what? How many freeze supporters know the intricacies of arms control? To dwell on them is to miss the point.
>
> The problem is not nuclear but political. The freeze movement members are not lobbyists pressing for a specific piece of legislation. They are people, ordinary citizens pressing for something much less intricate. They want to put nuclear restraint back on the track, to give diplomacy, and peace, a chance. The wonder is that the Reagan Administration seems so determined to take the other side.[5]

18–24 April 1982 was Ground Zero Week, a nationwide campaign that included rallies, films, foot races, lectures, and debates. Roger Molander, who was on Carter's National Security Council staff, founded Ground Zero to educate Americans about the danger of nuclear war. Molander was not, however, in favor of a freeze. He thought that an immediate weapons freeze was too simplistic. "Arms control is complex. . . . It's not good to encourage people to think that nuclear holocaust can be avoided by simple technical fixes."[6]

Nevertheless, Molander's efforts fueled support for the Freeze movement. Ground Zero's educational events were organized in 750 communities and on 450 college campuses, helping to build the Freeze movement whether or not it was intended to do so. It was not just that when anything happened of an antinuclear nature, the Freeze was credited. The newly concerned were gravitating in large numbers toward the Freeze campaign, seeing in it an outlet for concrete action.

Response from Reagan and the Right Wing

As the movement was building at brushfire speed, so were its power-ful adversaries in the Christian religious right, in the administration, and on Capitol Hill. It seemed as though everyone was weighing in, declaring their position on nuclear arms in general or on the Freeze movement in particular. The Freeze had become a dividing line be-tween the various social and political forces, polarizing the mood and content of public discourse. The freeze legislation, congressional supporters, and the movement itself were pitted against both the White House and right-wing religious and political groups. In this climate, the Reverend Billy Graham shocked both sides by defying critics and traveling in early May to the Soviet Union to participate in a religious leaders' meeting on nuclear arms control.

Eugene Rostow—then director of the Arms Control and Disarma-ment Agency and formerly a member of the Committee on the Present Danger—wrote a memo to the White House urging President Reagan to counteract Ground Zero's week of activities with op-ed articles, administration statements, and television appearances. Rea-gan seemed to ignore Rostow's warnings, but the memorandum was published on May 9 in the *Washington Post.*[7]

The administration did announce on the same day, however, a new plan for reductions in warheads, to be negotiated beginning 29 June. Longtime peace and labor activist Sid Lens warned the Freeze move-ment about the Reagan arms proposal and urged the movement to respond:

> If this sounds bizarre, it is exactly the kind of scenario anticipated—and pro-posed—by Paul Nitze [present U.S. negotiator in Geneva] when he wrote the historic document NSC 68 in 1950. NSC 68 said that the U.S. must negoti-ate with the Soviets because world opinion demands it. Negotiations, how-ever, must be a means of "building strength"—using the failure, in other words, as an excuse for accelerating the arms race. In fact, Nitze's 1950 docu-ment says that the U.S. must be prepared to withdraw its own offers if the Soviet Union accepts them but refuses simultaneously to change its political system.[8]

The Freeze and congressional supporters responded—as mentioned earlier—by pointing out the differences between Reagan's use of the word *freeze* and the politics of the movement's freeze proposal. But clarifying the political differences was further complicated by the movement's need to respond to escalating right-wing attacks.

12 June 1982: Largest Demonstration in U.S. History

As Ground Zero Week and other grass-roots efforts on ballot initiatives and educational programs were building the nationwide movement, national organizers for the 12 June rally in New York's Central Park were checking last minute details for what would be the largest demonstration in the history of the country. While the rally was to make several political demands, its call for a freeze dominated news reports. A wide, even fractious, coalition had organized the rally, but by now the press covered nearly every peace-related event.[9] To the media, the rally was yet another indicator of the growing power of the Freeze movement.

The march of a million people through the streets of Manhattan to the rally in Central Park, punctuated the growing potential of the Freeze movement as a political force. While Washington announced that it was immune to such tactics, evidence shows that by June of 1982 the movement was of more than mild concern to the president, central figures in his administration, and luminaries in the right wing.

The groups who came together to organize for the 12 June demonstration represented a wide range of political perspectives and a larger political agenda than that of the Freeze alone. There were major confrontations and conflicts within the coalition. The views within the 12 June coalition were not only in conflict but sometimes even contradictory. For instance, the demonstration took place on the occasion of the Israeli invasion of Lebanon, causing groups to split over whether any mention of the massacres of Palestinian refugees in the Sabra and Shatila refugee camps should be mentioned. In the end, the issue was not addressed either in the demonstration's literature or from the platform. No agreement could be reached, and so there was silence. Nonetheless, the press and the public's attention was captured by the demonstration; the growing concern over the threat of nuclear war and President Reagan's policies caused the rally to be represented as primarily a demonstration in favor of the Freeze.

The Freeze became synonymous with the peace movement, even though the movement was larger than the Freeze coalition. So if the Freeze sneezed, the peace movement caught a cold.

Whatever any group did, the Freeze would be credited in the press. Funding came to the more visible Freeze coalition and, as a result, established organizations suffered. Those who had submerged their organization's identity to support the coalition lost funding. Those who chose to step away from the pack and distinguish their organizations by developing other strategies and a separate identity in the media gained visibility as a result of their organizational individualism. But the potential impact of a coordinated movement was eventually eroded as the media, politicians, and the public were bombarded with mailings and competing messages. If the Freeze campaign folded, that would not be the end of the peace movement. But the psychological impact at the local level would hurt.

Washington, D.C. Office Established

Meanwhile, the Freeze movement was faced with organizational strategy questions. While organizers believed strongly that the central office should be based in the middle of the country—because the Freeze proposal was a legislative one—it was soon apparent that the Freeze would need someone to represent it in Washington. The Second National Nuclear Weapons Freeze Conference in February 1982 had recommended that the executive committee and the strategy task force hire a D.C. liaison. The task of the liaison would be to "cultivate, assist, and coordinate" the enthusiasm of congressional Freeze supporters. As Randy Forsberg stated in her original memo, however, it was *not* the campaign's intention to put a resolution before Congress prematurely.

Numerous discussions and memos between Randy Forsberg, Betsy Taylor (then director of Nuclear Information and Resources), Mike Jendrzejczyk, and myself revealed our concern that the new D.C. position reflect the new peace politics that we were trying to create. We were all concerned that the D.C. Freeze contact would be able to work with the Washington peace groups without being pulled into their traditional way of organizing. It was finally decided that the primary role of the congressional liaison should be to coordinate, on behalf of the Freeze campaign, the Washington groups committed to the Freeze, members of Congress and their staff, and local campaigns. Specifically, we envisioned that the congressional liaison would strengthen the impact that local campaigns could create at the congressional district level. Thus, we were not intending to take away any local power but instead to extend the effectiveness of local groups.

The Freeze set up a Washington legislative office in July 1982. Reuben McCormack was hired as the director. Until the office was established in Washington, the coordination of the Freeze movement's legislative work had been done by Kehler, Forsberg, and Chris Paine. National lobbyists for other peace groups had participated heavily during this initial period.

The D.C. office worked with the other Washington groups through such sessions as the Monday Lobby and the disarmament working group of the Coalition for a New Foreign and Military Policy. But as the Freeze office became the point of contact for the media and the politicians, tensions among these groups developed.

COLD WAR CHILL HITS THE FREEZE MOVEMENT

By the time of the Freeze movement, the right wing had been institutionalized and promoting cold war politics for forty years. By 1983 the American Security Council (ASC), for instance, was supported by 230,000 members and the American Conservative Union (ACU) claimed to have more than 325,000 supporters.[10] The right wing's decision to mobilize its forces to defeat the Freeze movement was yet another sign of how powerful the Freeze had become.

The Freeze was affected by the ongoing marriage between the right wing and the government. For example, the eighties' wave of red-baiting began in June 1980 with the publication of an article on the Institute for Policy Studies, written by Rael Jean Issac for *Midstream.* According to Frank Donner, Issac's "highly slanted" article was widely reprinted and also inserted in the *Congressional Record* by Congressman Larry McDonald.[11] This was the first in a series of allegations against the peace movement that were recorded in the *Record.*

In March 1982 the European protests became even more visible as 250,000 people in Bonn, 350,000 in Amsterdam, 400,000 in

Madrid, and 200,000 in Athens gathered to protest the deployment of cruise and Pershing II missiles in Europe. When John Barron, a senior editor at *Reader's Digest*, made his case against the Freeze, he claimed that these protests were Soviet-inspired.[12] This was a particularly outrageous assertion because the European movements were obviously motivated by self-interest; that is, the citizens of those countries did not want a U.S.-Soviet conflict to be resolved on their soil. Barron would persist, however, in his claims.

In April 1982 *Human Events*, "the national conservative weekly," published a rehash of a memorandum that John Rees, a longtime, hard-line red-baiter, had given to Larry McDonald in February 1982 for publication in the *Congressional Record*.[13] The memorandum— which Rees felt so clever about having dug up—was to philanthropist Stewart Mott from Mott's aide, Anne Zill. According to Donner, "it was nothing more than a description of the organizational components of the peace movement, with an introduction on its transformation from a rather despairing campaign into a creative, energetic enterprise, but Rees managed to give it a heavily subversive slant."[14] Rees's report set the pace for more allegations. Several articles concluded from absolutely no evidence that there was heavy Soviet infiltration and control of the Freeze movement. Frequently, these articles would quote internal memoranda of various Freeze groups.

It was not long before the administration line included some smearing remarks. In April the State Department accused the World Peace Council (WPC) of being a major instigator and influence in the Freeze. "The WPC claims to be funded by contributions from national peace committees, donations to its World Peace Fund, and special collections. The evidence, however, strongly suggests that the bulk of its expenses are met by the Soviet Union."[15]

In May, an article by Vladimir Bukovsky, a Soviet political dissident, appeared in *Commentary*. Bukovsky accused the peace movement of naivete:

> One of the most serious mistakes of the Western movement and of its ideologists is the obdurate refusal to understand the nature of the Soviet regime. ... After several decades of listening to what they believe to be "anti-Communist propaganda," they have simply got "fed-up with it." They ascribe everything they hear about the East to a "cold-war-type brainwashing" and make no attempt to distinguish what is true from what is not. This attitude, which I can only describe as a combination of ignorance and arrogance, makes them an easy target for any pseudotheory (or outright Soviet propa-

ganda) that happens to be fashionable at any given moment. Besides, baffled by endless and contradictory arguments among the "specialists" about the nature of the Soviet system, the leaders of the peace movement believe they have found a "new approach" which makes the entire problem irrelevant.

He also accused the Soviets of involvement in the European peace movement:

Just as it did in the 1950's, the movement today probably consists of the same odd mixture of Communists, fellow-travelers, muddleheaded intellectuals, hypocrites seeking popularity, professional political speculators, frightened bourgeois, and youths eager to rebel just for the sake of rebelling. There are also the inevitable Catholic priests with a "mission" and other religious people who believe that God has chosen them to make peace on earth right now. But there is also not the slightest doubt that this motley crowd is manipulated by a handful of scoundrels instructed directly from Moscow.[16]

Also in May, the Heritage Foundation (a conservative Washington think tank) released a "backgrounder"[17] that, according to Frank Donner,

called for a massive nationwide anti-Soviet campaign to check the growth of the peace movement. It urged an all-out effort and the expenditure of many millions of dollars to mobilize "a corps of speakers to travel to the towns, cities and campuses across the United States" to blunt the freeze drive. . . . [It] also called on NATO and "its affiliated public support organizations" to mount a similar campaign in Europe to disseminate "information concerning the links . . . between known Communist front groups and the 'independent peace groups.'"[18]

Both the administration and the right wing heeded the recommendations of the Heritage Foundation. Groups such as ACU and ASC spent millions of dollars fighting the Freeze. By the fall of 1982, the Washington Legal Foundation, another conservative organization, would be organizing at the local level and dispatching a corps of speakers to defeat the Freeze.

During preparations for the 12 June rally, the right wing stepped up its campaign against the Freeze. The Reverend Jerry Falwell joined this crusade by signing a direct-mail letter that included a "Moral Majority Petition Against the Nuclear Freeze": "Here in America the 'freeze-niks' are hysterically singing Russia's favorite song: *a unilateral U.S. nuclear freeze*—and the Russians are loving it!" This petition was the first of several "mirroring" tactics that the right wing used against the Freeze. Later tactics were the introduction of antithetical legislation and the organization of local anti-Freeze groups.

The June issue of ASC's *Washington Report* was devoted to the Freeze movement. The ASC also published "How Realistic Is the Nuclear Freeze Proposal?" by Gilbert Stubbs of MIT. *Reader's Digest* came on the scene in June with an article on how radicals influence antiwar groups. Its author claimed that a successful Freeze movement would make the United States "an isolated second-rate power."[19]

On the eve of the 12 June rally, *National Review* columnist John P. Roche sounded the alarm: "What we are witnessing is an extremely primitive but nonetheless frightening campaign against nuclear buildup."[20] *Wall Street Journal* and *American Spectator* articles were also published immediately before the 12 June Freeze demonstration,[21] both being "clearly intended to discredit the demonstrators by subversifying the rally's principal sponsors."[22] War Resisters League (WRL) leader David McReynolds responded immediately to Dorothy Rabinowitz's allegation in the *Wall Street Journal* that WRL was a "nominally pacifist group . . . whose chief energies are today spent advancing the cause of world revolution."[23] Although the *Journal* printed McReynolds's letter, it deleted one of the most important sentences: "This is simply and categorically untrue—either Rabinowitz knows better and was lying, or she is incompetent and therefore misleading."[24] The Fellowship of Reconciliation (FOR) also denounced Rabinowitz's charges in a letter to the *Journal*.

In October 1981 the State Department had issued a report, "Forgery, Disinformation, Political Operations." Its July 1982 update focused more specifically on Soviet "front groups" in the United States and Europe:

> Front groups are nominally independent organizations that are controlled by the Soviets, usually through the International Department of the Central Committee of the CPSU [A footnote says that other international fronts include the International Institute for Peace and the Women's International League for Peace and Freedom.] These organizations have long sought to build support for Soviet foreign policy goals. In recent months the main thrust of front activity has been to try to see that the peace movement in Western Europe and the United States is directed solely against U.S. policy and that it avoids any criticism of the Soviet nuclear threat.[25]

The Freeze flourished in spite of all these attacks. In August a freeze was narrowly defeated by a House vote of 204–202. The resolution voted on had been nonbinding; a victory would have been a limited one. Still, the administration and the right wing viewed even a nonbinding resolution as a threat. It was remarkable that the vote on a freeze proposal was so close, considering the sentiment against it in the administration, in right-wing organizations, and in some wings of the Congress. Despite the efforts of hundreds of corporate lobbyists opposed to a freeze who twisted congressional arms at the last minute, the freeze proposal lost by only two votes!

The red-baiting intensified in the months prior to and after the 1982 elections. Attacks came from Republican leaders in the House and Senate and, again, from the president himself. Buttressing the anti-Communist line with claims of U.S. military inferiority, the administration played on the ambivalence in American public opinion: that is, the dual fear of nuclear war and the Soviet Union. One administration strategy was appealing to NATO to help get the press on its side. Editors from *Foreign Policy, Foreign Affairs, Harper's, New Republic, Washington Quarterly,* and *International Security* were among those "American opinion-makers" sent by NATO on "free junkets to Europe to be briefed on such subjects as the hidden backers of the European disarmament movement."[26]

The Washington Legal Foundation started local organizing against the Freeze. It offered suggestions on how to "defrost the freezeniks." But of all the red-baiting, probably the most outrageous was the Senator Jeremiah Denton's outburst in late September on the Senate floor.[27]

Responding to an amendment offered by Senator Dale Bumpers of Arkansas (and cosponsored by a bipartisan group of thirty-five senators) proposing that 10 October be proclaimed National Peace Day, Denton lashed out at the Freeze movement and several peace groups. He made a strategic error (from the right wing's perspective!) when he implicated the group Peace Links in this smear. It so happened that Betty Bumpers—wife of Senator Bumpers—was the head of Peace Links. Denton's allegations were swiftly and harshly rebuked. The counterassault ended with Senator Gary Hart shaking his finger at Denton and proclaiming, "Shame on you!" This didn't stop Denton, however, from putting forty-five pages of "documentation" on the evils of these groups into the *Congressional Record,* including a wide variety of peace movement papers (such as minutes of meetings that were unrelated to his allegations).[28]

The third and most infamous of the *Reader's Digest* red-baiting articles was published in October: John Barron's "The KGB's Magical War for Peace." He claimed that "the KGB has induced millions upon millions of honorable, patriotic and sensible people who detest communist tyranny to make common cause with the Soviet Union."[29] This article became one of the cornerstones of Reagan's arguments against the Freeze. Its allegations were undocumented.

By October, Reagan had joined the red-baiting of the movement. Speaking before an Ohio veterans' group on 4 October, Reagan accused Freeze supporters of being "inspired not by the sincere, honest people who want peace, but by some who want the weakening of America and so are manipulating honest people and sincere people." When asked in an interview about the European peace movement, Reagan said, "Oh, those demonstrations, these are all sponsored by a thing called the World Peace Council, which is bought and paid for by the Soviet Union."

ORGANIZING FOR LOCAL REFERENDA
AND RESPONDING TO RED-BAITING

The Freeze was faced with two challenges. It had to gear up for the November referenda, but it also needed to respond swiftly and strategically to the red-baiting. The movement needed to take careful action so that the administration would not regain control of the agenda by scaring off the public and discrediting the Freeze's agenda. On 5 October, the national coordinator, Randy Kehler, released a press statement in response to Reagan's allegations of the previous day:

> We are disappointed by President Reagan's statement in Ohio. . . . The President's unfortunate remarks show his lack of understanding of the nationwide freeze campaign which is supported by the majority of Americans from all walks of life, including Republicans and Democrats. . . . President Reagan was right when he said the U.S.-Soviet nuclear freeze movement is "sweeping across the country." What he does not understand is that freezing the nuclear arms race would enhance our national security and strengthen our economy. This is the common-sense approach most Americans support.

It was important for the Freeze campaign to lend reassurance and tactical advice to local organizers, who were also searching for an appropriate response. Education was particularly needed at this time; the public needed to learn that Reagan's red-baiting was a tactical weapon, designed to defuse the movement. Kehler sent a memo to local organizers on 11 October 1982 with the following advice:

> I want to reiterate that we on the national staff and Executive Committee still feel very strongly that it would be a grave mistake for the Campaign, either locally or nationally, to become defensive and risk changing the focus of the debate from the question of nuclear weapons to the question of patriotic credentials. . . . We want you to know that various people within the National Campaign and others who support the Freeze are trying to come up with ways of countering the *Digest* article by reaching the same general audience with pro-Freeze information. This includes attempts to have articles published in other magazines and to get Freeze advocates to appear on a range of television programs.

Most of the press was opposed to Reagan's new McCarthyism. A 6 October *Washington Post* editorial criticized Reagan and supported the goals of the Freeze on the one hand:

> Mr. Reagan was wrong. The notion that the some who want to weaken America are manipulating the many who want peace is a misstatement and a smear. . . . The intention of the freeze leaders is not to "weaken" this country. It is no fairer and no more conducive to civil debate to impugn the patriotism of their cause than it is for some of them to suggest that the president is gunning the country over a nuclear precipice.

On the other hand, the *Post* bought into the Soviet-front mythology about peace groups:

> Senator Denton got the rebuff he deserved. It is true, however, that one Peace Links advisory group, Women's International League for Peace and Freedom, is a Soviet front and another, Women Strike for Peace, has connections to a second front, the Women's International Democratic Federation. They have the right. But why does Peace Links abide the taint that even the slightest connection to a Soviet stooge group imparts? Its judgement is in question. Mr. Denton should have left it at that.[30]

The *New York Times*—which, in April, had been lukewarm to the Freeze—finally acknowledged that the Freeze was a legitimate voice in national security debates and that the smearing campaign was unacceptable:

> The charge that those who demonstrate opposition on vital issues of national security are either the dupes of enemies or directly disloyal revives an ugly strain in the American political character. . . . But the matter is more serious even than violating the reputations of fellow citizens. The purpose of such ugly defamation can only be to prevent debate, to abridge the rights of individuals and to cheat the nation of a rational choice of policies. . . . We say shame on you, too, Mr. President.[31]

National leaders of the Women's International League for Peace and Freedom and Women Strike for Peace responded promptly to the *Post* allegations with "detailed, documented refutations."[32] ACLU also protested the smear. The letters to the *Post* from these groups were printed on 9 October and resulted in an editorial retraction that admitted there was not sufficient evidence in "the available public record" to support its allegations. The *Post*'s ombudsman, Robert McCloskey, noted that the *Post* had relied too literally on a State Department report.[33]

But the right wing persisted. Its next move to counter the massive victories on nationwide Freeze referenda was a 9 October direct-mail letter from ASC's president, John M. Fisher, which made the following allegations:

> The KGB has privately taken a lot of the credit for nuclear freeze victories such as the 3 to 1 landslide vote for the nuclear freeze in the state of Wisconsin in mid-September.
>
> KGB leaders tell the Kremlin that their orchestration of the nuclear freeze movement through the World Peace Council is their greatest disinformation success . . . [which would not have been possible without] the intensive coverage of the freeze by the TV networks.

Another right-wing tactic was to introduce counterresolutions in Congress. These legislative proposals used freeze language in order to co-opt the Freeze concept. In the summer of 1981, ASC's Coalition for Peace through Strength had introduced the so-called Peace Through Strength Resolution (H. Res. 163), which had over 225 House sponsors. In the 9 October 1982 direct-mail letter, ASC reported that

> the TV networks haven't reported even the existence of our Peace Through Strength Resolution which has been passed by thirteen state legislatures,

127 national organizations such as the American Legion and VFW; sponsored by a majority of both Houses of Congress; and endorsed by the State Department, the Department of Defense and President Ronald Reagan.

ASC also launched a strategy that it had used before to influence public opinion about the SALT II Treaty—a television documentary:

> So, we have produced a new TV documentary called COUNTDOWN FOR AMERICA—with the full and enthusiastic cooperation of the Department of Defense.
>
> COUNTDOWN FOR AMERICA features exclusive interviews of such leaders as Secretary of Defense Caspar Weinberger, Chairman of the Senate Armed Services Committee Senator John Tower (R), Senator Sam Nunn (D), and Louis Giuffrida, Director of the Federal Emergency Management Agency.
>
> And, we have an exclusive interview with Major General Richard Larkin on the KGB's involvement in the nuclear freeze campaign.
>
> We've already leased transponders on two satellites for a total of eight feeds to transmit this documentary to every TV broadcast station and cable TV station in America.

The National Clearinghouse sent a 20 October memo to referendum campaign coordinators about possible responses they could make to the "Countdown for America" documentary. First, they recommended that campaign workers survey their local television stations and urge them to not show the movie. Second, the Clearinghouse recommended that fair time under the "fairness doctrine" of the FCC be demanded. The national organizers lastly urged that local people not respond directly to "Countdown for America" but instead use the broadcast time to make the case for the Freeze, either by showing films on the Freeze or by presentations from local Freeze leaders.

By mid-October, the administration's campaign to defeat local Freeze resolutions on November ballots was well under way. Top-level personnel were deployed to speak out against the Freeze. By its own count, The State Department made 77 speaking trips on nuclear issues between 1 April 1982 and 30 September 1982 and sponsored 220 associated "events." Seventy-six percent of the trips and events took place in referendum locations.[34] One highlight of that campaign included the appearance of Robert McFarlane—the second-ranking official at the National Security Council—on a local radio station debate!

The right-wing campaign frequently took on a patriotic bent, often trying to claim the higher moral ground. Several influential, Catholic administration officials became active in the campaign to defeat the Freeze. Senior administration officials said that these Catholics were "offended by the leading role that several Catholic bishops have taken in the freeze movement."[35] Among those "offended" were National Security Advisor William P. Clark, chief negotiator for the Arms Control and Disarmament Agency Edward Rowny, and three brothers—John Lehman, Secretary of the Navy, Joseph Lehman, chief spokesman for the Arms Control and Disarmament Agency, and Christopher Lehman, director of strategic nuclear planning for the State Department. Christopher Lehman said, in an unsolicited interview at a suburban Detroit newspaper, "I'm no theologian, but others far more expert have concluded there is such a thing as a just-war doctrine, that self-defense is morally acceptable, that nuclear deterrence is morally acceptable. . . . I don't take a backseat to anyone on being a moral person."[36]

The State Department funded about half of these speaking tours and events. (Local sponsors financed the rest.) Retired Rear Admiral Eugene J. Carroll, Jr. raised a cogent question about these State Department trips: "[Is it] appropriate for the State Department to spend taxpayer money in Arizona and other states on a state-ballot issue."[37]

By the time of the November 1982 elections—in 53 referenda (in 9 states, plus the District of Columbia, and in a total of 43 towns, cities, and counties), in 446 New England town meetings, in 370 city councils nationwide, in 23 state legislatures—over 11 million individuals stopped, thought, and said the arms race should be stopped in its tracks. It was the closest thing to a national referendum in the history of the country.

The California referendum was one of the largest successes for the Freeze. In February 1982, the one million readers of the *New York Times* had been confronted with the California campaign's full-page ad declaring, "Only one person can prevent a nuclear war. You." Even Reagan mobilized government forces in an attempt to defeat the California resolution; high-level administration officials were sent to speak against it across the state. But the Freeze still won, with 52 percent of the vote. Considering that California voters also elected a Republican senator and a Republican governor and voted down all the other statewide referenda, the Freeze victory was a remarkable achievement.

After the Vote: Administration Attacks Continue

During a 12 November 1982 press conference on foreign and domestic matters, Reagan was asked to elaborate on his recent statements about sincere Americans being manipulated by foreign agents; he was also asked for evidence. He responded:

> Yes, there is plenty of evidence. It's even been published by some of your fraternity. There was no question but that the Soviet Union saw an advantage in a peace movement built around the idea of a nuclear freeze, since they are out ahead. . . . I want to emphasize again that the overwhelming majority of the people involved in that, I am sure, are sincere and well-intentioned, and as a matter of fact, they're saying the same thing I'm saying. And that is we must have a reduction of those nuclear weapons, and that's what we're trying to negotiate in Geneva. . . . There has been, in the organization of some of the big demonstrations, the one in New York, and so forth, there is no question about foreign agents that were sent to help instigate and help create and keep such a movement going.

On 23 November, Reagan restated his belief that the Soviet Union was ahead of the United States militarily. Just as a similar statement by the president had generated heated response in March and April from Senate hawks like Henry Jackson, it did so again. James Schlesinger (former defense secretary and then the secretary of energy) said, "It is unwise for the President to declare that the U.S. is in an inferior position. Indeed, in regard to strategic forces particularly, the issue is much too ambiguous at any rate." But the polls showed that the Reagan strategy of emphasizing the Soviet threat was working with the American public.

At a 10 December press conference—one month after the November elections—Reagan spoke against a freeze, using information from the October 1982 *Reader's Digest* as his primary source, but also citing several "rather well-documented articles that have appeared in print with regard to, let us say then, participation in the peace movement by the Soviets." (Similar allegations had appeared in *National Review, Human Events, American Spectator, Barron's Weekly*, and the *Wall Street Journal*.)

In Janury 1983, the television program "60 Minutes" and *Reader's Digest* both leveled charges at the churches—especially at the National Council of Churches (NCC). Rael Jean Issac wrote of the NCC: "Critics charge that it supports Marxist-Leninist movements in the Third World . . . and that it has become obsessed with the alleged inherent injustices of America."[38] Both "60 Minutes" and *Reader's Digest* quoted the Institute of Religion and Democracy, which alleged that church money was going to a number of political organizations, among them the governments of Cuba and Vietnam.

FOR quickly responded to these allegations:

> It is a tragic indication of the Cold War hysteria in which we live to note that, paralleling these charges of communist subversion in the West, an independent peace group in the U.S.S.R. and Solidarity in Poland are charged with being inspired and supported by the CIA. Atlanta's mayor Andrew Young rightly observed to the NCC Governing Board: "Russians think the Polish Church is run by the CIA; the U.S. thinks the church in El Salvador is run by the KGB. Nobody wants to give credit to Jesus Christ." What the Cold Warriors of both East and West do not grasp is that biblical religion condemns injustice and oppression, whether of the Right or of the Left, just as it condemns nuclear weapons whether they are produced by capitalists or communists.[39]

THE FREEZE AT THE CROSSROADS

Despite the State Department's nationwide blitz, the Freeze got 11 million votes. If the State Department was prepared to deploy top-level officials, such as Robert McFarlane, to local communities in an attempt to defeat the Freeze, the administration obviously was viewing the movement as a serious threat. With the right-wing attack in full throttle and a new bipartisan struggle raging in Washington, it was clearly the movement's moment to push.

The infrastructure was in place for the movement to use the visibility and credibility of the Kennedy-Hatfield resolution and other legislation to expand its grass-roots base. The rapid growth of the movement was enhanced by Reagan's early response to it, the high prominence given it by Kennedy, and the solid organizing done by its founders. But as campaign director Randy Kehler told the *New York Times*, "I feel like I'm on a comet, but I don't know whether I'm leading or on its tail."[40]

The freeze resolutions introduced by Kennedy and Markey in 1982 were troubling from a movement perspective because they were nonbinding. They also put the movement in a supplicant's position toward the president and reinforced the negotiations-as-usual by proposing that a freeze could be a negotiating position around which a treaty might eventually be agreed to with the Soviets, rather than an independent step taken by the United States. There were other possible choices, but the Freeze leadership was not prepared to press for alternatives. By not proposing alternatives, by taking the route advocated by allies on the Hill instead, the Freeze gave Congress a cheap vote. The legislators could call on the president to do something and identify themselves with growing public concern about the president's policies, without having to take decisive action themselves. For the politicians, it was a win-win scenario.

For the Freeze, however, the legislative activity was potentially confusing to its supporters and threatened to unravel the movement's fundamental critique of the arms race. At that time, however, the enormous power and public attention that Senators Kennedy and Hatfield would bring to the Freeze movement seemed worth the compromise. With the introduction of the Kennedy-Hatfield resolution, the press attention skyrocketed and the grass-roots network expanded like a brushfire. In Randy Forsberg's judgement, the compromise was a smart, though not uncomplicated, move.

> I don't think we compromised away too much at an early stage. In fact I feel like it was the other way around. We started out with a clear call. It was translated into kind of a call that was fuzzy and then we went through the process of converting the extremely weak political formulation into a stronger formulation that was closer to what we wanted.[41]

Chris Paine continued as an advisor to both the campaign's national director, Randy Kehler, and to Kennedy's staff. Throughout the campaign, Paine was viewed by Kehler as an indispensable support: "You know I was a real neophyte in terms of arms control negotiations and whatnot. . . . Randy [Forsberg] and Chris were obviously far, far more sophisticated than I . . . I turned to them all the time because I just didn't have that background and I respected where they were coming from."[42]

Paine's technical expertise was undoubtedly helpful. As an arms control expert, he wielded enormous and unofficial influence over the direction and politics of the movement as a key advisor to Randy Kehler. Paine consistently advocated the more cautious and more traditional arms control approach.

While Chris Paine brought technical depth and a command of the scientific details to the Freeze, he was less experienced in movement building. The respect for him on the Hill was a real asset to the campaign, but that very access to his congressional allies caused him to advocate an insider strategy, diverting the Freeze away from tactics that might have escalated the debate. The name of the game became compromise: reaching for the lowest common denominator acceptable to all sides as opposed to challenging the deep structures of cold war and arms race logic. By playing the insider strategy at the expense of building its political power, the movement eventually became domesticated—a lapdog for Washington's realists. Clearly, a sophisticated relationship to congressional allies is central to the task of changing policy. The question is, What is a sophisticated relationship?

Kennedy, Markey, and other key Democratic supporters were not necessarily committed to making a freeze policy; they suported it in large part as a vehicle for their own political careers and as a way to prod the administration. Kennedy was hoping to launch a presidential bid, and Markey's staff viewed the Freeze movement as a base upon which the congressman could also build a national political reputation. That's politics. But Markey and Kennedy also deserve credit for taking the initial risk of supporting the Freeze. Markey, in particular, was one of the first politicians to support a freeze and put staff time into promoting it on the Hill. He did this even though his congressional district is heavily dependent on military spending. Markey took a political risk, which is rare in Congress.

Markey did gain national visibility when the movement took off the way his advisors had thought it would. In 1982, Markey established a PAC, the U.S. Committee Against Nuclear War. The committee was founded to "use the political system to stop this madness by helping elect members of Congress committed to freezing the arms race."[43] Markey's PAC raised $1.3 million by October 1986, but spent only 3 percent of these funds ($40,000) on supporting pro-Freeze political candidates. Markey later founded another PAC called the National Committee for Peace in Central America. Like the Freeze PAC, very little money raised by the Central America PAC made its way to candidates. Steve Waldman, an editor of the *Washington Monthly*, commented in a *Washington Monthly* article:

> At first glance even Markey doesn't seem to benefit from the arrangement. What's the point of a PAC that doesn't give out money? Mailing lists. The 1.7 million contributions have allowed Markey to build a bank of names of people who not only support his cause but have responded to a personal entreaty from him. He is, as one direct mail specialist put it, "sitting on a pretty valuable commodity." He has tapped it to run for re-election to the House and to run for the Senate in 1984—a campaign in which he made a point of rejecting PAC money as corrupting and tied to special interests.[44]

Waldman examined the nature and amount of average contributions to Markey's Central America PAC and noted that it "was not supported by wealthy financiers out to buy influence, but by people contributing small amounts to a cause in which they believe."[45]

What Markey did is perfectly legal. He did what almost any of his colleagues would have done if they could have anticipated and jumped atop a wave of public concern. This is what American politics is all about. But those in the Freeze movement believed that the political system works the way it is supposed to work theoretically; they believed that their political supporters shared their passion and commitment to stop the nuclear arms race.

As early as June 1982, two presidential aspirants, Edward Kennedy and Walter Mondale, had endorsed a freeze, which a Democratic pollster Patrick H. Caddell described as a concept that had caused "a firestorm that goes beyond comprehension."[46] The Democratic party endorsed the freeze at its midterm convention, after having rejected it in 1980. "Averell Harriman, the elder statesman of this party, brought the Democratic National Committee [DNC] to its feet for ovations today as he called for support of the nuclear freeze concept."[47]

But the softness of politicians' support for the Freeze was already apparent. At the same DNC meeting, Walter Mondale provided a twenty-three-page commentary on the issues he considered the most important to the Democratic party and to the country. This document did not include any mention of a nuclear freeze.

John Glenn, who would also become a presidential candidate, distanced himself at this meeting from the freeze by saying a freeze must be "verifiable" and should be part of an arms control policy.

In other words, a nuclear freeze was embraced by the Democratic party at the same time it was being used by presidential hopefuls to distinguish themselves on the issue in the eyes of voters.

This reflected the confusion among presidential campaign pollsters about how to read the Freeze movement. Matt Reese, an experienced Democratic operative, said, "It's a strong issue whose birth was secret. I didn't see it coming. I'm not smart enough to know how to use it yet."[48] Another Democratic polltaker, Peter Hart, speculated that the Freeze would have "greater impact in terms of turnout than anything else."[49]

Meanwhile the president's polltaker noticed that President Reagan's efforts to shift public opinion away from viewing him as trigger-happy were working.

> Richard Wirthlin says he has found a sharp rise, since April, in the percentage of Americans who think Mr. Reagan wants to reduce arms and a decline in the percentage who think he wants to build as many bombs as he can. The shifts followed Mr. Wirthlin's advice to Mr. Reagan to begin speaking out on arms control.[50]

In spite of such qualified assessments, most savvy politicians realized early on that supporting the Freeze brought a valuable campaign asset—volunteers. Adam Clymer of the *New York Times* was told "of a Boston-area Congressional candidate getting 14 volunteers from a high school after discussing the freeze there. . . . That's more high school volunteers than anyone is getting on any other issue."[51]

The Price of Progress

The American political system has become not so much about substance, leadership, and action, but about appearances, perceptions, and image making. There is a fundamental disjunction between social change movements on the one hand and political parties and politicians on the other. Each group operates with its own set of rules. They can cooperate and share some goals; but until the peace movement gains the political sophistication to differentiate between window dressing and serious political action, it will be taken for a ride by politicians.

Did the Freeze trade away its own substance when it agreed to the language in the early legislation? Were there alternatives? I believe the answer is yes. The Freeze could have used its early popularity and political viability to insist on the original language and go for binding legislation in 1983. It had the necessary visibility, Reagan was on the defensive, and grass-roots pressure would never again be so easily mobilized.

While the close cooperation with politicians brought the Freeze visibility, credibility, and respectability, by late 1982 it was losing its voice, by which I mean its own independent way of speaking to the press and to the public when movement views diverged from those of politicians. The Freeze lost its political and moral voice by allowing its decisions in the critical early months (and later, during the 1984 elections) to be more or less dictated by its elite supporters. It became very difficult to take risks—to find a way to challenge our friends on the Hill—when we allowed their political constraints to become our own.

Access to prominent Democrats or Republicans should not be confused with political power, that is, the power to hold those same people accountable. There remains today an unclear and troubling relationship between the movement and the Democratic party. It is not too late to debate, discuss, and resolve that relationship.

The problem was not only fearing risks but dealing with the belief of some in the Freeze campaign that a shortcut into the power structure had been found. The Freeze's access to so many politicians became confused with power. Campaign representatives could get appointments; leaders were getting called and courted by major political figures. But that access was not transformed into the power to commit those politicians to what the movement proposed as an actionable measure: a nuclear freeze.

Through its grass-roots organizing, the Freeze movement had caused the shifts in the administration's rhetoric. It forced Reagan to develop an arms control policy, or the appearance of one, and gave the Democrats an issue to use against Reagan. The proliferation of arms control measures and the partisan struggles that followed their introduction in Congress confirm that public sentiment demanded action on the issue of nuclear war. But the support of prominent arms control experts and former government officials imposed constraints on how the movement could present itself and its goals to the public and to the press. What began as a timely movement behind a radical proposal to break out of the trap of negotiations was domesticated when its agenda and message were narrowed to accommodate its most conservative supporters.

It is critically important to understand that the Freeze movement's supporters in Congress and in the arms control community saw and treated the movement, for the most part, as a *protest* movement and not as a *political* movement. The tension between the Freeze and its elite supporters—more than any of the other dilemmas the Freeze faced—caused the movement to lose its power to hold decisionmakers accountable and shape the political discourse. It was a fundamental mistake to believe that Democrats were seriously committed to the movement's goals.

The Freeze campaign had no clear strategy for dealing with the media. When the major political figures spoke to the national press about the nuclear freeze proposal, the Freeze did not pay attention to the impact that politicians' words could and would have on the movement. As it turned out, the movement was treated like a parade with politicians fighting to get out in front and lead it. While politicians and, by extension, the national media viewed the Freeze as a "symbolic statement"—an unorganized and spontaneous outpouring of fear of nuclear war—movement insiders thought they were developing a sophisticated and methodical political force. Although the Freeze was gaining momentum, this representation of the movement in the press marginalized it by both generalizing and trivializing its demands and its political message.[52]

Once again, the Freeze was faced with a significant challenge. It was no longer sufficient to simply respond well to press queries, address substantive issues knowledgeably, and fight off red-baiting. Now the movement needed to shape and define its own image in the press and with the public. A sophisticated media problem, to be sure.

The second wave of media attention—the inevitable scrutiny for flaws and internal divisions—came upon the movement as quickly and unexpectedly as the first wave of positive coverage had. It is important to recall that at this time the Freeze leadership was negotiating with powerful and "soft" supporters in Congress, trying to keep the grass roots mobilized, trying to get the message of the Freeze movement across to the broader public, and fending off highly funded right-wing and administration attacks. With the media searching for cracks in the movement, the Freeze faced quite a formidable set of challenges as it looked toward 1983.

5 EXTERNAL AND INTERNAL CONFRONTATION

On the whole, the attacks against the Freeze did not work in the ways they were meant to; this was largely due to press opposition to the red-baiting and to the swift response of the movement and key leaders in Congress. The tolerance for McCarthyism is very low in political circles. Senator Denton's attack on Peace Links and Betty Bumpers broke the back of the red-baiting campaign as Senator Gary Hart and others rose to the floor of the Senate to castigate the shameful tactics of Senator Denton and his cohorts.

Nonetheless, the Freeze was diverted politically. The right-wing assault was effective in resurrecting the specter of Communism. That reassertion of cold war politics into modern political discourse may have been overdone by the president at first, but through repetition cold war logic eventually prevailed.

Although the movement held strong and did not become too defensive, it also did not take this critical opportunity to go on the offense. But a cold war chill had made the Freeze movement shudder. The arms control debates were effectively disciplined by cold war politics as President Reagan claimed that Congress would be giving the advantage to the Soviets—and was getting soft on Communism—if they did not give him the full range of military programs he had requested as bargaining chips. The hold that cold war thinking has over the everyday political debate in Congress would eventually become more evident to national Freeze leaders as one congressional vote after another was deferred whenever the president invoked the Soviet threat.

The Freeze did not use the opportunity presented by the attacks to stress that this new debate was about national security and that the U.S. international role should be the focus. It missed its chance to deepen the public debate. Instead, the movement responded to right-wing criticisms by saying that the debate was not about ideology but about the threat of nuclear war. This response contributed to the debate's focus on the technical issues instead of the political issues.

In spite of the unified response to the right wing, four different perspectives on how to respond to cold war tactics were emerging within the movement; they were never formalized, but did, I believe, represent the political analyses of different camps.

Fears of pro-Soviet charges caused some in the movement to make anti-Soviet arguments for the Freeze. These people argued that the Freeze would hinder Soviet weapons developments, and would therefore be bad for the Soviet Union and good for the United States. This was the "national security" argument for the Freeze, and it emphasized the hardware approach. A second group, provoked in part by this anti-Sovietism, promoted the view that the United States had initiated the arms race; they saw the Soviet Union as being caught in a dynamic for which it was somehow less responsible. Again, this group emphasized the hardware approach, but did not account for Soviet political policies in Eastern Europe and in the Third World.

A third perspective—with which I identify—advocated that the Freeze become much more vocal on the East-West relationship and that it also develop a political program that would allow it to confront cold war politics at home, while sending the Soviets a clear signal that the movement was politically independent. The issues of the technological arms race and the foreign policies of both superpowers could also then be addressed. The fourth perspective represented a pragmatic view that the issues described above were beside the point, because the Freeze was a bilateral proposal. Nothing would happen unless both sides agreed.

These "positions" became apparent over time as issue after issue was debated and decided upon by the executive and national committees. These differing, and sometimes conflicting, points of view

were all represented among those of us on national Freeze committees and were never debated or resolved.

NATO COUNTRIES DEBATE DEPLOYMENT
OF EUROMISSILES

International events now provided a serious challenge to the Reagan
administration and opened up a pivotal organizing opportunity for
the Freeze. These events were centered around the debate within
NATO countries about whether to follow through on the December
1979 decision to deploy cruise and Pershing II missiles.

It is important to recall the political context in which intermediate-
range nuclear forces (INFs) had been proposed. Some Europeans felt
that the U.S. commitment to the defense of Europe was in danger of
crumbling. West German Chancellor Helmut Schmidt had taken the
major role in raising questions about NATO nuclear policy. He feared
a decoupling between the United States and Western Europe with
respect to U.S. extended nuclear deterrence on the Continent. INFs
would demonstrate the U.S. strategic and military commitment to
putting itself at risk in the event of a Soviet conventional attack.

The deployment of INFs in Europe was also part of the implementation of the military doctrine of "flexible response," which calls for
the early and simultaneous use of conventional and nuclear weapons.
The weapons themselves—particularly the Pershing IIs—were capable
of hitting command and control centers in the Soviet Union within
six to eight minutes; this was a serious technological step toward
implementing a policy of launching a preemptive first strike. The
new missiles were also called "theater" nuclear missiles, and Europeans began to understand that Europe could become the stage for a
superpower "limited nuclear war." It was this danger that helped to
ignite the massive European protests.

By October 1979, Soviet leader Leonid Brezhnev had offered to
halt the deployment of Soviet SS-20 missiles. The Soviets had deployed 170 intermediate-range nuclear forces in response to the 162
French and British intermediate-range nuclear weapons aimed at the
Soviet Union. Their view was that, by reducing their arsenals to the
level of these forces, parity would be restored. But the United
States calculated geopolitical factors and numbers differently. Two
months after the Soviet offer, NATO voted to pursue deployment of

INFs and to also pursue negotiations for the elimination of weapons of this class on both sides.

While the United States and the Soviet Union planned to begin the INF negotiations in Geneva in October 1980, they both proceeded with new deployments. The Soviets deployed several hundred more SS-20s, eroding any potential impact of the Soviet's offer to halt their deployment. And the United States built and prepared to deploy the cruise and Pershing II missiles.

On 1 April 1982, Brezhnev announced the Soviet suspension of SS-20 deployment in Eastern Europe and suggested a freeze until an accord could be reached. In December 1982, the new Soviet president, Yuri Andropov, proposed a plan for reducing Soviet INF weapons. If the United States would not deploy any cruise and Pershing II missiles, the Soviets would reduce the number of SS-20s aimed at Europe to 162—again, to match the number of French and British missiles. In response to Andropov's offer, Reagan proposed the so-called zero-zero option, whereby both sides would get rid of all weapons in this range. "Zero-zero" was the kind of offer that made Reagan look good to those segments of the American and European publics that were relatively uninformed about its implications, because it gave the appearance of radical reductions. At the time, it was safe to assume the Soviets would reject an offer on grounds that they would give up more; reciprocity and equivalence were essential from the Soviet perspective. (By 1986, General Secretary Gorbachev resurrected the zero-zero option as a part of changing Soviet thinking.)

Andropov responded to Reagan's zero-zero option by reiterating his first offer: reducing to 162 SS-20 missiles in deployment in exchange for U.S. cancellation of the 572 cruise and Pershing II missiles. The zero-zero option had called on the Soviets to withdraw *all* INFs, that is, those aimed at both the West and China, not just those aimed at Europe.[1]

The situation in Europe was intensifying by December 1982. The administration was having trouble managing the Allies; NATO leaders were publicly calling on Reagan to get on with the INF talks. Peace movements throughout Western Europe were gaining ground. The administration was being pressured by the Allies about the NATO missiles, while it continued to promote its zero-zero option.[2] In West Germany, the Greens had won some seats in the Bundestag. West German Social Democratic leader Hans Jochen Vogel called on the United States to make a compromise offer to the Soviet Union.

The administration was clearly still on the defensive on the Euromissile issue, even though it had initiated an offense against the Freeze and the Democrats.

The Soviet offer was meant to appeal to the European peace movement and to European public opinion. Both the U.S. and Soviet options, however, were unacceptable to the peace movements in Europe, which wanted their countries to withdraw unilaterally from the commitment to deploy new missiles and also wanted the Soviets to withdraw their missiles. Clearly, the United States and the Soviet Union were attentive to West European public opinion. But the administration continued to pursue a hard line with the Soviets, while the Freeze movement coped with the domestic fallout from months of intensive attacks by the White House and right-wing groups.

In early 1983, Vice President George Bush went campaigning in Europe on behalf of Reagan's zero-zero arms control proposal. In response to questions about whether sticking to Reagan's plan would ever lead to an agreement, Bush claimed the moral high ground while walking past Europeans protesting the proposed new U.S. missiles: "Let's be not only more idealistic but also more determined to reduce and eliminate this category of weapons. We have the strong moral position and people ought to be carrying signs about that."

During the INF negotiations, U.S. negotiator Paul Nitze and Soviet negotiator Yuri Kvitsinsky discussed a compromise package during the famous "walk in the woods" near Geneva. It would have allowed retention as well as reductions of certain INFs on both sides. But both sides rejected the proposal.

In early November 1983, Great Britain voted to go forward with the deployments, and the first missiles were delivered on 14 November. Then, on 22 November the West German Bundestag gave final approval to the planned deployments, which began at the end of the month. On 8 December, the Soviets responded to the U.S. deployments by withdrawing from the INF negotiations.

Freeze Relationship with European Peace Movements

Those of us who wanted to confront cold war politics and explore East-West relationships wanted to join European peace leaders such as E. P. Thompson and Mary Kaldor, along with the majority of independent West European peace movements, to work on achieving "détente from below." This program envisioned the gradual dissolution of the Warsaw Pact and NATO and, therefore, an orderly return to peace and democracy for both East and West. European peace movements assume that their governments can not be counted on to create the "new Europe." Instead, activists assume that they must take the initiative by building relationships with free thinkers and independent movements in the Communist bloc countries.

Melinda Fine, Mike Jendrzejczyk, and I represented the Freeze at meetings of the International Peace Coordination and Cooperation (IPCC). IPCC is made up of West European peace movements that share a desire to remain independent from political parties, a commitment to nonviolence, and a determination to organize for peace and disarmament through the main institutions of society. There was near unanimity among these West Europeans on the program of "détente from below"; that is, they believed it was critical to make contact with independent peace groups in the East and to also engage in ongoing dialogue with officials and semiofficial peace committees from these countries.

The Soviet Peace Committee and the peace committees from other Communist bloc countries attempted for a long time to become the Eastern counterparts to the Western movements. How to relate to the Eastern peace committees was, and continues to be, a point of controversy within the West European movement and in the United States.

The West Europeans felt that it was important to relate to the Communist bloc Peace Committees, even though they did not consider these committees the counterparts to Western groups because they were quasi-governmental. On the other hand, the Eastern independent groups may have lacked the freedoms and vehicles in their countries through which to influence debate and policy, but they were much closer to being the counterparts of Western peace groups. The West European solution was to maintain formal relations with Eastern Peace Committees in settings apart from the annual meetings of European Nuclear Disarmament (END), where strategy and movement planning takes place.[3] END is a British-based organization that sponsored the statement of principles written by E. P. Thompson and Mary Kaldor. This statement animated the politics of movements throughout Western Europe.

The U.S. peace movement responded differently. Through AFSC, a request had come from the independent Soviet Group to Establish Trust: they wanted to make contact with Freeze leaders. There were divergent views in the Freeze movement on how to respond to this request. Some feared that any contact with the Eastern groups would lead to charges of Communism and collaboration with the Soviets. Others feared that supporting Communist bloc dissidents would inadvertently reinforce cold war politics. And finally, those of us who were working closely with the West European movement felt that to challenge cold war politics, it would be important to be in touch with these groups. But the Freeze campaign could not reach consensus and therefore decided on the narrowest interpretation of its work and its mission. It decided not to relate formally to either the official or independent Eastern groups. Instead, the movement would stick to its agenda of fighting within the United States for the bilateral freeze proposal. This decision revealed once again the movement's inability to address the international politics of the East-West conflict and the arms race.

Although the Freeze never fully integrated international work into its strategies, from the beginning it had an international "caucus" that kept up international peace movement contacts and did some very important organizing. The 1979 AFSC trip to Moscow had encouraged organizers to make the Freeze into a full-scale campaign. Forsberg and Sommaripa had recognized that international work would be a critical part of Freeze organizing, and the first national conference set up an international task force, which Terry Provence chaired.[4]

The Freeze campaign did decide to devote more of its resources to international work when it hired Melinda Fine in 1983 to be the international coordinator. Fine had worked closely with Mike Jendrzejczyk and me on European peace movement issues in her previous work at the Institute for Defense and Disarmament Studies (IDDS). That collaboration continued when she assumed her position with the Freeze. Fine was particularly helpful in getting the campaign to take quicker action on stopping the deployment of the cruise and Pershing II missiles. At the time of the 1986 nonproliferation treaty review conference in Geneva, Melinda Fine, in cooperation with the British Freeze campaign, organized the first international conference on the Freeze. Throughout the 1983–85 period, she almost single-handedly coordinated U.S. cooperation with a wide range of European peace groups and government officials. Representatives from opposition parties in West Germany, Great Britain, France, Italy, Belgium, and the Scandinavian countries—among others—contacted the Freeze. Many prominent international figures endorsed the Freeze, including the heads of state of Greece, India, Mexico, Tanzania, Argentina, and Sweden.

Despite all of this, an internationalist perspective never flourished in the decisionmaking committees of the Freeze. Perhaps if it had, the Freeze would have been better able to differentiate the realities of U.S.-Soviet conflict from the sources and uses of cold war rhetoric to domesticate the movement. The movement might also have been better equipped to deal with the missile deployment issue and with the political opportunities that greater U.S.-European cooperation would have offered. Lacking an international program, the Freeze was implicitly saying to itself, and to other movements, that it thought it could stop the arms race without challenging the cold war.[5]

The movement invoked the bilateral nature of the Freeze proposal to prove that the movement was equally critical of the Soviet Union for perpetuating the arms race. Bilateralism began to function as a shield against the cold war, enabling the movement to sidestep the centrality of changing the superpowers' political relationship if disarmament talks were to succeed. This avoidance only deepened the hardware focus of the movement's efforts and further embedded the freeze idea in the trap of arms-control-as-usual.[6]

The Freeze inability to name the larger problem—identifying the political context within which it was working—would seriously effect its potential to achieve change. Because it could not come to consensus on how to work internationally, the Freeze reverted to a completely domestic strategy.

THE THIRD NATIONAL NUCLEAR WEAPONS FREEZE CONFERENCE

As the movement prepared for the 4–6 February 1983 national conference, it needed to respond to Reagan's red-baiting, to the imminent deployment of cruise and Pershing II missiles in Europe, and to the administration's attempts to breathe new life into the MX missile. This was a time of critical political opportunity. The Reagan

administration was beginning to bow to the heightened public awareness of its nuclear war fighting strategies. The European peace movements were putting serious pressure on their leaders to withdraw
their support for the deployment of cruise and Pershing II missiles.
In turn, NATO leaders were putting pressure on Reagan to return to
the negotiating table.

At this time, the Freeze had a fully mobilized and aware grass-
roots base. But national coordination was needed to deepen public
understanding of the issues and avoid being diverted by Reagan's red-
baiting. Freeze legislation was in Congress and due to come up for a
vote again. The pressure was on.

The strategy committee prepared its first draft strategy paper with
these issues in mind. As chair of the strategy committee, I suggested
that the following dilemmas facing the movement be put to the national conference for discussion and debate: the "sloganization" of
the Freeze; the political loophole that provided for members of Congress; the trap of bilateralism; broadening Freeze involvement in all
social, political, and economic sectors; deepening understanding of
the Freeze as a serious disarmament proposal; implementing a freeze;
and increased efforts to set the terms of arms control and disarmament debate.

But the national conference never had the opportunity to debate
these points. Conflicts among the national leaders often halted the
effort to develop a larger political agenda. In particular, Randy
Kehler and I frequently disagreed about the direction, timing, and
needs of the movement. As national coordinator, he was finally responsible and had to make the decision about direction. Kehler and
other staff members had to bear the daily tugs and pulls; the narrow
and focused course seemed best to them.

Thus, the strategy paper that was finally presented to the national
conference was much more limited and did not address the concerns
outlined in the draft strategy paper. It outlined three national political goals: pressure Congress to support the Freeze; cut off funds for
testing new weapons (tied to mutual restraint by Soviets); and lay
the groundwork in 1983 to make the Freeze a decisive factor in the
1984 elections. Randy Kehler spoke before the national conference
and sang the gospel song, "Keep Your Eyes on the Prize." With that
refrain, Kehler rallied the participants behind what he felt was the
best direction for the Freeze: to stay focused on getting a bilateral
freeze. The other issues and disputes should be left for later.

There was an attempt by others in the campaign, however, to get back to the original agenda for which the Freeze was intended. The issue of what the Freeze stood for was debated in full force at the third national conference. In the hope that the Freeze's agenda would be broadened, various groups and constituencies within the campaign brought in resolutions on the Martin Luther King, Jr. Anniversary March and on the relationship between military spending and the U.S. economic crisis. Conference participants were also challenged by Jim Wallis of Sojourners, who introduced a resolution calling for the abolition of all nuclear weapons.

A heated floor debate ensued in response to Wallis's abolition resolution. Rather than argue it out at the conference—which would have been logistically impossible—the resolution was referred to the strategy committee. Instead of voting on the abolitionist resolution, the strategy committee recommended later that year that the national committee vote on a substitute resolution on long-range goals of the Freeze campaign. Jan Orr-Harter outlined the committee's reasons:

1. Such a vote is unnecessary. No local Freeze campaigns or national organizations in the Campaign have requested the Freeze Campaign to take such a stand.

2. Though all Strategy Committee members involved in the discussion are themselves abolitionists, they were not able to reach consensus as to how to vote on the Wallis resolution. They therefore felt that the National Committee also would not be able to reach agreement and that such a division would not help us at this stage of the campaign.

3. We are not sure that the key sentence in the Wallis resolution is fully true: "The ultimate goal of the Freeze Campaign is the abolition of all nuclear weapons." First, when endorsing the Freeze, no one has ever been asked to also endorse abolition. We feel that a bilateral, verifiable nuclear weapons freeze is the goal of the Freeze Campaign. Second, abolition is only one of a variety of "ultimate goals" that Freeze supporters may share, ranging from abolition of nuclear weapons to abolition of hunger to abolition of all weapons to creation of a different kind of world.

4. The Strategy Committee believes that the "first step" clarity of the Freeze Campaign constitutes the political "edge" or "bite" which such a goal as abolition cannot have at this point. Many organizations which have passed abolitionist and other such statements appreciate the Freeze Campaign as a focused political vehicle toward their ultimate goals.

The national committee then authorized the strategy committee—at its request—to gather ideas from national organizations and local

Freeze campaigns about the possible goals and programs of the Freeze. The commission they created was mandated to present a written report to the executive and national committees prior to the 1984–85 national conference so that action could be taken at that conference. The commission would be instructed to

> explore such possible goals as the bilateral abolition of nuclear weapons, a Freeze on proliferation of nuclear weapons, economic conversion, a transfer of funds saved to human needs and/or other steps toward a more peaceful world, and looking at the relationship between nuclear and conventional weapons.

The national committee did discuss the proposal. Following that meeting, ballots were sent out to national committee members. But the process was circuitous and slow; after all, it would be a year and a half before the Freeze conference would deal with this issue again. While people thought that it was necessary to begin defining Freeze goals and programs for the future, they also believed it had to be a slow and thorough process, leaving open as many options as possible. Again, a long-range vision and the deeper problems of national security were seen as a priority for the Freeze's agenda, but leadership and action were not forthcoming. By the time goals were set, the momentum of the campaign would be gone. Because of that lost momentum, there would be even more serious conflict over whether the movement should clarify a broadened political program or work even more narrowly on short-term campaigns, such as a comprehensive test ban or a cutoff on SDI funding.

Structural Problems in the Campaign Surface

The low status and powerlessness of the original strategy task force contributed to the Freeze's difficulties in establishing its political agenda. The 1982 second national conference had approved a recommendation by the executive committee that such a task force be formed, but it was seven months until the strategy task force actually held its first meeting.

The first problem—that of actually getting the group going—was a reflection of its lack of priority in the campaign. The seven months during which the strategy task force was being formed were some of the months it was most needed. Legislation was being introduced, and preparations for the 12 June rally were under way. The public momentum was high, and the campaign needed a very clear plan if it was to take advantage of this momentum and be ready to escalate the movement's demands if policymakers did not respond sufficiently. The executive committee planned strategy during this period, but it was also responsible for the administrative details of running the campaign. The national committee met only twice a year, was larger than the executive committee, and was even less able to function as a source for timely political analysis and strategy recommendations. Thus, it was hoped that a separate task force would do what neither the executive committee nor the national committee were equipped to do.

But even when the strategy task force did get under way, it could only advise the campaign and make recommendations. In other words, *committees* had power; *task forces* did not, even though the strategy task force was supposed to meet much more frequently than either the bimonthly executive committee or the semiannual national committee. Inevitably, this structure produced conflicts. The strategy task force would meet for long hours, debate ideas, and make proposals, but in the end they had no power to make their proposals the campaign's strategy. Instead, the executive committee was still mandated to make the final decisions. This created tension and frustration between the members of the strategy task force and the executive and national committees. Task force members recognized the need to turn ideas into decisions and action quickly. But strategy proposals lost their potency when they all had to be referred from the strategy task force to the executive committee, then to the national committee, then to the national conference, which would finally approve or reject the proposals, then send them back to the strategy task force for implementation. As these proposals rolled over from one committee to another, moments of opportunity kept slipping away.

In an attempt to resolve these problems, cochairs of the executive committee and the strategy task force were invited to attend each other's meetings, and a number of the strategy task force members ended up also being on the national committee. In June 1983, the strategy task force was given the status of "strategy committee," but it was still only responsible for reviewing strategy ideas and making strategy recommendations to the executive committee, the national committee, and the national conference.

At an August 1983 retreat, the strategy and executive committees examined the campaign's structure and recommended that a subcommittee look at structural problems in more detail. The subcommittee recommended that the executive and strategy committees be abolished and replaced with a new coordinating committee. Although these ideas were floated at both 1984 national committee meetings, no changes were made at that time.

1983 LEGISLATIVE STRATEGY DEBATED

By the time of the third national conference, and during national committee meetings of that time, the dominant and hottest debates centered around legislation.

There were two main problems with this shift of focus. The first lay in how the Freeze handled the pressures exerted by congressional staff at Freeze meetings and in the direction the legislative work took as a result. The second problem was the effect on the grassroots momentum.

As the focus began to be more and more on Washington, the campaign moved away from emphasizing grass-roots action. Local organizers were called upon to lobby their congressional representatives; in March 1983 local Freeze activists converged for a lobby on Washington. But that vital flurry of grass-roots activism—from the gathering of petition signatures in 1981 through the organizing of referenda in 1982—suddenly slowed down. People had fewer ways to participate. The grass-roots campaigns were left to do whatever types of local organizing inspired them, although the national campaign did make suggestions through the "local organizers mailings."

The Freeze movement debated three competing legislative strategies for 1983. The first strategy was to work on abolishing certain weapons systems that would erode parity, while continuing to push for the comprehensive freeze proposal. The second position was held by those who felt a comprehensive freeze proposal was not only the first priority but that it should be binding; they also opposed spending any resources on cruise and Pershing II missiles. The third strategy, advocated by Markey aide Douglas Waller and Kennedy aide Jan Kalicki, was to pass the nonbinding resolution first; binding legislation could follow. They also believed that individual weapons systems should not be taken on as part of the national strategy.

Of the three options originally presented to the third national conference, none was distinctly chosen. But the campaign did decide to pursue two legislative strategies in 1983; one was focused on stopping the deployment of cruise and Pershing II missiles; the second was working toward nonbinding, comprehensive, freeze legislation.

Cruise and Pershing II Missile Debate

The Freeze proposal was in part a solution to the problem posed by the deployment of new first-strike weapons systems. It was intended to comprehensively circumvent the next round of the arms race. If passed, freeze legislation would be a way to halt the development of all new weapons systems at once, enabling the movement to stop going after weapons systems one at a time.

But as the movement was confronted with the deployment schedule and appropriations debates for the cruise and Pershing II missiles, organizers questioned what the priorities of the campaign should be. "While the goal may be to achieve a freeze, how can we allow the further development of new weapons systems?" was a question frequently asked. While nonbinding freeze legislation was being pursued at this time, it did not seem likely that *binding* legislation would be in place soon enough to stop the Euromissile deployments scheduled for fall 1983. No deadline had been attached to the comprehensive freeze. The campaign was faced with the dilemma that the Freeze proposal seemed less and less potent as each new increment of the arms race developed.

Nevertheless, the Freeze was slowly and tortuously building a strategy to deal with the Euromissiles. There was strong support at the grass-roots level for taking on the missiles. Europeans had toured the United States, and Freeze activists had spoken throughout Europe. Freeze representatives had attended every major European strategy meeting. The Greenham Common women were weaving their own web of U.S. contacts as they sued the United States to stop the deployment of cruise missiles in Great Britain. There was a widely held feeling among Freeze activists that it was politically important, and a matter of expressing solidarity with their European counterparts, to work to stop the missiles. The first-strike nature of the new weapons also gave organizers a sense of urgency about stopping deployment.

At an April 1982 meeting in Bonn, Mike Jendrzejczyk and I (representing the Freeze movement) agreed with European peace movement leaders on a proposal that the movements on both sides of the Atlantic could support; it would call for a delay in deployment while negotiations were taking place.[7] The delay was a reasonable demand *if* the negotiators were negotiating in good faith, which would be made evident in the following year. This proposal bought the movement some time. It entailed neither unilateral disarmament on the part of the United States nor staying confined to the bilateral box that had trapped us. After a one-year delay, deployments would continue if the negotiators had not reached an agreement.

But Waller and Kalicki still lobbied heavily against the delay strategy on the grounds that the movement would be charged with unilateralism. The delay strategy was in fact a partial and practical application of the principle they had agreed to at the Atlanta national committee meeting in June 1982; that is, that the campaign should call for a "negotiator's pause" on new weapons while negotiations proceeded. Their opposition to the delay strategy was clearly a product of Washington politics; this strategy surpassed the limits of what they felt they could press for in Congress. Nonetheless, the grassroots pressure to adopt a Euromissile strategy was strong. At the 1983 national conference, participants resisted the congressional lobbying consideration and adopted the delay strategy recommended by the strategy task force. As adopted, the strategy included gathering 5,000 signatures from each of 435 congressional districts; pressing for a congressional amendment to withhold funding for the new deployments; and mass demonstrations.

Even though the grass-roots base voted for a Euromissile strategy, in the months that followed both the Freeze national leaders and cooperating congressional representatives would fail to implement the strategy mandated by the conference.

1983 Congressional Freeze Resolution

The changes in strategy due to the influence of Doug Waller and Jan Kalicki were more evident in the national conference's decision-making on the Freeze legislation. Waller felt that the Freeze was facing a peril engendered by its own momentum. Most Freeze leaders agreed, but how to handle that dilemma was not a point of consensus. According to Waller:

> The press angle in the spring and summer of 1982 was the gaining momentum of the freeze movement. By the winter that was old news. The new story would be any slippage in the freeze's momentum, no matter how slight, which, in turn, might justify a prediction in the press that the movement was waning. The second problem arose with the freeze movement itself. In a nutshell, the movement's leaders started believing too much in their own predictions that victory in the House was a foregone conclusion. The result: considerable pressure began building within the movement to increase the political pressure on Congress.[8]

That was how things looked from inside the congressional cloakroom. But from the movement's point of view, it was time to put added pressure on Congress if it was to translate support and public awareness into political power. Therefore, movement leaders proposed that Freeze strategy be escalated by introducing binding freeze legislation, as well as legislation calling for a delay in the deployment of cruise and Pershing II missiles.

But congressional aides disagreed. Debates on legislative strategy ended up centering not around the political progam of the Freeze but around what was acceptable to members of Congress. In its 1983 debates about whether to oppose the MX missile or take action to stop funding for the deployment of Euromissiles, the Freeze met determined opposition from Waller and Kalicki. Congressional support would dissipate, they claimed, if the Freeze tried to go for anything but the *sense* of the Kennedy-Hatfield resolution: a bilateral halt to the nuclear arms race. In their view, a binding step and the specific details could come afterwards. Claiming the Freeze would be attacked for unilateralism, Waller and Kalicki worked the conference as though it were the floor of the House, lobbying and bargaining with Freeze leaders.

The Freeze was having enough trouble reaching consensus within its own ranks. The critical "partnership" with Congress increased the Freeze's problems in setting the political agenda because it was not an equal partnership. Aides Waller and Kalicki argued for accepting the "realism" of Washington politics. While the Freeze needed to listen to congressional allies for advice, it was always resisting the insiders' efforts to wholly determine Freeze choices. Strong grassroots groups insisted on not deferring to the judgments of Waller and

Kalicki. For example, the Massachusetts delegation consistently opposed going for anything less than a comprehensive freeze; it even advocated specific language for such a freeze. The Massachusetts delegation was among the first groups to push for binding legislation.

But for the fledgling movement, the power imbalances proved to be too great. More often than not, the Freeze made decisions under the guidance of its congressional representatives that seemed pragmatic but that ultimately eroded its clarity of purpose and political power. Even when the decision was made to press for a Euromissile funding cutoff, the campaign could not implement the strategy by itself since it was up to congressional leaders to introduce language they could support. The staff that were given the task of implementing strategy decided by the grass-roots were also constrained by the more conservative cooperating organizations, which did not agree with the national conference decision. The 1983 legislation strategy sat in limbo during the most important months for action. The Freeze chose the path of respectability and accommodation to Washington realism. It was decided that the campaign would continue to pursue nonbinding legislation, as it had done the previous year.

Attack and Accommodation: Reagan's Strategy

In spite of these internal debates, any Freeze legislation was viewed by the administration with alarm.

By March of 1983, it was becoming evident that the red-baiting tactic was not working to stop the progress of the Freeze. But in one last effort to use this tactic, President Reagan made his infamous "evil empire" speech on 8 March: "I would agree to a freeze if only we could freeze the Soviets' global desires. . . . In your discussions of the nuclear freeze proposals, I urge you to not ignore the facts of history and the aggressive impulses of an evil empire."

On the same day, the *Washington Post* published an open letter, in the form of a one-sixth-page ad, from the Reverend Jerry Falwell:

> I for one refuse to sit back and wait for the Soviets to enslave us or to destroy us in a rain of nuclear warheads.
>
> . . . . What would happen if the President of the United States received a call on the "hotline" some day, and the Soviet President said: "Give up or be destroyed."

> If our President said no, it could mean that more than half our people would be incinerated in a nuclear attack. If he said yes, the United States would no longer be the land of the free and the home of the brave.
>
> . . . . Now I can predict what will happen when this letter goes out. The "antis" and the "ultras" will start screaming: "There goes that warmonger again. He won't be satisfied until we have a nuclear showdown."
>
> I've endured that kind of abuse before. And I will now.
>
> It is incredible, but those of us who believe in peace through strength—which means moral as well as military strength—have to put up with this kind of abuse. So be it.

Administration officials were now trying to use the "moral majority" as a base for opposing the Freeze. Falwell was chosen as the religious spokesperson for this mission. As the head of Moral Majority, Falwell had already taken an active stand against the Freeze. He was eloquent and charming, and he had a following in the fundamentalist community.

President Reagan called Jerry Falwell to the White House. On 15 March, they met for over an hour, during which time Falwell agreed to take the anti-Freeze crusade out to local citizens around the country. Several days later, he was briefed by the National Security Council about his mission. Falwell was to present the president's case for the Soviet threat and America's fading military strength.

Falwell immediately hit the road. According to the *Washington Post*, during one of the first weeks of his campaign,

> . . . he logged some 10,000 miles crisscrossing the country. . . . His present formidable travels across the nation have a single, well-orchestrated, well-financed political purpose. As he would put it, he's rallying support for the president's nuclear arms policy of "peace through strength." Others, less charitable, would say he's selling the bomb.[9]

The cooperation between the right-wing religious groups and the state was made overt.

In late March, the FBI released their report on Soviet "active measures." Prepared at the request of the House Permanent Select Committee on Intelligence. The FBI determined that the Soviet Union did not "directly control or manipulate" the American nuclear freeze movement: "Based on information available to us, we do not believe the Soviets have achieved a dominant role in the U.S. peace and nuclear freeze movements, or that they directly control or manipulate the movement."[10] While Republican representative C. W. Young tried to qualify this report by noting that the most damning material was still classified, no further evidence substantiating the claims of Soviet infiltration ever came to light.

The president and the right wing quickly changed their tune. They no longer made claims about Soviet infiltration. The president seemed to be making some accommodations to the Freeze movement by shifting his focus from criticism of Freeze protestors to outlining the "danger" of the Soviet Union. Senator James McClure announced that Reagan was about to accuse the Soviets of treaty violations:

> To save his defense budget and undercut the nuclear freeze movement, President Reagan soon will have to accuse the Soviets publicly of violating arms control agreements with the United States, Senator James McClure (R-Idaho) said yesterday. . . . The Senator told reporters that he saw his role as preparing the public for disclosures he expects Reagan to make soon.[11]

But McClure inadvertently exposed the political uses that Reagan intended to make of these accusations, and the strategy was temporarily abandoned. Within a week, another news story announced that, according to administration officials, the president had "backed away for now from suggestions by conservatives in Congress and within the administration that he publicly denounce the Soviet Union for purported nuclear arms control violations."[12] The officials said that the administration would be "exceedingly careful" about accusing the Soviets of treaty violations; he explained that the administration wanted to avoid the appearance of using such accusations to justify new nuclear missile development and deployment programs.

The time eventually came when Reagan could use the accusation of Soviet violations as part of his offensive strategy against the movement. By mid-February 1984, he accused the Soviet Union of seven definite or probable violations of arms control treaties. By that time, however, he had also returned to the negotiating table.

Accusations of Soviet treaty violations was an old trick. Accusations of "missile gaps" and "windows of vulnerability" had frequently been used by the Reagan administration to drum up public support for a new round of missiles. Senator McClure's statement had unabashedly acknowledged this trick.[13]

But the Freeze persisted. On 23 June 1983, the House Foreign Relations Committee approved the Freeze resolution by a vote of 27–9! The committee resisted administration smear statements by announcing that *U.S. citizens want a freeze.*

As Reagan accommodated to the movement, no matter how marginally, the movement should have escalated its demands and tactics. If anything has become clear about the Reagan administration—and to a large extent, about the right wing as well—it is that their strategy is to go on the offense when attacked and to use every liberal accommodation as an opportunity to push their political demands further.

The Freeze ably defended itself against attacks, but did not use the attacks as opportunities to elaborate its political program. Furthermore, it did not claim victory, as it should have, when Reagan shifted his rhetoric in early 1983. The movement should have exploited these opportunities to point up the contradictions between his policies and his rhetoric. The victory in the November 1982 elections had been a similar opportunity; Reagan could have been confronted with the movement's public mandate and called upon to take specific steps within a clear time frame. The 12 June demonstration could have had a much greater political impact if, instead of merely conveying the general message of public support for a freeze, it had been aimed directly at such a set of timely political demands. No decisionmaker felt the political heat that these actions could have generated.

The 12 June rally and the November referenda were powerful means of recruiting public support for the Freeze. Clearly, politicians felt pressure from their constituencies. But if the Freeze had escalated its demands and called on Reagan and Congress to initiate a freeze with the Soviets before the 1984 elections—the president by going to Geneva and Congress by using the power of the purse if the president refused to act—then the outpouring of action and support from 12 June 1982 through March 1983 might have produced a greater measure of power for the Freeze. Had the movement been more visibly escalating pressure and demands for action, the movement's involvement in the 1984 presidential election in particular might have been more potent.

1983 LEGISLATIVE STRATEGY CO-OPTED

Those at the 1983 national conference who had opposed the Euro-missile strategy—on the grounds that it would divert the campaign's attention from the pursuit of comprehensive freeze legislation—continued to haggle at the national committee meetings and to pressure national staff into making a change in the 1983 legislative strategy. Randy Kehler proposed a compromise that led the campaign in a very different direction than had been decided at the national conference by proposing a new "No Freeze, No Funds" strategy at the June national committee meeting. The movement remained focused on passing the nonbinding Freeze resolution.

On 7–9 March 1983, 5,000 Freeze activists had converged on Washington, D.C. for a citizens' lobby. They delivered 885,000 petition signatures to members of Congress. Freeze supporters from New York State descended upon their senators' offices and stayed until the senators agreed to meet with them. One thousand Freeze supporters marched single file into Senator Alfonse D'Amato's office to protest his refusal to talk with Freeze representatives. He eventually met with them. D'Amato was like other members of Congress who were previously either uninvolved or only marginally concerned with nuclear weapons policy. Now they had to play catch-up to a "citizen-expert" community in their home districts.

According to a report prepared for the House Foreign Affairs Committee by the Congressional Research Service:

> Some considered the House action [on the Freeze resolution] wholly politically motivated and the debate hollow because of the probability that President Reagan would veto the resolution even if the Senate ever passed it. Nevertheless, the resolution was seriously debated at length in Congress, enabling Members and the public to gain greater understanding of the U.S. strategic arms and arms control policy involved. Moreover, the strong popular concern reflected in the debate gave a new impetus to the Strategic Arms Reduction Talks [START].

On 4 May 1983, the House of Representatives approved the freeze resolution (M. J. Res. 13) by a vote of 278–149. The Freeze created a debate in Congress that not only advanced the education of our representatives but raised new questions about the role of Congress in the arms control process.

House Votes on MX and Midgetman Missiles

At the same time that the House was debating and voting for the freeze resolution, key Democratic leaders were collaborating with the administration to use the House freeze vote as part of a strategy to get the MX and Midgetman missiles approved by the House. Congressman Les Aspin was elected to Congress at the age of thirty two and had been on the Armed Services Committee for some time. By 1983, the forty-four-year-old Aspin was for the first time chairman of an armed services subcommittee, Military Personnel and Compensation. One House Democrat said, "Being chairman of a defense subcommittee means you are now dealing with a constituency out there—the Pentagon. It means being able to deliver favors to your colleagues, but in order to do that you've got to have the support of the Pentagon. . . . They need you and you need them."[14] Elizabeth Drew analyzes what might have driven the congressman:

> Aspin is seen by some of his colleagues as wanting the approval of the community of defense intellectuals; and the less charitable of his colleagues suggest that a strong motivation for Aspin is that he wants to be Secretary of Defense someday. To reach such a goal, one cannot have been simply a critic of the Pentagon. . . . In any event, Aspin was ready to play a role in helping the Administration get the MX approved.

Aspin worked closely with his old friend James Woolsey, a member of the Scowcroft Commission, which had been appointed by President Reagan to study the best way to get congressional approval of the MX missile.[15] Woolsey was an advisor to the SALT talks and had been a member of Nixon's NSC staff and Carter's under secretary of the Navy. Drew characterized Woolsey as "an old friend of [Robert] McFarlane's and a defense conservative."[16]

Aspin coordinated meetings between key Democrats, Brent Scowcroft, Woolsey, and the rest of the Scowcroft Commission. Congressman Albert Gore was one of those consulted who later said he felt confident that the commission realized the importance of the Midgetman missile and that arms control would be stressed in the commission's report. And indeed it was. Besides stressing arms control, the report also described the MX as a "transitional weapon," and it recommended the deployment of Midgetman single-warhead missiles. The report was fashioned to be acceptable to Democrats on the Hill, to the Pentagon, and to the White House.

The MX was argued for in Congress as a weapon that would demonstrate our "political will" to the Allies and, more importantly, to the Soviets. Sometimes the MX was also presented as a bargaining chip; at other times, it was labeled a "necessary" part of nuclear-force modernization. The Democrats, particularly Congressman Albert Gore, simultaneously pushed for the Midgetman and represented it as "stabilizing single warhead weapon."[17]

Support for the MX was traded in Congress for the Midgetman missile and a greater commitment to arms control negotiations. Some bargain. The American people got the vulnerable MX and another $44 billion weapon system in the Midgetman. The MX was once called the "illegitimate child of the SALT II"; now a second bastard was born, thanks to Democratic liberals' support for "arms control."

The story gets worse. Aspin then worked closely with Assistant Secretary of Defense Richard Perle to orchestrate the various votes so that congressional support for the symbolic freeze would actually translate into votes for the MX and for Midgetman research and development. According to Aspin:

> Everyone was looking to cut money for defense; if the Scowcroft report was up first it would sink. We had a vote on the budget resolution, and people could vote to cut the defense budget there . . . and all the doves could vote against [Kenneth Adelman, whom Reagan had nominated to head ACDA] and the House could vote on the freeze. . . . People will then have voted three dove votes. The usual pattern around this place is that people begin to get a little uncomfortable if they've gone too far one way and start looking for a way to pop back the other way.[18]

Just as Aspin had predicted, "a number of people who had supported the freeze were eager to cast a vote that would blur the picture and protect them from the charge of being 'unilateral disarmers.' The vote on the MX gave them a chance to do that."[19] Aspin recruited congressional allies to support this position among House Democrats; Congressmen Norm Dicks, Albert Gore, and Tom Foley joined the effort. In essence, the Democratic liberals, fearful of looking dovish, used congressional confusion over the meaning of the freeze to push through the Scowcroft Commission recommendations, which had come up as a package: funding for the MX, funding for Midgetman R&D, and a new emphasis on arms control. As Massachusetts Democratic Congressman James Shannon (now that state's attorney general), said:

> There are some guys around here who will take any position they need to become players on a big issue. The driving force for a lot of guys here is not consistency but their profile on defense. You get a lot of Democrats worried about having looked "weak" on defense in 1980 who feel that the pendulum has swung back but don't have confidence that that's going to last, and, having voted for the freeze, they want to cover their other front. And this process allows them to do it.[20]

In addition, the Democrats led the campaign to make the new emphasis on arms control part of administration policy. Arms control could then do in Congress what it had done to public opinion; that is, control the opposition to nuclear arms under the cover of negotiations and bargaining chips.

While the Freeze had accommodated to Markey and Kennedy's strategy of first passing their resolution and then going after something with political bite to it, the movement's impact on this process would prove to be a mirage. This was underscored as the House went on to vote for the MX, Midgetman R&D, and the largest military budget in the nation's history—all within a week. The Freeze began to seem more and more like a paper tiger.

Freeze Stymied by Internal Divisions

June 1983 was a critical time for the Freeze campaign. It was now evident that the campaign was unable to move forward on the decisions made by the national conference. Two major strategy decisions had been made: to pursue the delay strategy on Euromissiles and to pursue nonbinding legislation on a comprehensive freeze. Since the nonbinding legislation had been voted on by then in the House, now was the time to press Congress to make good on its word by pressing it to abolish some of the weapons systems that the Freeze had been designed to prevent.

But the campaign remained trapped by its almost religious commitment to bilateralism. The rigid bilateralism adopted by the Freeze made any step contingent upon both superpowers moving simultaneously. The "Call to Halt" had included a provision for independent initiatives; but the activists' memories were dim on this approach. Despite the cleverness of the delay resolution in getting around the bilateral problem, the debate went on about whether the campaign should take a position on Soviet reductions of intermediate-range missiles, so as to preserve the Freeze's *bilateral* nature. The conference statement had included "pressing for reductions in Soviet missiles," but the delay strategy was not contingent on Soviet action. By allowing the fear of unilateralism charges to dictate its actions, the Freeze undermined a crucial fact: that parity already existed, even without the deployment of cruise and Pershing II missiles. This obsession with bilateralism was eventually resolved, but it was still a diversion of energy, which needed to be highly focused on organizing around the Euromissile delay resolution.

While the failure to effectively implement the Euromissile strategy was attributable in large part to the national leadership, it was also somewhat due to the unwieldy process by which the power for taking action was handed from the national conference to the strategy committee, then to the executive committee, on to the national committee, and back to the strategy committee—over a period of several months. This process diluted accountability.

It was not until the fall of 1983 that the campaign would finally implement the approved legislative and political strategy on Euromissiles. Randy Kehler made the delay strategy a more prominent part of his work. Still, the national offices of FOR, AFSC, and IDDS had to do much of the work of organizing the demonstrations, putting together the delegation of prominent European politicians, and releasing the plan put forward by Willy Brandt at the time of that visit. The plan—originally proposed by activists at the Bonn meeting in April 1982 and distributed 17 October 1983 as the Brandt Plan—called for a delay in deployment in addition to "a total halt by the U.S. and U.S.S.R. to all nuclear-weapon testing and deployment that can now be verified by existing national means."

On the occasion of Willy Brandt's U.S. visit—to meet with members of Congress to discuss the delay in deployment strategy—Senators Kennedy and Hatfield agreed to introduce the delay legislation. They got forty other senators to sign a 17 November letter to President Reagan, asking him to make an offer to the Soviet Union of deferring the current U.S. deployment for six months if the Soviets simultaneously agreed to reducing and dismantling at least 20 percent of their SS-20s targeted on Europe. A further condition would be that both sides make their best effort to negotiate major reductions of their intermediate-range nuclear forces during this six-month period. Legislation was also introduced in the fall of 1983 proposing to suspend deployment funds for one year. It was too late to have an impact.

U.S. deployments began, and Soviet deployments continued. Ironically, by 1986 Soviet General Secretary Gorbachev would revive Reagan's zero-zero option by making several accommodations. The question then became, would Reagan accept his own offer? As soon as an INF agreement seemed near, however, criticisms poured forth from European allies and congressional leaders.

A 1983 FREEZE PROGRESS REPORT

While it remains important for Freeze leaders to have an understanding of the technical issues of arms control—so that we are intellectually prepared to defend our positions—by 1983 we got swallowed up by the technical arguments. The Freeze got trapped into a narrower debate and increasingly became accessible only to those already expert or interested in the details of arms control. The public's interest was diverted and diffused.

The arms control approach led the Freeze into a cul-de-sac, making the movement apolitical and amoral. By blaming hardware and technology—emphasizing, in effect, that we are somehow the victims of technology and not able to shape it or determine its uses—the Freeze blurred the fact that *people* make the decisions, design the weapons, and manage the policies for which these weapons are the instruments. Because the Freeze movement did not have a firm definition of the problem—a specific vision of the future it was working toward—it abdicated the very moral and political ground on which its appeal to the American public had been based.

A Faltering Educational Strategy

The fight to inaugurate a new way of thinking about security in the nuclear age might have sustained the movement, by providing a durable framework for a new political discourse. By having this intention, the Freeze did begin on a path of enormous importance. But the Freeze's ability to carry on a sophisticated educational strategy was severely hampered by its narrow political vision and goals. The Freeze was diverted into a piecemeal information campaign; it responded to legitimate inquiry about related issues but did not develop the new way of thinking about security that could have put the movement's short-term projects into a new political context and could have answered that important question, What comes after the Freeze? Instead, educational work was either supplemental to the Freeze proposal—or tangential to that proposal and therefore beside the point.

The Freeze asked people to follow it away from the brink of nuclear war. It raised many questions about closely related issues. It first posed a problem—and suggested a first-step solution—then raised a series of follow-up questions that it was not prepared to answer.

Still, the Freeze movement was viewed by many progressives as one of the few viable political movements on the horizon. Many saw it as a potential vanguard for a broader political force within the Democratic party. Ironically, the Freeze was compelled to narrow its agenda and, at the same time, to become a political base for the many who were disaffected from politics after Reagan's election. The Freeze consistently juggled these two opposing pressures, trying to accommodate both. Its sympathies compelled it to emphasize "outreach" to new constituencies, to dedicate significant resources to building relationships, for instance, with labor and people of color.

Faced with the requests and proposals that went along with seeking endorsements and the support of other movements, the Freeze not only opted for a narrow political focus and limited action strategies but it added new items to its "educational" agenda in almost pin-the-tail-on-the-donkey fashion. Education was no longer a vibrant movement-building tool.

As a result, the Freeze was viewed by the press, the public, and the politicians as not understanding the political realities it was designed to question. This meant, for example, that President Reagan could propose a "Star Wars" defense system as not only a technological fix to the problem of the nuclear threat but as a morally superior solution. He could condemn nuclear deterrence and propose the abolition of nuclear weapons, two positions on which the Freeze was muzzled. In other words, the Freeze could not develop its messages and demands to keep pace with the very political shifts it successfully stimulated. The president was not so constrained. He co-opted the movement's moral and political ground.

The Freeze had intended to mobilize the inherent popular fear of nuclear war as the first step in educating American citizens about the arms race and the larger problem of militarism. By galvanizing that fear of nuclear war, it began to help people deal with the danger in a mature way—by offering the meaningful actions of involvement in the movement and support for a freeze. As the original organizers correctly predicted, much of the Freeze's beauty was its simplicity and accessibility; many of its successes can be attributed to the fact that it was understandable and seemed to offer a positive way out of the nuclear trap.

Yet the Freeze (as well as Helen Caldicott and the physicians' movement in particular) has been accused of generating and trading on fear. The Freeze movement was indeed built on a negative agenda insofar as it emphasized survival over other authentic human values. By emphasizing survival as its most important goal, the movement's moral authority was undermined.

Time after time, those involved in the Freeze said, "The issue is survival," and, "The Freeze is about survival." In my view, this is where the Freeze movement is most vulnerable to charges of negativity and of focusing more on the public's fear than on the public's ability to take charge of the social, technological future. In operation, the difference is subtle, but philosophically and politically, it is pivotal to the movement's future. Perhaps this point is best illustrated by the campaign's slogan "The Freeze: Because No One Wants a Nuclear War." The April 1980 national Freeze demonstrations organized by FOR and AFSC's Rocky Flats Action Group had as their slogan, "Freeze the Arms Race: The Future in Our Hands." When the official slogan of the Freeze movement was chosen, some local campaigns opted for the latter.

In his book *The Minimal Self*, Christopher Lasch comments on how the peace and environmental movements' message contributed to their unraveling. "If survival is the overriding issue, people will take more interest in their personal safety than in the survival of humanity as a whole. Those who base the case for conservation and peace on survival not only appeal to a debased system of values, they defeat their own purpose."[21]

The nuclear weapons debate has been conducted from two competing views of survival. The peace movement argues that survival after even a minimal use of nuclear weapons is impossible, that the survivors will envy the dead. Advocates of a nuclear buildup argue that we can fight and survive a nuclear war, that the threat of nuclear war is worth the risk if the alternative is giving up our freedoms and our way of life, that the risk of war is low, given the enormity of the threat.[22] This circuitous logic leads those who try to focus on the possibility of nuclear war and the magnitude of the threat into pushing the public toward fear responses. As survival is made *the* issue, the layperson is left swimming in facts and more than likely drowning in feelings of confusion and helplessness, susceptible to quick fixes or official reassurances, no matter how unrealistic they may be. Dr. Carol Nadelson writes that psychological reactions to being put in the middle of this survival debate can be increased narcissism and selfishness, escape fantasies, and looking to an authority figure to solve the problem.[23]

While the Freeze helped to break down the "psychic numbing" for many, its focus on survival may have contributed to the effectiveness and the appeal of Reagan's "Star Wars" solution. The president addressed the fears, accepted popular disbelief in deterrence theory, and offered a "vision of the future which offers hope." He envisioned a world free from the threat of nuclear war by making nuclear weapons obsolete. Making civilians the targets for nuclear weapons was "immoral," according to the president. Standing on the moral ground built by the Freeze movement, Reagan proposed the psychological fix as well as the technical fix. "Star Wars" is an escape fantasy, presented by the reassuring authority figure.

The Freeze imagined itself as a movement putting forth a positive program, offering people a solution to the problem it highlighted. But the Freeze was increasingly seen as negative not only because of its emphasis on survival but because of its inability to offer a long-term positive vision and interim policy paths toward that vision. The energy and the nearly ferocious commitment that new activists brought to the Freeze were rooted in their own fear as well as the value they put on human life. Its political vision and deeper value message was either lost or unarticulated, creating a vacuum that eroded both the moral clarity and the intellectual strength of the Freeze over time.

Coping with Elitism

The Freeze was enormously successful at getting all segments of the American population mobilized. In the 1982 referenda, people of color widely supported the goal of freezing the arms race. Although endorsements came from numerous labor, Black, and Hispanic individuals and organizations, the Freeze organizers—as was true of peace movements since the turn of the century—were predominantly white, professional, religiously based, and middle-class; many were from the established peace organizations.

At the local level, some efforts were made to achieve a better gender and racial balance. For example, the committee running the California referendum drive agreed to step down to make room for newcomers and to achieve a better gender and racial balance. But the emphasis on fear and survival inevitably shrunk the Freeze's base of support, by not showing that the Freeze was affirming positive values and working toward economic and social advantages for all.

Harvard psychiatrist Robert Coles has written a piercing critique of elitism in the Freeze movement.[24] Specifically, he tells the story of a family that was outraged by Helen Caldicott's speech to the graduating class of Salem State College in May 1982. Caldicott spoke of the imminence of the nuclear threat; she claimed that everyone had nuclear nightmares, that the world was sick, and that we were all victims of psychic numbing.

The family was outraged by the accusation that they were psychicly numb and also by having to listen to this doomsday message on the day their son was graduating, which was for them a joyous occasion. Coles quotes the father:

> We come there to see our son get a college degree—the first person in our family to get one—and she's there telling us the world is sick, sick. She said it's "terminal." I remember. And she said we're sticking our heads in the sand—she didn't say that, she said something that meant that, that we're all numbed out, I remember. Everyone but her and her friends. How does she know? What gives her the right to think every single person in that hall isn't as worried as she is about a nuclear war? . . . And if we had the Goddamned gall to want some other kind of message on the day our kid was getting his diploma, and getting ready to have the first office job of anyone in this family, I'll tell you, then tough luck for us—and aren't we the dopes and the blind

fools to expect that, when any day now the nukes will go off and that'll be the end, and here we are, whistling Dixie! . . . Will you tell me who in hell is in favor of those Goddamned bombs? If we could get rid of every single one of them tomorrow, if every nation got rid of its store of them and we could all be sure none would be built afterward, that's what we'd all want. You bet![25]

Coles refutes the data on psychic numbing: "Who has interviewed whom to ascertain the presence or degree of this numbing?" He asks us to consider what else we might be numb to:

Dr. Caldicott, for example, reminds us that "two-thirds of the world's children are malnourished and starving." But how often do many of us who worry about nuclear war think of those children, and what are we doing to better their lot? Giving half of our fat physicians' fees to Oxfam? Giving up our second homes, our BMWs, our ski vacations? Are we, living pleasant lives, thereby "numb" to the manifest death of thousands of children—and enormous tragedy unfolding every day, never mind the speculative one of nuclear war? The man I have quoted here worries all the time that he won't be able to pay his bills. He lives at the edge of things in ways some of us well-to-do liberals never stop to consider. Are we "numb" to him and millions like him and their fates?[26]

Coles finally asserts:

It is a near "mathematical certainty" that the freeze movement shall never succeed so long as we, its supporters, fail to make common cause with working men and women—people for whom survival will still be an issue even after the last bomb has been dismantled.[27]

Internal Communication Problems

By July 1983, one year after it had opened, there were numerous problems in the D.C. legislative office. The director, Reuben McCormack, reportedly had troublesome relationships with Congress and with other Washington peace groups: abrasive with the former and excluding of the latter. The problems this created deepened and McCormack eventually resigned.

His assistants, Chap Morrison and Pat Harman, carried out the work of the office while a new director was sought. A vacuum of leadership developed in Washington. Harman and Morrison had no authority in the eyes of other lobbyists, so Randy Kehler tried to fill in when and where he could on the Hill. But he did not replace McCormack for several months.

We hoped that a change in staff would bring the D.C. office back into better relations with other Washington peace groups and clarify communications between all parts of the Freeze coalition. The problems in Washington added to the tension between that office and the St. Louis headquarters. The St. Louis staff felt that the emphasis on legislation was pulling the Freeze away from the original model—grass roots–based power developed through education and local action strategies such as the referenda. Tactically, the Freeze could not find other actions like the referenda to localize the debate even further.

The campaign's communication problems were only exacerbated by Randy Kehler's need to return to western Massachusetts. Kehler decided that his position as national coordinator would be for only one year, because his family did not want to make a permanent move to St. Louis. The Freeze executive committee decided instead to allow Kehler to remain national coordinator and to set up yet another office in western Massachusetts.

There was a lot of ambivalence about this decision, and with good reason. The campaign was already having enough troubles with leadership; stationing the national coordinator away from the rest of the campaign made little organizational sense. Kehler acknowledges that this was a significant mistake on his part: "To have the head of your campaign isolated in a little office a thousand miles from your staff is total insanity. It's hard to understand why anybody, including myself, ever thought it could work or agreed to it."[28]

Dwindling Emphasis on Grass-roots Organizing

While some local organizers were seeking autonomy, most were looking for greater direction. In 1983, Steve Ladd of the California Freeze campaign coined the term "optionitis" to describe the dilemma of some local groups: too many action possibilities and not enough direction from the national campaign. Jim Driscoll, at that time program coordinator of the Albany Friends of the Freeze, also called for more national direction and, in a 1 October 1983 letter to the strategy committee, pointed out the growing confusion at the local level:

Please let's have a simple, clear task for all of us to work on. Most local people (that is non-career activists) want that kind of leadership from the National Campaign. It is the activists who keep talking local option and participation. The five-hour-a-week volunteers want to know how to spend that time most effectively. A two hour consensual discussion about priorities does not meet that criterion and yet that is what most local groups are stuck with *every month* as a result of these fragmented and shifting messages coming from St. Louis.

The 2–4 December 1983 national conference would respond to these concerns by identifying three "citizen pressure objectives" for 1984, as outlined by Randy Kehler in a 21 November 1983 memo: congressional district lobbying, participation in the 1984 election process, and nonlegislative-electoral citizen actions. The conference outlined two kinds of activity meant to meet these objectives. "Freeze Fridays" held on the first Friday of each month would encourage Freeze supporters around the country to publicly demonstrate their support by engaging in a strategy committee-recommended action on that day. The conference also designated 5 October 1984 as a "Day of Concern." This final Freeze Friday, designed to "affect the political climate, both before and after the elections," would be held to "keep the issue of stopping the nuclear arms race foremost in the public mind." When Randy Kehler presented these recommendations, he noted that "it has now been seven or eight months since we had such a unified national objective that called for massive grassroots outreach." Those seven or eight months may have been critical ones in the loss of Freeze momentum.

Irreconcilable Political Differences

Political differences among the various groups making up the Freeze coalition were evident from the time of the first national conference in 1981. By 1982, Freeze committee members and national staff recognized that these differences were affecting the movement's ability to set its political agenda. A gathering 13-16 May 1982 at the Blue Mountain Center in New York discussed the different points of view. It proved impossible to agree on political aims and definitions for the Freeze:

> Instead, the idea that the national freeze campaign can serve as a floor, or least common denominator, had a strong appeal. If the freeze is the floor, then other organizations must be to the left of it or ahead of it, pressing for radical disarmament and linking peace with justice. . . . The "freeze-as-floor" approach helped the groups avoid wrangles over when and how hard the campaign should hit intervention in El Salvador, American imperialism elsewhere, nuclear power, the conventional arms buildup. The consensus was that leaders of the national freeze must remain flexible and very attentive to how far grass roots support goes on these issues. . . . The ambiguity of the national freeze movement was seen as a good thing, to be preserved, not attacked.

But what did this mean for the organizations making up the Freeze? One retreat suggestion was that these groups should be "testing the ground" for the Freeze. Mike Caspar suggested that "others in the movement have to be pushing more extreme goals, more forcefully." Randy Kehler agreed with these views: "Somebody's got to be out ahead. If the Freeze is the farthest ahead, we'll only be able to step back, in the inevitable compromise."[29]

But the Freeze-as-floor approach never worked. To pursue a strategy, the Freeze had to be *for* something. And that something had to be agreed upon. As the Freeze seemed to decline, differences in politics became more apparent. Struggles for personal power were more frequent and less civilized. The cohesion of the organization was devalued as these political differences sharpened and some with sectarian points of view tried to take over leadership. Camps developed in the campaign. There were those who wanted to keep the Freeze narrowly defined as an arms control group. Others saw the Freeze as a vanguard political movement, that is, a constituency to be moved behind one or another political candidate. (Later in the campaign, Mondale supporters would line up against Jackson supporters.) New racial and political lines were drawn by the different camps. What held the Freeze coalition together became more and more fragile and politically volatile. Only short-term campaigns provided the cohesion and the opportunity for the Freeze to try to sort through its political directions and set itself on a new course.[30]

As the Freeze became more narrowly defined and more focused on legislation, groups with broader political agendas were forced out or dropped out. National organizations were marginalized and left out of decisionmaking. This happened in part because newer local Freeze activists wanted more say in the national campaign's direction. Eventually, the nominations committee and the executive committee decided to decrease the number of slots for national organizations on the national committee and increase the number of slots for local representatives to one slot for each of the fifty states.

Leadership and Power Struggles

As the prominence and visibility of the movement grew, the inevitable competition and power struggles emerged. Motives became suspect, and with suspicion came a dampening of creativity and leadership. Making proposals was often viewed as making a "power move," and the Freeze became something to "protect." Second-guessing and rumor competed with open, honest dialogue. The organizing model of the Freeze was originally designed to be deeply political and to send a message about a new sophistication in the peace movement; but the antileadership ethos muted the campaign's public voice and eroded the social dynamics within the campaign.

When the visibility of the movement faded, some turned their frustration inward. The price of taking leadership became even more costly. Those who took initiative were viewed with suspicion. When leaders rose to speak and offer ideas, they were silenced. When they remained silent, they were equally condemned for lack of leadership. The Freeze staff was buffeted around by these mixed signals; they chose a consultative and facilitative style in some instances and were compelled by organizational and political realities to take leadership in others. The Freeze movement was particularly hard on its staff, and it "used" leaders poorly.

Overt confrontations between Randy Forsberg and Randy Kehler in national committee meetings seemed to give others permission to jockey for power. Partially in response to this, leaders and staff focused on developing elaborate consultative processes that attempted to include everyone. Those who were historically responsible for the organization pulled back, out of commitment to the principle of sharing responsibility and power. They did so out of self-protection as well. Taking leadership could get you on the endangered species list. The Freeze lost as a result. Other individuals who could have helped to provide continuity and a collective memory for the Freeze were also forced out.

The fixation on process and the bureaucratized definition of democracy—which involved everyone at every level of decisionmaking—grew as trust was eroded among leaders and within the Freeze's various committees. Status and access to key staff become scarce resources; cooperation and collaboration deteriorated.

The structure for relations among the committees, the task forces, and the staff caused some of these difficulties. In particular, it was often unclear who should be the decisionmaker for what. According to former Freeze staff members Barbara Roche and Pam McIntyre, the increase in staff at the Clearinghouse contributed to unclear divisions of responsibility between task forces and staff. The staff gradually assumed more and more of the jobs originally done by task forces. In June 1983, the nominations task force proposed that some of the task forces become permanent advisory committees working with staff members. It was recognized that staff positions had become more central to the everyday decisionmaking of the campaign.

This process of redistributing responsibilities from task forces to advisory committees and staff may have alleviated the problem of unclear responsibilities. But is also hastened the transformation of the Freeze from a coalition to an organization, with emphasis put on paid staff and not on coordination with the groups and recruitment of volunteers.

The Freeze became more and more involved with maintaining its own elaborate structures and decisionmaking processes. The focus on organizational strategy competed with the development of political strategy. Randy Kehler and other national staff felt these pressures. For those faced with tough choices, great pressure, and limited resources, the only way to build a movement with political clout seemed to rest in keeping the grass roots mobilized—by whatever means possible—and in keeping the Washington "arms control lobby" coordinated around a common legislative agenda. Kehler and the other campaign staff advocated a broad educational program and a narrow strategic focus. As Kehler notes, this was a compromise meant to appease those who wanted to "broaden" the consensus, on the one hand, and those whose political agenda was most narrowly defined, on the other. This solution emerged as much from Kehler's management style as it did from internal and external pressures on the campaign. Although the internal dynamics described above were made worse by external pressures. These pressures came from Democratic party and arms control supporters as well as from everyone's competing visions of what the Freeze was leading toward. Kehler and the national staff functioned more as mediators than as political leaders.

While each of us in a leadership position had a principled commitment to building a grass-roots, democratic organization, Kehler's temperament and leadership style—seeking broad input and solutions that accommodated views along a wide spectrum of opinion and belief—may have been more appropriate for the campaign in its early stages. His warmth, dedication, and personal commitment provided social cohesion, particularly when the campaign was young and relatively uncomplicated. He and the other national staff set a tone that people respected.

In the midst of conflict and tough choices, however, mediation and broad consultation could inform but not substitute for a decisive, risk-taking voice. Kehler, the other staff, and the campaign itself were caught in an organizational style that fostered participation, but created a significant leadership vacuum—one that, once recognized, nearly everyone tried to fill. "Participation" did not necessarily lead toward decisions, much less toward timely ones. Those with the most information seemed to hold back, emphasizing process. Yet in the end, they were compelled to act. Inevitably, their decision would then offend someone.

While power issues are expected—and, of course, better dealt with if expected—these issues were all the more problematic for the Freeze because of the movement's own cultural tendencies. Certain organizational behaviors within peace movement culture can take on pathological proportions. These behaviors include: ambivalence about power itself, resulting in a conflict between those who reject it and those who are intimidated or charmed by it; inherent mistrust of leaders; a clear projection of the anger and alienation that some members feel about society onto the movement itself; a related negativity about the dominant culture and no identification with the United States as "our" country; blurring of both values and positive visions of the future; fierce individualism and the internalization of an atomized culture, even while rejecting it.

Many people were aware of these problems and sought to resolve them. Unfortunately, this attention to the problems reinforced the turning inward throughout the time the campaign needed to be most responsive to the flurry of activity it had initiated with the public and in Congress. As time went on, the Freeze frequently turned to consultants to help it address these problems. At an August 1983 retreat, two consultants from Collaborative Change Associates, Peter Woodrow and Suzanne Terry, were hired to facilitate sessions and give feedback. On the one hand, Woodrow and Terry observed a tremendous amount of good will, dedication, and commitment. They also noted that the campaign had maintained its commitment to an organizational structure based in grass-roots groups and leadership. On the other hand, they saw high competition and noted several areas of group process that needed improvement. They particularly noticed a resistance to leadership: "People get chewed up as facilitators of small groups and chairs of committees." They felt that, in general, Freeze members were ambivalent about the role of leaders and thus gave them mixed messages. Woodward and Terry observed "general confusion (somewhat clarified as a result of the retreat) about which items need full democratic consideration, which need some form of consultation, and which can be decided by fiat and by whom. You have made a start on this one, but need to continue to learn."

Regarding power struggles, Woodward and Terry concluded:

A central conflict within the organization is the unacknowledged struggle for power and status. The Freeze as a movement has gained national recognition and power. There is confusion right now about how best to make use of that power. There are those within the organization who have strong opinions about how the organization should move—and want a personal role in shaping the organization. As a first step, this conflict needs to be surfaced in a constructive manner. The power brokering will go on and is probably healthy, but must be managed well in order to keep it from destroying the whole endeavor.[31]

6

1984
The Electoral Window
of Opportunity

The Freeze movement had generated significant trouble for the Reagan White House. His bellicose, anti-Soviet rhetoric had gone too far, arms control was stalled, and there seemed little hope that things would improve. Public outrage had gotten through to the president and his pollsters, and he was finally forced to make some accommodations.

REAGAN RETURNS TO NEGOTIATING TABLE

On 17 January 1984, Reagan called on the Soviets "to return to the negotiating table and join him in forging a constructive working relationship. . . . We will never retreat from negotiations. . . . The fact that neither of us likes the other system is no reason to refuse to talk. . . . We will negotiate in good faith."

Most notable about this kind of talk was the complete absence of anti-Soviet rhetoric; Reagan was no longer portraying the Soviet Union as the "evil empire." Indeed, in early February he spoke as a man of peace:

While our governments have very different views, our sons and daughters have never fought each other. We must make sure they never do. I hope the lead-

145

ers of the Soviet Union will work with us in that same spirit. . . . If the Soviet Government wants peace, there will be peace. . . . We are meant to be one family of nations. . . . We who are leaders in government have an obligation to strive for cooperation every bit as hard as our athletes who reach within for the greatest efforts of their lives.

The administration justified this position on the grounds that the U.S. military buildup had advanced and America was now able to bargain from a position of strength. The *New York Times* commented on the change: "All that military spending has changed the psychology of negotiations. Well, maybe. But what has changed much more clearly is politics. Mr. Reagan knows, for instance, how many millions of Americans are deeply concerned about the arms race."[1]

Reagan did not put forward any modifications to the U.S. bargaining positions. He would go as far as returning to the negotiating table, but he had no coherent arms control program that would make his claim of "negotiating in good faith" credible. Even administration strategists admitted that Reagan's decision to return to the negotiating table was politically motivated; the *New York Times* noted that excerpts from the 14 January speech were released on a Sunday in advance of a Democratic presidential candidates' debate in New Hampshire the following week. Former Vice President Walter Mondale said, "Once again, President Reagan is trying to deal with the politics of a problem instead of the problem itself."

Later, the president would use the 1984 Summer Olympic Games as a dramatic and unifying arena for rallying American citizens behind their country. Desperate to feel good about ourselves as a nation, we were caught up in the pageant imagery, and the Olympics became an important symbol for those who cling to the "America is Number One" rule of foreign policy. In cooperation with numerous corporations, such as ITT, the U.S. Olympic Committee organized a run across the country with the Olympic torch passing from one runner to the next, rippling the national pride from coast to coast.

Meanwhile, Soviet officials were under pressure from their own military to station new weapons in response to the 572 cruise and Pershing II missiles to be deployed by the United States in Europe. They also knew that they had to counteract the effects on international opinion of shooting down Korean Airline 007 in the late summer of 1983. Yuri Andropov had been replaced by Konstantin Chernenko.

The Soviets initially dismissed Reagan's friendlier tone as "verbal camouflage," covering the administration's "militarism, enmity and war hysteria," according to Soviet spokesman Andrei Gromyko at an international conference in Stockholm. Later, the Soviets would also have political reasons to stop their own bellicose rhetoric. In early 1984, however, it served their purposes to remain hostile to Reagan, to not respond to what they perceived as the president's election year rhetoric. From the Soviet Union's point of view, it was a matter of watching American politics and making a move at the most opportune moment. If U.S. public opinion and the Democrats kept the heat on the president, he would be more likely to make concessions toward the Soviets and arms control.

Reagan's accommodations—returning to the negotiating table, cooling off his anti-Soviet rhetoric, and forming bipartisan commissions such as the Commission on Strategic Forces—seemed to take the wind out of the Democrats' sails. Reagan's belligerence toward the Soviet Union and his relentless military buildup had provided the Democrats with ammunition for three years. When Reagan began to make cosmetic concessions, the Democrats' task became more difficult, but in a sense this change was also their window of opportunity. Now was their chance to challenge traditional arms control. They could have argued that returning to Geneva was not enough and pressed for an acknowledgement that there was already essential parity between the United States and the Soviet Union. They could have promoted confidence-building measures to enhance the spirit of cooperation needed to proceed with disarmament. But Democrats were just as constrained by election year politics as Reagan.

FREEZE PLANS FOR 1984: A DUAL STRATEGY

The preprimary days were another period during which the Freeze could have asserted some independent political power behind its goals. Having watched the Freeze legislation become a purely symbolic statement—or worse, a cheap vote by members of Congress and one that they used to get new weapons approved—the movement attempted to devise strategies that would escalate the costs for decisionmakers. One strategy was to introduce binding legislation, that is, legislation with the force of law. Concurrently, the movement also formed a freestanding PAC called "Freeze Voter '84," the purpose of which was "to create such a potent grassroots force that current incumbents and potential challengers at the national level dare not ignore the Freeze issue."[2]

The Freeze movement felt that it could mobilize a grass-roots organizing base that would compel candidates to adopt its position and lead to the election of a president who would implement the freeze. The 1984 presidential election was an important turning point for the campaign. Peace advocates suddenly felt renewed optimism; if we could replace Ronald Reagan with someone who was sympathetic to the Freeze, we would be one step closer to actually achieving a freeze. Thus evolved the slogan, "If You Can't Change the Politicians' Minds, Then Change the Politicians!" Such a strategy would require a coordinated effort, political consensus, and strategic agreement among the Freeze leadership.

But ousting Reagan would be no easy feat. Despite the fact that Reagan had been responsible for slashing social welfare programs, getting the largest military buildup in cold war history, and implementing policies that protected the rich and hurt the poor, he was a popular president. He was perceived as a strong leader; also, the economy was looking stronger, at least for the short term. Reagan's decision to return to the negotiating table and his announcement of the "Star Wars" space-based defense system as the solution to our nuclear weapons fears had somewhat defused the public concern.

The Freeze decision to form a separate electoral arm meant that the movement was now pursuing a dual strategy, with two separate organizations. The campaign would continue to work on legislation in Congress, and the PAC would work to elect candidates who supported the Freeze. This raised all sorts of structural and organizational problems, besides the obvious problem of pursuing a full legislative effort and doing grass-roots electoral work at the same time. Nonetheless, organizers were determined, and that determination seemed to provide national and local activists with an endless store of energy. The Freeze's move into elections was welcomed by all as a step toward gaining political power.

Freeze Voter '84

Freeze Voter '84 grew out of Project '84, an exploratory subcommittee of the strategy committee. After studying Federal Election

Commission (FEC) laws, Project '84 had proposed that the Freeze form a separate, freestanding PAC. Because Freeze Campaign, Inc. was a nonprofit organization, with a tax-exempt education fund, it had had another choice: to form a PAC as part of the Freeze campaign. This choice was not feasible, however, because solicitations could be made to members only. The Freeze had no membership in that formal sense. (Although in its early stages it could have developed one of the largest memberships of any peace organization.)

Freeze Voter '84 had its own offices, staff, board of directors, and local networks. Because it was separate from the Freeze, many individuals were called on to set aside work on the campaign's new and complicated legislative program. Local groups formed state PACs affiliated with Freeze Voter '84, with some individuals trying to keep up the pace demanded by pursuing both strategies. Legally, the two efforts had to be kept separate. Coordination and communication between the two campaigns was not allowed by FEC regulations.

Resources were scarce, and now competition for the same organizers and the same pool of donors added to the organizational complexity. The development of Freeze Voter '84—from the initial strategizing to making the PAC operational—followed many of the same patterns and encountered many of the same problems of the overall Freeze campaign. Freeze Voter '84 began with a grand strategy, a plan consistent with its goal of developing a long-term, grassroots base of supporters. It was envisioned that this base would continue to become more politically adept and would be able to hold politicians accountable to their promises. This would be only the first of many elections the movement would participate in as it sought to change policy over the long run. But as the plan was implemented at the national level, it suffered from the Democrats' use and misuse of the Freeze as a political weapon and from internal conflicts on its board of directors and with its national staff.

The Project '84 task force had created three working groups: delegate selection, voter registration, and targeting. The preliminary work of these groups included the distribution of a questionnaire to each group on the local organizers mailing list. The questionnaire was designed to determine the strength of the Freeze campaign by geographical area and by congressional district. It asked the groups if they had plans to reach out to less organized congressional districts and if they thought that a national organizer could facilitate their work. The questionnaire revealed significant enthusiasm among grass-roots organizers for working in the elections, particularly because this would represent a "get tough" approach for a frustrated network of determined activists.

There were two dimensions to the electoral strategy proposed by the original task force. One was to elect a president, senators, and representatives who were willing to "support and propose a Freeze in a meaningful and timely way." The second dimension was using the elections to build the movement: "Project '84 must be careful that, upon completion, it leaves a legacy of having assisted in overall campaign growth and avoided 'burning bridges.'"[3]

The national committee approved this electoral strategy and elected a board of directors for Freeze Voter '84. The board was mandated to be the major decisionmaker for the PAC. Its first meeting was in July 1983, with the agenda of hiring an executive director. The process was slow, but eventually Bill Curry was hired.

Curry had run unsuccessfully for Congress in 1982, after having served in the Connecticut state legislature. He was a brilliant speaker and adept at political maneuvering. But Curry was much better as a political candidate than as the head of Freeze Voter '84. While he shared the progressive political vision and beliefs of his colleagues in the Freeze, Curry was controversial among some of his staff and with members of the PAC's board. He was in particularly strong conflict with Randy Forsberg and Carla Johnston, both of whom called for his resignation during the last several months of Freeze Voter '84's campaigns. Members of the staff were split, with some actively seeking to have him replaced and others remaining loyal to him, even while acknowledging his administrative weaknesses.

The conflicts were substantive. Curry was committed to Mondale and was candid about that when he interviewed for the job. From that position, he was expected nonetheless to carry out a wide-ranging program: building an organization to accomplish the everyday tasks of getting out the vote, recruiting volunteers, setting up candidate forums, and so forth, while also strengthening and flexing the movement's political muscle. Such a tall order required a great deal of flexibility from an executive director.

The Search for a Candidate

Freeze Voter '84 was in search of a presidential candidate. The Freeze commanded serious attention from most politicians, who knew that the movement represented volunteers and also that it was important to be "good" on the freeze idea. As the nine Democratic presidential hopefuls climbed on board, they each sought to distinguish themselves on the issue. All except Askew had officially endorsed the Freeze by February 1984.

But while the Democrats intended to use the peace issue to build their campaigns, most of them had no real intention of challenging national security policies. The fundamental disagreement between the Democrats and the Republicans was not over whether to stop and reverse the arms race, but rather over which weapons should be "modernized." Like their predecessors, they were willing to manage the arms race, but not to end it. One needed only to scratch beneath the surface of both Mondale and Hart's positions to see that their arms control objectives were quite different from the movement's. While Senator Hollings claimed to support a freeze, he also supported force modernization, the Jackson-Warner amendment, and the Nunn-Cohen build-down resolution. Senator John Glenn backed both the freeze legislation and the Jackson-Warner amendment. And even California's Senator Alan Cranston—whose record on nuclear policy was excellent—supported the B-1 bomber, probably because it was built in his state. Everyone claimed to support a freeze (or at least their interpretation of it), but by the winter of 1984 it was an easy issue to support. The Freeze had been reduced to a symbolic expression of public sentiment, no longer a political force behind a serious policy proposal.

The Freeze needed to highlight the differences between the candidates' positions and the Freeze's agenda. In an attempt to test the depth of each candidate's commitment to the Freeze, a questionnaire was sent to each of them. The questionnaire outlined the Freeze's immediate goals; it asked technical questions about the candidates' views on modernization of weapons and solicited their opinions on the so-called quick freeze (discussed later in this chapter) and what it should include. The questionnaire cover letter spelled out what the Freeze was seeking in a presidential candidate:

The way to draw a positive profile of difference from Reagan and tap the wellsprings of popular American support for the freeze is to announce, *clearly and unequivocally*, that the new Democratic administration will make a good faith effort to reach a verifiable, bilateral halt in the production of all types of nuclear weapons. In other words, the new administration will seek effective new means of verification; will institute the broadest possible bilateral moratorium on verifiable items at the outset of negotiations; and will seek a bilateral freeze that covers not only the first-strike MX, but also the first-strike Trident II and Pershing II, any exorbitantly expensive, unnecessary, and more threatening new bomber, unnecessary, destabilizing new cruise missiles, and improvements in tactical nuclear weapons that make them better suited for nuclear warfighting—and their Soviet counterparts. This is the sort of "new leadership" that the public seeks.[4]

But the questionnaire failed to address the deeper political questions of foreign policy. It did not ask candidates to state their positions on issues such as intervention, conventional arms, the role of nuclear weapons, foreign arms trade, or the conflict in the Middle East and the appropriate U.S. response to it. Candidates were not queried about the diplomatic initiatives they would take for dealing with cold war tensions and, ultimately, breaking through cold war structures. In other words, candidates did not have to define the foreign policy that these weapons were intended to implement.

Some Freeze Voter '84 board members expressed concern at the outset about whether such a litmus test could really determine hard support for a freeze. Should voting records on related issues or the candidates' public positions be measures of their commitment? Should the specificity of their plan for implementation of a freeze be the indicator? Or should the movement take the word of Mondale and Hart supporters with access to high-level campaign staff in measuring the support of those candidates? The political consensus among PAC activists about how to rate political candidates' commitment to the Freeze as both a policy and a movement soon dissolved. Most politicians had covered themselves by voting for the nonbinding legislation and could use the charge of unilateralism to defend their votes for individual weapons systems. The movement's political test did not pin down anyone.

The Freeze also tried to meet with all of the candidates. Mondale and Cranston were the most receptive. In January 1984, the Freeze joined with other groups—including AFSC, SANE, Physicians for Social Responsibility, and the Coalition for a New Foreign and Military Policy—to meet with Walter Mondale and question him on the arms race, the Freeze, certain weapons systems, foreign and military policy, and defense spending levels. A similar group eventually met with Senator Hart and had a discussion much shorter and less detailed than the one with Mondale.

Mondale was well prepared and thorough in his understanding of the issues:

Mondale showed the gifts of a longtime campaigner but they did not ring false in what he clearly regarded as a sympathetic but somewhat skeptical group. He also showed that he knows the details of arms race/arms control matters—dates, votes, performance characteristics, treaty provisions, arguments and counter-arguments, articles by arms control leaders, and daily developments. . . .

More important, Mondale made somewhat more specific commitments on a range of negotiation and arms control points than we had generally expected. He emerged with a credible stance for restraint, sound judgment, and a serious quest for peaceful alternatives to the Reagan arms build-up and Cold War tensions.

. . . The most important issue in the election, he said, was to bring to the Presidency "new policies for a safer world."

Mondale spoke well about his intentions to change the whole context and tone of U.S./Soviet relations and to build up a sustained dialogue with the Soviet leaders. He regretted that press coverage of the campaign tends to filter out complex issues of this dimension and importance, insisting that he spoke every day about the dangers of the arms race and the need to talk with the Soviets rather than bully them.[5]

Neither Mondale nor Hart, the two front-runners, stood out. John Isaacs of the Council for a Livable World thought either candidate would be acceptable. Others knew that Hart had changed his position on the Freeze for political purposes and that he had used the movement particularly well in New Hampshire. Still, even they believed that Hart had a better chance of beating Reagan than Mondale did, and a camp favoring Hart developed within the movement. Some of those with contacts inside the Mondale campaign argued that Mondale was genuinely committed to the Freeze and that his record demonstrated he would be a better candidate for the Freeze. Some had notions that they might find jobs in a Mondale administration; others testified to his sincerity on the Freeze and other progressive issues. The Mondale camp developed.

In the preprimary days the two front-runners were trying to outdo each other on their peace positions. In mid-March, Hart placed an ad in the *New York Times*, promising that, if elected, he would initiate a test ban: "On my first day in office I will call for a six-month suspension on testing of all nuclear weapons as the first step toward negotiating a comprehensive test ban treaty."[6] That same week, Mondale had already promised the same thing: "I would initiate a six-month moratorium on underground nuclear testing and challenge the Soviets to respond in kind."[7]

The debate on arms control became more acrimonious. When Hart claimed that he had supported the Freeze since it was first introduced in March 1982, Mondale pointed out that this was simply false. During a March debate, Mondale also criticized Hart for supporting build-down in its early days. "Without mentioning his original sponsorship of the build down plan, [Hart] said he voted against it when it came to a vote in the Senate."[8] Unfortunately, as the debate heated up it also became less meaningful. The candidates focused on when the other did or did not support a particular system, but they did not delve into the underlying issue of how national security policy should change.

It was true that Hart had not supported a freeze and had supported build-down in the early stages of each proposal. When the Freeze resolution was first introduced in the House in March 1982, Hart claimed to "sympathize with those who argue 'enough is enough.'" He agreed that "the logic of a freeze is compelling in its simplicity." He would not, however, endorse a freeze at that time, although he ended up voting for it in October 1983. But in 1982 he argued that it did not go far enough: "A bilateral agreement to halt the testing, production and deployment of nuclear weapons would not, in and of itself, significantly reduce the likelihood of nuclear war." "Mr. President, I am today submitting a resolution expressing the sense of the Senate that the Government of the United States initiate, without delay, negotiations with the Soviet Union to prevent the use of nuclear weapons."

Hart's STOP (Strategic Talks on Prevention) resolution was his main response to the Freeze between 1982 and 1984. There were many problems with STOP and with its focus on preventing the *use* of nuclear weapons. First, the resolution threw the problem back to the president and the negotiating table, which guaranteed that nothing would happen. Second, STOP did not deal with the spiraling arms race, which would continue to increase the chances of war and drain the national budget. Hart's STOP proposal was another form of cooptation. Masquerading as a proposal that would prevent nuclear war, its objectives would do very little toward that end, particularly if the resolution was dependent on Reagan for implementation.

Hart joined the chorus of those who said, "Yes, we must stop nuclear war!," and then introduced plans that, for the most part, maintained the status quo or allowed further developments in the arms race.

Hart did make a proposal in the early 1980s to freeze plutonium production, which was one of his most practical and serious arms control proposals. It would have been a major contribution if he had committed serious staff time to it and made it a priority in his work on the Senate Armed Services Committee.

He also remained supportive of the Midwest protest against the MX missile. His initial arguments against the MX—and, in particular, against Reagan's 1982 dense-pack basing proposal—centered around the missile's infeasibility. He pointed out that the MX offered no long-term solution to the problem of intercontinental ballistic missile (ICBM) vulnerability and was excessively costly. The various basing modes proposed by the Air Force came under increasing ridicule by the public and press. By July 1983, Hart was taking an even stronger stand against the MX, arguing that it was an outgrowth of nuclear war fighting policy and should be opposed

> because it is designed not to deter a nuclear war, but to fight and win one. . . . Our national security depends as much upon our diplomatic successes as upon our military strength. Our security increases with our competitiveness in international markets and declines with our increased reliance on raw materials from unstable countries. National security is the aggregation of how secure each of us feels, and, more importantly, the manner in which each of us is secure. . . . Do not make this decision; do not build this missile.

Although Hart was initially reluctant on the Freeze but not on build-down, his faithfulness on the MX issue and his legislative proposal to freeze plutonium production made him an attractive candidate to some in the peace community. Still, the Freeze would need to put pressure on him.

The candidates who were most solid on the Freeze's positions, however, were Alan Cranston, Jesse Jackson, and George McGovern. Some in the movement supported Senator Cranston as the best Freeze candidate. But Cranston's candidacy was short-lived. Though he had been a senator for twenty-five years, his name recognition was less than Hart's or Mondale's or Jackson's. By the end of the Super Tuesday primaries and caucuses, Cranston was faring poorly. He withdrew his candidacy.

But Cranston remained committed to the Freeze after he was no longer a presidential candidate by continuing to work on the peace platform. He met several times with a committee of peace representatives throughout 1983 and 1984 and eventually put together a "peace plank" that was debated and voted on at the Democratic National Convention in July 1984. The peace plank thoroughly addressed the issues. It called for both serious weapons reductions and longer term goals, which included working "to end big-power military intervention in Third World countries" and promoting "the peaceful resolution of civil wars and other conflicts by mediation and diplomacy, and [reducing] the international arms trade."[9]

Both Jackson and McGovern were solidly pro-Freeze; both brought support from other constituencies, including progressive movements. But McGovern was in the race to raise the issues; he was not considered a serious candidate. Some gravitated toward the Rainbow Coalition and the Reverend Jesse Jackson's campaign, arguing that this was the best political foothold for the Freeze in 1984. Additionally, Jackson was at least a real player at the Democratic convention.

But Jackson's strategy seemed to be one of pushing a progressive political platform rather than building a campaign structure capable of organizing state by state. Although the Rainbow Coalition was more than a rhetorical device, it was not able to become as politically sophisticated as Mondale and Hart's campaigns. However, his political stance on foreign and military policy issues made it obvious to everyone that he was providing real vision and leadership. Jesse Jackson's anti-Semitic remarks and unwillingness to disassociate himself from Louis Farrakhan made it hard for many Freeze leaders to support his candidacy.

In the final analysis, the Freeze did not have a Freeze candidate; it was unprepared politically and as an organization to choose just one and throw its weight behind that person in any meaningful way. This inability to choose a candidate became the functional expression of its structural problems vis-à-vis decisionmaking. Further, it revealed the movement's lack of standing in real world power politics, that is, its inability to assert control over the political debate and its confusion about how to get a freeze. Just as reading the cloakroom politics on the Hill had been difficult, it was equally tricky for the movement to make its mark in the highly stylized and personalized process of presidential politics.

Freeze Voter '84 had agreed from the start that it would not endorse a candidate until after the national conventions, reasoning that it was important to get all the candidates from both parties to move as far as possible on peace issues *before* endorsing one of them. But given who the Republican candidate was, it should have been clear that this strategy would leave the Freeze disempowered. In spite of Freeze Voter '84's delay strategy, individuals were jumping on certain candidates' bandwagons, as were different state Freeze groups, making this strategy even more vacuous. Its circularity also became apparent as support for the Freeze became common currency—and subsequently, devalued currency.

The Freeze movement, presidential hopefuls soon learned, could not deliver in any coordinated way. The fact that Freeze Voter '84's top staff person was committed to Mondale sent informal signals that undercut whatever formal strategy the PAC might have had. The commitment of various board members to Hart did likewise. Meanwhile, it became apparent to all that the Freeze as a movement would never be able to endorse a candidate. Unclear standards, personal preferences, and private promises and ambitions—mixed with the reluctance of local groups to endorse one candidate—turned the Freeze "endorsement" into a free-for-all. A national movement was up for grabs, and the national staff and board of Freeze Voter '84 had little to offer that a presidential campaign could not go out and get on its own. The candidates knew that the way to get the peace constituency was to go after it state by state and, in effect, ignore the national movement leaders. The peace movement representatives believed to be capable of "delivering" the peace constituency were the ones who gained "access" to candidates or their top advisors. A candidate would use the national freeze leaders who endorsed him to convince state peace groups to work for his presidential campaign. While Freeze Voter '84 was able to master the technical skills of electoral work, it could not develop a political sophistication to influence presidential politics in a meaningful way. The record in the Senate and congressional races (discussed later in this chapter) was a different story.

Binding Legislation

The campaign's decision at the December 1983 fourth national conference to go for binding legislation was controversial and revealed once again the weakness in some parts of the campaign structure. One constituency had pushed as early as February 1983 for binding legislation on cruise and Pershing II missiles as well as on a comprehensive freeze. Randy Kehler's annual national coordinator's message, delivered in December, reflected the growing consensus for escalating the demands on Congress—a consensus, however, that may have finally come a year too late.

> First, for a piece of legislation to be voted on by Congress, the Resolution places too much emphasis on action by the President. . . . Second, the Freeze Resolution is not connected to the all-important budget-authorization-appropriations process by which nuclear weapons continue to be funded. . . . Third, a strategy which talks only about immediate negotiations, rather than an immediate freeze, is not likely to capture the imagination and enthusiasm of large numbers of people—nor will it address the increasing risks of nuclear holocaust as a result of this new round of weaponry. . . . For all these reasons, we are rapidly moving toward a revised national strategy which emphasizes congressional rather than presidential initiative, the funding process rather than legislative resolutions, and an immediate halt or moratorium at the beginning of the Freeze negotiating process rather than at the end of it.

This freeze concept, it was hoped, had legislative "teeth."

But before the new proposal made it to the Freeze conference floor, several disagreements emerged within the Freeze leadership. The Freeze had met resistance in the arms control community on the issue of verifying a freeze on production. While most people within the Freeze believed that it was possible to verify a production freeze, many were afraid that it would be hard to get congressional support for binding legislation that included it. They were anxious to achieve a victory; others felt that not to include a freeze on production subverted the overall freeze idea and was also a capitulation to mythologies within the arms control community. Those with weapons facilities and radioactive contamination threatening their communities had particularly strong feelings about the exclusion of a freeze on production.

This indirect pressure from the arms control community led to the development of several proposals, which covered the spectrum of views. When the fourth national conference convened, three options were presented for debate, out of which a national policy objective was to be developed by the end of the weekend.

After hours of small group discussions, the strategy synthesis group narrowed the field to two options, to be voted on at the plenary session. The first option became known as the "quick freeze":

> The Campaign will press Congress to enact parts of a comprehensive freeze, such as suspending funds for the testing of nuclear warheads and for the test-

ing and deployment of ballistic missiles, provided the Soviet Union halts the same activities. It is widely recognized that these activities are currently being monitored by both countries with confidence.

The second option was to work for the quick freeze, as defined above, but to also

press Congress to suspend all funds for all testing, *production* and deployment of nuclear warheads *and their delivery systems*, provided that the Soviet Union halts the same activities. *This Congressionally-legislated comprehensive freeze shall be verified by national technical means.* (Emphasis added)

The first option passed. The Freeze movement was chopping its own proposal up into even smaller pieces at a time when it was also proposing the primary political strategy of entering the 1984 elections.

The process of debating and subsequently implementing the new legislative proposal raised three significant issues: 1) the Freeze movement's readiness to allow the politicians to control the political agenda, 2) the Freeze's inefficient and untimely strategy-making process, and 3) the Freeze's inability to resolve its internal controversies quickly and positively.

PROBLEMS OF NATIONAL COORDINATION

There was nothing new about the agenda-setting issue. The Freeze still could not figure out its own long-term agenda—distracted this time by concerns over 1984 electoral strategy—and was still being trapped in the arms control box.

In addition, the Freeze's procedures for making national strategy remained, as often as not, untimely and inefficient. Two months after the legislative strategy decision was made by the national conference, the national committee was still wrestling with it. Putting the responsibility for fine-tuning strategy details onto the national conference contributed to this problem. Many people also felt it was unrealistic for the conference to decide national strategy in the three days allotted to it, particularly when strategy-making needed to be flexible and responsive to changing political circumstances. The entire process of finalizing national strategy actually took several months.

All conference attendees were sent the strategy draft papers in advance. They would then send their suggestions to the strategy committee. As time went on, however, this process became unwieldy. The strategy committee had decided that it could not circulate all of the proposals. There were too many. The campaign committees sifted through all the strategy ideas and then made strategy proposals out of them, which were circulated to conference attendees. Each committee would mention the proposals it had considered in its final strategy paper. Based on all the proposals, the conference would then decide the overall strategy. But the national and executive committees were left to figure out the details of implementation—although the Clearinghouse staff would actually end up figuring out most of them.

The structure task force recommended to the December 1984 fifth national conference that certain steps be taken to alleviate this structural problem: that the Freeze become a membership organization; that state and local Freeze organizations develop democratic decisionmaking in order to elect their representatives to the national committee; that the national committee become the equivalent of a board of directors for the Freeze; that the national conference continue to be held only yearly, with its emphasis on movement building and education. The underlying assumption in this proposal was that, by regularizing state and local groups and building a membership organization, more people could participate in decisionmaking at the local level than was possible at the national conference. Yet the "board of directors"—elected by and therefore representative of the grass roots—would be small enough to make decisions efficiently. That was the strength of this recommendation—which was missed by most voting delegates because it was not fully explained.

The recommendation was rejected. A smaller board, even if widely and democratically elected, was viewed as a move toward centralization rather than toward streamlining and broadening participation. Delegates favored a national conference where the 800 or so participants would continue to make the final decisions for the campaign. The delegates agreed to explore the idea of making the Freeze a membership organization, but only a few other changes were made. The strategy committee was abolished; the executive committee was empowered to form subcommittees to deal with short-term and long-range planning; and it was agreed to keep the decisionmaking structure the same.

It was impossible for the executive committee to communicate the substance and theory behind the task force's proposal to a gathering of 700–800 people. To complicate that task even further, the committee was given some ten minutes to outline its thinking, and a representative of an opposing caucus was given equal time to argue against the recommendations. These proposals had grown out of a long and expensive committee process.

In 1984 the executive committee had scheduled a retreat and performance evaluations. A structural analysis was done at the retreat, and an ad hoc structure committee was subsequently formed to evaluate the structural problems and make recommendations. Helena Knapp, who chaired this committee, pointed out in a subsequent memo that people tended to blame the structure rather than take personal responsibility.

> By mixing the structural and personal evaluation and analysis we have failed to do either of them well. Even if there are structural obstacles to doing the best possible job it is still possible to do a straightforward performance analysis of the quality of work done under the present imperfect conditions. We did not do that, preferring to blame on structural flaws some of our performance weaknesses.

As part of its evaluation, the ad hoc structure committee hired Burke Leahy Associates and Susan Gross to evaluate the Freeze's structure. In a 24 October 1984 letter to Helena Knapp, Dan Leahy summarized the Freeze structure and how it led to problems of competition:

> The structure of the national Nuclear Weapons Freeze Campaign is characterized by a multiplicity of national participatory groupings (i.e. executive, national, strategy & ad hoc committees) and forums (i.e. task forces, conventions) which have no clear lines of authority over organizational decision-making and resources nor any clear lines of formal interrelationships.
>
> This arrangement while involving diverse individuals will act to inhibit any clear *organizational* direction. More importantly, it will obscure any easy understanding of HOW decisions are arrived at. *Thus those individuals who know the informal power relationships can exercise inordinate control within the participatory groupings.* (Emphasis added)

Leahy suggested that the Freeze implement better grass-roots control by: writing a clear description of the formal national structure, as legally defined in the bylaws; clearly defining Freeze membership; and organizing national office that promotes local groups and their interrelations instead of keeping local groups focused on national institutions (Congress, the presidency, or the media).

The vacuum in leadership was never more keenly felt than during this period of reassessing the structure of the campaign. No clear directions were offered because the national leadership was split. The campaign's policy of "national coordination with local self-determination" was laudable, in principle, but in practice several problems arose. Whenever individuals or groups of individuals wanted to do something differently, or break away from decisions they disagreed with, they frequently invoked this principle. The national strategy's cohesion was dependent on local participation. Whenever the principle of "local self-determination" was invoked, cooperation threatened to unravel. A spirit of fierce individualism overruled national coordination.

A prime example of this problem was the 1983 debate about pursuing a quick freeze versus a comprehensive freeze, a debate that went on into 1984. A major reason for the decision continuing to be questioned was the Massachusetts contingency's dissatisfaction with it. Several Massachusetts organizers felt that not including a freeze on production would be giving in to the myth that production is not verifiable.

So throughout January and February of 1984, these organizers contacted their congressional district representatives to declare mutiny on the national strategy. "Quick freeze" and "comprehensive freeze" camps staked out their territory in Massachusetts. Statewide meetings were held to persuade Massachusetts Freeze supporters that they should go ahead and advocate comprehensive legislation, despite the national strategy decision to do otherwise. Meanwhile, national organizers were nervous. They knew a divided campaign would be a disaster.

In February 1984, George Sommaripa, a leader in the Massachusetts Freeze movement, asked the national committee to pass a resolution encouraging Massachusetts to pursue with its congressional representation the possibility of a congressional suspension of funds on the testing, production, and deployment of all nuclear weapons, as long as the Soviet Union reciprocated. This resolution was tabled. Then Jan Orr-Harter, a national committee member and leader in the Presbyterian church, introduced a resolution that praised Massachusetts for its hard work but encouraged the state's organizers not to pursue a legislative program different from the national strategy.

This resolution was also tabled. Finally, the national committee reaffirmed local self-determination with national coordination; it also reaffirmed the original December 1983 conference decision to press Congress to enact *parts* of a comprehensive freeze via funding cutoffs. Once again, these two competing views were not resolved.

The policy of local self-determination with national coordination reached a breaking point. Massachusetts persisted in its advocacy of comprehensive legislation. The tragedy was not just that Massachusetts pursued a different organizing strategy, but that its organizers attempted to change the national conference strategy by raising its local organizing to the level of national legislation. This was accomplished by getting Massachusetts Congressman Nicholas Mavroules to introduce comprehensive freeze legislation soon after the Freeze campaign had quick freeze legislation (the Kennedy-Markey Arms Race Moratorium Act) introduced.

The campaign became seriously divided. Massachusetts represented a strong base of local support. New ideas had frequently been tested in that state; in fact, the first freeze referenda were held in western Massachusetts. From the start, one of its representatives, Edward Markey, and one of its senators, Edward Kennedy, were key congressional leaders for freeze legislation. In addition, *all* of the Massachusetts congressional delegation supported the Freeze. So when Massachusetts defected from the national Freeze's agenda, the strategy controversy and the movement's leadership conflict intensified.

A considerable amount of national staff time was spent trying to resolve this internal struggle. That time could have been spent on building public support or lobbying Congress. Instead, those activities slowed down. The issue was rehashed over the phone lines between the national office and the Massachusetts offices. National leaders Randy Kehler and Randy Forsberg were called to several Massachusetts meetings held to present the various sides of the argument. The national committee discussed the problem at both its February and June 1984 meetings.

This controversy weakened and confused the Freeze's relationship with Congress. Congressional Freeze supporters were pushed and pulled by the campaign; now the congressional *advocates* were being lobbied by the various factions of the campaign! It was a heyday for congressional adversaries of the Freeze and for those sitting on the fence. They could just sit back and watch the infighting.

The Freeze movement already had its work cut out in getting congressional support for the new quick freeze legislation. The political stakes were high enough in passing binding legislation. It was the Freeze movement's job to put pressure on House members so that the political stakes would be even higher if they did *not* endorse the legislation. But without local unity around this one specific demand, these efforts were doomed to fail as congressional supporters and other political elites could not help noticing the lack of unity in the movement about its definition of a freeze and about what it could or could not achieve.

By the end of the summer, the two pieces of freeze legislation floating around Congress—the Kennedy-Markey quick freeze bill and the Mavroules comprehensive freeze legislation—were destined to go nowhere in 1984. Congressional advocates continued to seek their colleagues' support, but less than enthusiastically. Congressman Markey recruited about 100 cosponsors, but Kennedy mustered up only six in the Senate. Even though both did not expect the quick freeze legislation to succeed, Senator Kennedy made another effort to get the freeze passed in fall 1984, by adding an amendment— identical to the nonbinding Kennedy-Hatfield freeze resolution of 1982—to the Debt Limit Increase Bill. But Senator Howard Baker made a motion to table the amendment, which passed by a 55–42 vote.

FREEZE CONTRIBUTIONS TO 1984 DEMOCRATIC GAINS AND LOSSES

Mondale did take the Democratic nomination—an event that had been predicted from early on in the race. But Reagan was charismatic, with a tough image, against which it was difficult for Mondale to compete. This left the peace movement in a predicament again. The joke emerged, "Vote for Mondale; at least you'll live to regret it." But it is rather difficult to motivate people to work for a candidate who does not inspire them. Recalls Karen Mulhauser, who took a leave of absence from Citizens Against Nuclear War to work for Mondale,

> When I tried to get local activists to attend Mondale rallies with freeze signs, I inevitably had to spend several hours trying to convince them that there was a real difference between Mondale and Reagan. They often said they'd vote for Mondale but they couldn't "stomach" working for him.[10]

If Mondale could not beat Reagan, maybe Reagan could beat Reagan, by mobilizing those most opposed to him. The Democrats, other progressive groups, and the Freeze tried to build on an emerging demographic force that had the potential to defeat Reagan: the "gender gap." The Democrats were taking the gender gap seriously when Mondale chose Representative Geraldine Ferraro to be his running mate. The documented "feminization of poverty" had been exacerbated by Reagan's economic policies from the time he first took office. The effects of budget changes—including a $1.2 billion cut in AFDC funding and food stamp benefits cut by $757 million— were driving women to the voting booths. And polls showed that the gender gap was widening. A 1983 *New York Times*/CBS poll revealed that, while 46 percent of men approved Reagan's economic program, only 36 percent of women approved it. A February 1983 Gallup poll asked if the Reagan administration helped or hurt "people like yourself" and found that 60 percent of the women surveyed thought it hurt, while only 50 percent of the men thought so.[11]

At the end of 1983, a *New York Times* poll found 38 percent of women thinking that Reagan should be reelected compared to 53 percent of men so inclined.[12] Nevertheless, Freeze Voter '84 was aware that women had differing views on peace issues:

> What does emerge [from the polls] is that women are (and have traditionally been) more concerned with and opposed to war in general, but there is considerable slippage in that support when arguments focus on technical aspects of weapons systems, and discussion of solutions to the problem of defense spending, relations with the Soviet Union, or nuclear arms.[13]

To tap the political potential in the gender gap, Project '84, the original task force, had recommended that "women be targeted as a group in order to transform their generalized negativism about war into clear and consistent support for the Freeze and Freeze-related issues. We think that women are just beginning to realize their potential as political actors in society."[14]

Unfortunately, targeting women was never made a priority by Freeze Voter '84 in spite of this early recommendation. But some other groups did organize women for the 1984 elections; for example, the Women's Action for Nuclear Disarmament formed a PAC, and Eleanor Smeal and some of us from the peace and women's movements formed the Gender Gap Action Campaign. But the Democratic party did not devote enough of its resources toward getting women's votes, Geraldine Ferraro's nomination to the Mondale ticket notwithstanding. Meanwhile, White House pollsters and Reagan campaign operatives eroded the gender gap on war and peace issues simply by portraying the president as committed to arms control and negotiation with the Soviets, even as they grappled with the latest foreign policy albatross: the death of 241 Marines in Lebanon.

After the fall 1984 Beirut explosion, Democrats called for the withdrawal of Marines, striking a chord in public opinion. The White House responded by, once again, going on the offense rather than lingering in a defensive position. Since, by this time, reiterating the Soviet Union "evil empire" threat had lost its effectiveness, the White House struck up a new rallying cry—terrorism.

The bombing of the Marine barracks was a terrifying incident, and the Marine deaths were a great loss to many American families. This tragedy was the result of misguided actions by the Reagan administration. By transforming the attack on Marines in a war zone into a terrorist activity, at a time when attacks on innocent civilians were on the rise everywhere, the administration was overdramatizing the external threat to Americans in order to dilute the public opinion opposed to its Middle East policies. Blurring the line between civilian and military "targets," the administration was able to turn a military loss and foreign policy disaster into a renewed American determination to fight terrorism.

In a speech at the Center for Strategic and International Studies at Georgetown University, Reagan said, "Military force, either direct or indirect, must remain an available part of America's foreign policy. . . . We will not return to the days of handwringing, defeatism, decline and despair." George Schultz, speaking to the Trilateral Commission, struck a similar theme: A foreign policy worthy of America must not be a policy of isolationism or guilt, but a commitment to active engagement. . . . [The United States] has no choice but to confront state supported terrorism, with preventive and pre-emptive action."

To be against the presence of Marines in war zones—even in situations where they were sitting ducks—was to be "for" terrorism. The ideology of counterterrorism was born. It functions much the same way as the "cognitive regime of the Cold War,"[15] disciplining thought and action even though it is full of logical and factual errors. Reagan had gained the political initiative once again.

Reagan and Schultz were highly critical of Congress by this time, both for its stand on the events in Lebanon and for reminding the administration of the 1973 War Powers Act, which prohibited prolonged U.S. military intervention overseas without congressional approval. National Security Adviser Robert McFarlane suggested publicly that Congress should keep its criticisms to itself once the president had committed U.S. troops: "To call for a change in the policy [once troops are committed], can place Americans at greater risk."

Democratic response was sharp. House Speaker Tip O'Neill said, "The deaths lie on him, and the defeat lies on him and him alone. . . . He is looking for a scapegoat." Senator Alan Cranston added, "To suggest that we should not debate policy is to suggest a dictatorship." But *Newsweek* noted that "beyond rhetorical thunder . . . Democrats on Capitol Hill seemed to have little in mind—and on the campaign trail . . . an eerie silence prevailed."[16] But even if the president skillfully kept arms issues on the sideline—aided and abetted by the level of debate among Democratic candidates—suddenly he was hit broadside by a new round of public pressure.

The Freeze movement was having its effect on members of Congress, particularly on those facing reelection. Freeze Voter '84 was active in eight Senate races and thirty-seven House races. Republicans and Democrats alike felt compelled to put pressure on the president to break out of the stalemate with Moscow. Senators Charles Percy of Illinois and Howard Baker of Tennessee appealed directly to the president to initiate regular Soviet-American summit meetings. On 13 June, Representative Les Aspin told an American Stock Exchange conference, "This is arms control year. Everybody is for arms control. We have more arms control amendments on this bill than defense amendments." President Reagan responded to these pressures with an offer to "meet any time" with the Soviets.

Even though the president could not ignore their pressure, the Democrats were hampered by the lack of a coherent policy alternative to Reagan's new cold war rhetoric. As Jay Wink, the executive director of the Coalition for a Democratic Majority, noted, "If the Democrats embrace the freeze as policy, they will give the impression of playing fast and loose with national security and may jeopardize gains they have made over the Republicans in responding to public fear about the nuclear threat."[17]

The Reagan-Bush campaign went on the offensive in August when Bush attacked Mondale for being "so hot for an agreement right now that he will do almost anything to get it. We are not." Bush added that the president was nevertheless committed to major reductions in strategic weapons, intermediate-range weapons, and chemical weapons.

That same month, President Reagan tested his radio microphone by saying, "The bombing begins in five minutes."

Throughout September 1984, Mondale continued to emphasize arms control and foreign policy, and on 16 September he announced that he and Soviet Foreign Minister Gromyko would meet soon. At this meeting, Mondale would, among other things, "fix the spotlight on the issue of arms control." Mondale's staff still believed that Reagan was most vulnerable on arms control, and, in fact, the Democrats and the movement had finally made their point: the American people wanted talks with the Soviets and a genuine commitment to stop the nuclear threat. But the attempts of Mondale and others to make President Reagan's policies and words stick to him did not work. By mid-September, a *New York Times*/CBS poll showed that portrayals of Reagan as a dangerous warmonger were not convincing to the public: "Six Americans in ten agree with a principal theme of the Mondale campaign: that the United States should try harder to negotiate an arms agreement with the Soviet Union. But that same proportion, 60 percent, also believe that Mr. Reagan will make such an effort if he is re-elected."[18]

Within the Reagan administration, George Schultz, James Baker, and Robert McFarlane had overcome the arguments of Caspar Weinberger, Richard Perle, and Fred Iklé and persuaded the president to meet with Gromyko to propose a new forum for breaking out of the deadlock. Reagan did meet with Gromyko in early October, advancing what his aides called the RESTART proposal for new and broader negotiations. *Newsweek* suggested that, besides pressure from NATO, Reagan's decision to pursue negotiations may have been attributable to pressure from Congress, from which he was trying to obtain SDI and MX funding.[19]

In the last presidential candidates' debate, Mondale raised the issue of arms control and foreign policy. Two weeks after Reagan's landslide victory, a postelection poll revealed that "[Reagan] got even higher marks on the issue over which Mr. Mondale attacked him the hardest in the campaign, arms control. Two-thirds of the public and nine-tenths of his own voters said yes when asked 'do you think Ronald Reagan will make a real effort to negotiate a good arms control agreement with the Soviet Union?'"[20] Amazingly enough, 40 percent of Mondale supporters agreed with this prediction for Reagan's second term.

Lessons for the Future

If one looks at just the numbers, Freeze Voter '84 was a smashing success. In just over one year's time, its national office raised almost $1.5 million for the 1984 elections.[21] This figure is impressive when you compare the figures to the other "peace PACs":[22]

Council for a Livable World	$1,166,557
Peace PAC	67,791
Freeze Voter '84 (National)	1,490,549
Freeze Voter '84 (State PACs)	2,250,000 (estimated)
SANE PAC	251,452
WAND PAC	34,926
(Friends of the Earth) PAC	168,722

The Freeze Voter '84 fund-raising success is also remarkable because it was a newly formed PAC; only one other new PAC—working on social security issues—raised more than Freeze Voter '84 did in its first year. The success of the state PACs was particularly noteworthy.

But the important question is, Did the successful fund-raising efforts of Freeze Voter '84 reflect a growth in the Freeze campaign's political power? The Freeze, SANE's PAC, and others worked from an arms control record they had developed to determine who would be targeted for support or defeat in the 1984 races. Out of the eight Senate races that Freeze Voter '84 was involved in, four Freeze-supported candidates won. Of the thirty-seven House candidates it supported, twenty-four won. Both the Freeze Voter '84 staff and the politicians they had supported felt that the PAC had made a difference in the congressional and senatorial races.

But the movement's loss in Presidential politics must be seriously assessed. The critical lesson seems to be that the movement should not set out to influence a presidential election unless it is ready to endorse a candidate based on a specific and politically potent agenda, one to which it can hold that candidate publicly accountable. The movement's clarity about its goals and its ability to keep its agenda before the public and in the media should be indicators, for 1988 and beyond, of whether it has the basic strength to take on presidential politics. If clarity and visibility do not exist, the movement will do itself more harm than good. Others could once again define its messages, and internal conflicts over differing or unclear standards for measuring candidates could be as divisive as ever. Candidates could peal off one group after another until the movement finds itself experiencing the déjà vu of being split among a field of candidates, none of whom view the movement as a serious political force to be dealt with after election day. The movement must have real political power with which to demand political accountability for security in the nuclear age. Unless and until it has that power, it is best for it to aim at influencing the security debate locally, but to not claim a decisive influence on presidential politics before it has a realistic chance of that being a *positive* influence.

The Freeze can begin building on both its successes and its failures as it looks toward 1988 and 1992. More Freeze activists have entered electoral politics and have gained skills and political sophistication. If the movement can fuse a clear political agenda with independence from political parties—and assert its own voice through the media— then its hard-won technical skills in electoral politics might change the politicians and—finally—the security policies themselves.

7 THE HOPE IS IN THE ACTION

While the national campaign seemed unable to make the task of ironing out a long-range political strategy an organizational priority, the need for such a plan became more urgent at the local level.

1984 ELECTION AFTERMATH

The Detroit Freeze group presented a proposal to the 7–9 December 1984 Fifth National Nuclear Weapons Freeze Conference, "Campaign for Mutual Security: A Plan to Implement Our 'Longer-Range' Vision." The proposal reflected an understanding of the deeper problems of foreign policy that the Freeze needed to challenge. This local group also understood that the Freeze campaign was failing, partly because it lacked such a vision.

> The 1984 political campaigns showed how the freeze can suffer by being tacked on to a political outlook still based in the cold war. The arguments we make for the freeze have implications for foreign policy incompatible with the approaches of recent Republican *and* Democratic administrations alike. It's time we spelled this out, creating a general outlook for America in the world, with the freeze proposal as a centerpiece and model.

The draft strategy paper developed for the fifth national conference had called "for adoption of a set of long-range objectives for the

Freeze campaign which would move us toward a foreign policy based on the common security of nations." Pointing out that the strategy paper lacked any means for implementing such a long-range vision, the Detroit Freeze plan set out some goals:

1. Develop a set of principles which expands on the analysis which created the freeze proposal. We believe these principles should be based on the idea that in the nuclear age, our national security rests on the mutual security of nations.

2. Reach consensus nationally within the Freeze on some specific changes in American foreign policy which put these principles into practice.

3. Create materials to integrate the Campaign for Mutual Security into the work of the Freeze Campaign.[1]

But the conference did not approve the Detroit plan. Instead, they sent the task of setting long-range goals back to committee; that is, the executive committee was instructed to create a special task force to work on the problem.

The 1985 national conference approved, once again, "adoption of a year-long process to begin developing a long-term vision for the Freeze Campaign," including educational forums with local groups throughout 1986. But "specific aspects of this long-term vision will not be decided until next year's national conference, after the campaign has discussed the vision."

The sixth national conference did at least endorse the principles of "common security," as a guideline for the development of a long-range vision.[2] But the seventh national conference (which made 1986–87 strategy) did not follow through by including common security principles in its discussions of a long-range vision. That conference did vote on one long-term objective: "Enactment of a bilateral, comprehensive Freeze as an essential verifiable step toward lessening the risk of nuclear war; the phased mutual reductions of nuclear weapons, beginning with U.S. and Soviet ballistic missiles." The larger purpose of this objective was stated as "an end to the Cold War, sharp mutual reductions in conventional forces, conversion to a peace economy, and establishment of common security among the nations of the world." But there was no method suggested for achieving this goal, although one of the resolutions passed did mandate that a task force of economic conversion experts be set up.

While the Freeze had taken a strong position in 1983 on U.S. and Soviet interventions—and could have incorporated anti-interventionist principles into its long-range vision—its failure to actually address that issue meaningfully drove many Freeze activists into the Central American peace movement. There they could try to make the global connections in their work for one region, albeit without national coordination or political coherence from a larger peace movement.

Again, the Freeze could agree only on the Freeze proposal—the near-term step. By now, however, the Freeze was facing financial as well as political troubles. Following the December 1984 conference, the decision was made to close the St. Louis office, partly for financial reasons, but also out of a desire to consolidate the national headquarters, which by then was in three places. The closing resulted in some staff turnover and in bitter feelings on all sides; it forecast the organizational disintegration of the Freeze.

Legislative Fallout

In January 1985, some thirty national peace groups signed a joint statement congratulating President Reagan on his reelection and urging him to make progress on arms control. The statement was released to the press, but had little coverage. The media no longer considered the disarmament movement (now calling itself the "arms control" movement) a factor in the administration's policies. The grass-roots movement—which clearly had held the president's feet to the fire, extracting from him commitments to meet with the Soviets and pursue an agreement, making him abandon bellicose and provocative rhetoric—had made gains that its leaders were not prepared to capitalize on to rebuild a dispirited movement. The movement had succeeded as a protest movement but found itself, after the 1984 elections, no closer to changing policy.

The Washington Freeze representatives seemed unprepared to respond to the change in power dynamics. They and other Washington peace leaders reacted to Reagan's reelection by adopting the same posture as the Democratic party. The "lesson"—one the Democrats never examined throughout the Reagan years—was that a president so popular was not to be taken on directly. The movement could have taken credit for the minimal but hard-earned power it had achieved and then used it to launch a new offensive against the administration it so clearly had forced to change. Instead, it retreated even further on its agenda, by pursuing in Congress another symbolic, nonbinding resolution on a warhead test ban. Many in the Washington groups were following the lead of Senator Kennedy, who once again urged them to first pursue the cautious strategy of calling on the president to begin negotiations for a comprehensive test ban as a signal of his newfound commitment to arms control.

Around the same time, Representative Patricia Schroeder introduced legislation in the House that happened to follow more closely the strategy preferred by the Freeze's grass-roots activists: a binding bill that called on the United States and the Soviet Union to simultaneously stop testing, with Congress cutting off U.S. testing funds as long as the Soviets tested no warheads themselves. (This was an independent reciprocal initiative, similarly used by President Kennedy in the early 1960s to obtain the Partial Test Ban Treaty.)

Numerous groups and individuals had travelled to the Soviet Union during the 1984 election season to urge the Soviets to take some concrete, unilateral step. Such a step would force the second-term Reagan administration into delivering on its rhetoric or have that rhetoric exposed as election year posturing. By asking the Soviets to deliver on their rhetoric as well, the peace groups were asking the Soviets to display the seriousness of their commitment. On the August 1985 anniversary of the bombing of Hiroshima, just months after Reagan's inauguration, General Secretary Gorbachev, announced a six-month unilateral, testing moratorium.

The American peace groups were unprepared, however, to push Congress or the administration to move away—as world events seemed to be dictating—from symbolic legislation and toward support of the Schroeder bill, which would have put Reagan and Congress to the test. Passage of that bill would have enabled Congress to legislatively accomplish a test ban in the absence of leadership from the White House. The groups involved in the nonbinding legislation were strongly opposed to the Schroeder bill. Admiral Eugene LaRocque and Jim Bush of the Center for Defense Information advised Schroeder—as did I—to press forward in spite of opposition from groups like Greenpeace, the national Freeze campaign, and Physicians for Social Responsibility. By this time I was advising Schroeder on foreign and military policy issues after managing her 1982 and 1984 congressional races. I was contacted by Chris Paine, Jane Wales, Karen Mulhauser, and others, all asking me to pressure Schroeder into withdrawing her bill because they felt that it went too far. They argued that members of Congress were cautious and skittish on arms control, and that slow, incremental change was the only safe route to success.

But the grass-roots groups rallied behind the Schroeder simultaneous test ban bill and so, finally, did the national groups lobbying in Washington. When the Freeze national conference could not agree to adopt the strategy of civil disobedience at the Nevada Test Site, the American Peace Test—led by some local Freeze organizers and Nevada residents—took shape. The American Peace Test has an ongoing and sophisticated campaign that provided leadership and action on the test ban during this period when the national offices of most peace groups were foundering for direction.[3]

Schroeder's colleagues in Congress also came around eventually because of pressure from their constituents. The National Resources Defense Council had moved quickly on the issue of verification by negotiating separately with the Soviet government to place seismometers in the Soviet Union for independent monitoring of compliance. But another critical ingredient in the first round of successful votes on the legislation was the internal dynamic of Congress as the members returned from the 1986 elections. Les Aspin was facing a tough fight to remain the chair of the House Armed Services Committee. To garner the support he needed, Aspin was looking around for some piece of arms control legislation he could be behind and, fortunately, the test ban bill was it. Aspin, Representative Richard Gephardt, and others rallied behind the legislation, making it into a 1986 Democratic test of Reagan's commitment to arms control and a bargaining chip in the battle for House leadership.

The test ban bill, however, is still being punted around between Congress and the White House. One cannot help but wonder what the bill's fate would have been if the peace groups had been better prepared to push the administration or to take bold action in support of binding legislation in the context of a Soviet unilateral moratorium. The twin fears of pushing Congress and supporting anything the Soviets proposed paralyzed the movement during the very critical months in which this item on the Freeze agenda might have been accomplished, that is, during the Soviet Union's unilateral moratorium on underground testing. The inability of those groups that had promoted an independent step by the Soviets to mobilize timely support for a U.S. response was undoubtedly noted by the Soviets.

The Freeze Campaign Reorganized

In the fall of 1985, Jane Gruenebaum, Kehler's successor as national coordinator for the Freeze, initiated discussions on both the organizational future and the political agenda of the movement. At her initiative, a small group of individuals from the Freeze and SANE came together to address the question of how to sustain the national momentum of the movement in the short run and rejuvenate it in the long run. Cora Weiss (codirector of the Riverside Church Disarmament Program), David Cortright (national director for SANE), and Jane Gruenebaum met in New York to explore the potential for merging two of the largest peace organizations and thereby create a new momentum for the peace movement. The idea of a merger between SANE and the Freeze had been circulating for over a year prior to that meeting.

Gruenebaum had taken over the job of national director at its most difficult moment. There could not have been a riskier, more challenging job. All the frustrations, the disappointments, the longing to regain the momentum and the political dynamism of the first years of the campaign, were hers to assess and respond to. Gruenebaum was inheriting the confusion and all the shortcomings of the Freeze as well as its still latent political strength. She stepped into an almost impossible situation. People were feeling frustrated and were turning their frustrations and anger inward, onto the organization itself. Internal national office conflicts had nearly consumed the organization and had led to divisions within the staff and among the various committee members. The human and social dynamics within the movement were at an all-time low. Jane Gruenebaum resigned eventually, a casualty of the continuing dilemmas within the Freeze.

As the merger discussions gained momentum in 1985 and 1986, the discussion of long-range political and strategy goals was once again postponed. A "unity commission" was established with the goals of developing a long-range strategy as well as proposing and accomplishing the structural merger between the two groups. The commission was made up of SANE and Freeze representatives and a few at-large representatives. It did address long-term strategy in the "credo statement" it outlined. Even though the credo statement was broadly discussed—going through several transformations during the merger process—the commission focused mainly on organizational questions. How would the two organizations merge? What about finances? Who would be in charge? The discussions that were held with local groups in the fall of 1986 also centered on questions about the merger instead of a long-range political strategy and program. The Freeze and SANE voted to merge in December 1986 and January 1987, forming one peace organization with number of individual members and local chapters in the country.

In the spring of 1987, the Reverend William Sloane Coffin was appointed president of the new organization. His appointment indicates that SANE/Freeze is taking seriously the issues of leadership and political autonomy. Coffin brings to the organization a history of personal involvement in the antiwar movement and is a recognized political and moral leader in his capacity as senior minister at the Riverside Baptist Church in New York. But the future political leadership and long-term programs of the new organization are still in the making. Whether it will be able to learn from the past and build on the peace movement's successes—it is too soon to know.

THE POLITICAL IMPERATIVE OF THE NUCLEAR AGE: COMMON SECURITY

The early years of the Freeze and the recent comprehensive test ban campaign point once more to a central conclusion of this book. The Washington representatives of this new, large, grass-roots-based peace community need to adopt a more sophisticated advocacy relationship with the Washington power structure. Lacking this, its hard-earned political currency will be squandered. It is up to the leadership to draw moral and political lines with our friends and foes alike. Only the movement can break out of the conventional wisdom, propose bold initiatives toward an alternative security system based on radically new assumptions, and force decisionmakers to do more than pay eloquent lip service to the movement's goals.

The following operating assumptions are adapted from the Palme Commission Report and might form the core concepts for the development of an alternative security system.[4] The peace movement will need to refine and fight to legitimate ideas such as these, which can form a framework for working on incremental policy objectives. These ideas—and others formed by those in the new peace movement—must challenge the dominant national security discourse and coin specific new language for security.

Definitions of Common Security

1. *All nations have a right to security.*
2. *Military force is not a legitimate instrument for resolving disputes between nations.* Restraint should be the attitude underlying all international relations, not only to acknowledge that others have the right to live in a secure world but also to recognize that in the nuclear age the only real security will come through common action. Only when our enemy is secure will we be secure.
3. *The fundamental lesson of the nuclear age is that no nation can achieve security unilaterally.* The real unilateralists are those who advocate America's right to project military force as a determinant of security. Those who advocate security through military superiority and policies of rollback and confrontation with the Soviet Union widen the real window of vulnerability—the threats of confrontation, war, and escalation to the use of nuclear arms.
4. *Our "national interests" must be redefined so that they are truly in our interest and do not rely on the exploitation of Third World resources.* Dependence on the import and export of raw materials means that the United States cannot insulate itself from reliance on others, nor can smaller nations remain completely independent of the superpowers. Attempting to gain exclusive access to Third World resources through military means embroils us in local conflicts, undermines rather than strengthens our domestic economy, and thwarts the economic growth of developing nations.
5. *The Soviet Union's international role must be realistically assessed.* Until we do so, we will continue to exaggerate the Soviet Union's significance in other parts of the world and will waste our precious national resources on an arms race no one can win. We will continue to divert U.S. scientific talent away from solving our own social and economic problems. Working from distorted images, we will continue to miscalculate the Soviet Union's capacities and intentions and our heavy-handed reactions will continue to lose us friends

and allies around the world. Misreading local conflicts by transforming them into superpower confrontations is one of the easiest ways for a local conflict to escalate into global war.

6. *Each Third World nation has the right to choose its own political and economic course, and we should refrain from using indigenous conflicts as an opening for either Soviet or U.S. intervention.* We must recognize that local conflicts have local solutions, restraining our tendency to turn these conflicts into opportunities for expanding our influence. Using these conflicts for superpower intervention or influence expansion only ends up undermining U.S. and Soviet relations with the people of those regions, to whom the costs of economic and social development—in lives and resources—become exceedingly high.

Both the Soviet Union and the United States compete for political influence in areas such as the Middle East, Europe, and Latin America—exploiting local conflicts for their own purposes and using their own security interests as justification. Local conflicts are thus transformed into U.S.-Soviet confrontations through the imposition of cold war politics, arms sales, and the infusion of military advisors and aid. Local problems rooted in poverty, maldistribution of land, and religious, political, or cultural differences become the "theater" for superpower competition, which forces "resolutions" that intensify the polarization of these situations into East-West alliances. The local origins of the conflicts continue to fester.

7. *Our allies are autonomous, and they should be responsible for defining their own security needs and appropriate vital interests.* In so doing, our allies should be entitled to hold views that differ from ours without fear of economic, military, or political ramifications. Our allies should also shoulder the burden of costs for achieving their security needs. Such reciprocity and joint sharing of responsibility would strengthen rather than undermine alliance relationships.

8. *True security is reached not by amassing weapons but by restoring our social and economic integrity and devoting economic resources to the attainment of that integrity.* To pit increased military spending against maintaining the social and economic progress of our nation erodes the real basis for the security we seek. Massive arms allocations drain fundamental social investment, thus threatening the health of our people and undermining those democratic freedoms we seek to protect.

REBUILDING THE PEACE MOVEMENT

The movement must not only create this security debate, it must also have the organizational capacity to carry through a multifaceted strategy that keeps the mainstream public involved while also engaging elites in the debate over specific policy objectives for this new political program.

Laying the Groundwork

Social movements are invented and can also be planned and implemented. Particularly with the use of new communications technologies, a stronger peace movement can be built in the next fifteen years on the infrastructures of peace organizations, professional groups, and churches that emerged in the heyday of the Freeze. To do this, activists must debate and come to overt agreement about the role and nature of the movement—its structure as well as its program. They must decide whether their commitment to democracy is a means of opting into the political power structure or a way of opting out, that is, using the movement to make a symbolic statement of dissent from the larger political system.[5]

Finally, we must acknowledge the complexity of the issues we work on and the organizing obstacles we face. These recognitions are particularly difficult given the seduction of simple, fundamentalist solutions and explanations. The challenge is compounded by the intractability of policy issues, due to the interrelatedness of social, political, and economic systems and the bureaucratic momentum behind the arms race. Acknowledging these complexities will strengthen our will as we organize for the long haul.

Revamping the Education and Research Strategy

Organizing around alternative security policies requires sophistication as well as a popularized expression of the issues. In the next phase of the disarmament movement, we should build an exceptionally informed and deeply committed core group of local activists who are prepared to take this effort on for the next fifteen–twenty-five years of their lives.

The size, diversity, pluralism, and deep divisions in our society, the schooling most Americans experience, the nature of information systems and news reporting—all point toward the need for an on-going political literacy effort as an integral part of building a social and political force. A comprehensive analysis is not a substitute for thoughtful and strategically planned public debate.

Additionally, ultimate goals must be organized in a successive progression of achievable aims. Each victory must carry within it the seeds of future and more far-reaching changes. We must redefine short-term success and demand measurable progress toward our objectives. Transitional measures are steps toward a comprehensive political shift, which are consistent with that shift. On the other hand, incremental steps are designed to achieve specific policy changes but do not obviously lead toward deeper change.

Blending Local, National, and International Organizing

All politics is by definition local. This new phase of the movement needs to even more sharply articulate its preference for building the influence and power of strong, grass-roots campaigns. This demands, however, the strongest of national staffs and leaders. The more decentralized the organizing base for the movement, the higher a priority must be put on national strategy building and coordination. At the same time, locally based politics can succeed in this country only if it is coordinated with the support of elite opinion. Scientists, academics, church leaders, or other "authority figures" give us "permission" to trust our own instincts and judgment when we hear them legitimizing a concern or a way of thinking about problems normally reserved for "experts," but which we share. These "authority figures" reassure each other as well. In the late 1970s, for example, scientists urged religious leaders to provide moral leadership on issues of science, technology, and the future. Religious leaders were in turn both challenged to provide moral leadership and empowered to address issues of national security that they had avoided for decades. Similarly, when physicians began to organize in 1979 and teach us about the effects of nuclear war, they gave their imprimatur to what antinuclear groups had been arguing since 1974.

Just as the movement must have strategy for organizing both elites and the public, national activists cannot stop their imaginations or their organizing efforts at the borders. We must recognize and take into account the international context of our work. For example, West European peace movements had an enormous impact on U.S. opinion in the early 1980s. That impact could have been intensified by the Freeze if it had orchestrated European voices to overpower the administration's argument that NATO Alliance cohesion was dependent on the deployment of cruise and Pershing II missiles. A more recent example of international movement strategizing is that of church leaders from the Contadora countries asking U.S. religious peace activists to help their Central American counterparts in generating domestic pressure and support for the Contadora process.

Fostering Leadership

We need a "Manhattan Project" for the peace movement. The most influential and experienced national organizers who understand the local, national, and international nature of politics should be recruited and put to work on building a new strategy and political consensus. Good management skills in addition to commitment to democratic principles should be among the first qualifications of our national leaders. Furthermore, the movement needs the visibility and continuity of voice it gains from identifiable and empowered leaders and spokespeople.

The new organization needs to develop a sense of community through a shared sense of mission, a common and explicitly held belief system, and concrete community-building mechanisms such as group health and life insurance, credit unions, and so forth.

Perhaps most importantly, activists must pace and replace themselves. The recognition that the changes the peace movement is working for will not happen in our lifetime should help us organize our lives so that they are full and rich with everything that keeps us human. As we learn to pace ourselves and avoid burnout, we might consciously plan to replace ourselves. Nurturing younger activists might be taken on as a priority of older activists and organizations alike. Youth programs and outreach to college and high school students will keep the movement alive and growing.

Working with Constituencies

This new peace movement should stay out of the business of cynically calculating and packaging constituency strategies as its primary organizing mode. While the peace movement does need to learn how to communicate better with *all* Americans, it is always walking a thin line between having its goals overdramatized and simplistically packaged, on the one hand, and taking a "holier than thou" approach that dares rather than invites people to become involved, on the other hand. A movement that knows what it stands for will attract people of various backgrounds and will eventually reach a mix of ages, races, and classes because of the beliefs it embodies.

Participants should be asked to help shape the peace movement's direction, but in such a way that they can make personal decisions. The organization should be ever mindful of the moral necessity for individual choice and action, which creates a genuine community of shared concern. We all need to feel that we are significant and that we belong to something larger than ourselves. We need a movement that is professionally capable of working toward the goals we hold as individuals.

FROM PROTEST TO POLICY:
RENEWING THE VISION

The Freeze cannot be judged as simply a success or a failure. The story is more complex; like politics, it is that complexity that is important to explore. Social change does not happen according to a blueprint, or in a linear fashion. Rather, it is initiated and advanced in that moment when politics happens. It takes place as the actors involved read the dynamics and move in timely and appropriate ways to make that moment their own.

By taking as critical a look at the Freeze as an insider can, I have tried to point out the strategic and political choices that the movement faces. Some may find me too hard on our political allies. Others may think I have shortchanged the movement itself and am overcritical of so young and gangly an effort as the Freeze. In any case, my intention is to start a discussion about the lessons we must embrace if we are to change the direction of our country's national security policy and not merely stand at the periphery protesting.

As we oppose—and that is our responsibility—we must also propose. It is here that the Freeze broke new ground: proposing a concrete policy alternative that caught the imagination of the public and enticed politicians into paying attention. Holding the attention of both the politicians and the public over the time necessary to bring about change is difficult, but possible. The related challenge is to never stop proposing alternative security policies and to relentlessly claim our right to define what is in our national interest.

The problems explored in this volume remain troublesome. Yet the Freeze movement gave people a taste of its potential to influence policy. In spite of its difficulties with power relations and with maintaining a broad grass-roots base, thousands of people were empowered through participating in the Freeze.

The move from protest to policy was not accomplished in this first phase of the Freeze movement, which fell short of its goal of making a "mutual freeze on the production, testing, and deployment of new nuclear weapons and their delivery systems" into government policy. But given the nearly total integration of the national security state into the social, political, economic, and academic life of the country, and the years of bureaucratic momentum behind the arms race, the Freeze accomplished an enormous amount in just five years. The political accommodations of the president, the international pressure on the administration by U.S. allies, and the education of both the public and congressional leaders are all successes that can be claimed by the Freeze movement.

At this writing, President Reagan has not only met with General Secretary Gorbachev in Iceland, proposing the abolition of nuclear weapons, but he is also on the verge of signing a treaty to ban intermediate-range nuclear missiles from Europe. The INF agreement is a significant step toward disarmament, but it is nonetheless a small step on a very long path. The political implication of the treaty is that conditions may soon be ripe—if the European and American movements are prepared to take advantage of them—for redefining security, reassessing the threats in Europe, and beginning to press for negotiated reductions of conventional forces as well.

The Freeze and antinuclear public opinion are not the only factors leading to these historic opportunities. Significant changes are under way in the Soviet Union. The apparent seriousness with which Gorbachev is pursuing openness in his society and serious peace policies with the United States has global implications. Can the world's peace movements regain momentum and leadership during such periods of progress? Can they encourage the process and pose a consistent challenge to governments both East and West? Meeting these challenges is part of what it means to be more than a protest movement.

At the end of the Second World War, a new international system was constructed out of the chaos and destruction of Europe and Japan. That system may have made some sense in 1945, but it can no longer explain, much less manage, today's interdependent world. But interdependence is only half the picture. The other half is reflected in movements for national independence and in the nonaligned movement. The bipolar world established in the late forties—and the ideologies that have sustained the division of the world into U.S. and Soviet spheres of influence—is breaking apart. But rather than deal with these changing global realities, U.S. foreign policy continues to be based on the transfer of weapons and on building military alliances. Under the Reagan administration, public opposition to war in Central America, for example, was dealt with by privatizing arms sales, to the benefit of arms manufacturers and government officials working out of the White House basement. International law has been broken, the Constitution ignored. Negotiation, diplomacy, and security through economic relations have been all but cast aside.

The nations that come to terms with these new global realities will enter the twenty-first century with opportunity and promise for their children. But governments seem to learn slowly, or not at all, unless social movements force confrontation with new realities. Is the U.S. peace movement up to the task? The peace movement's silence during the Iran-Contra affair and the lack of principled leadership by Democratic leaders on the Hill demonstrate that events themselves will not generate public debate and organized opposition. Too many peace groups have looked for the politically safe standard established by the parties—usually the liberal end of the Democratic party—and have adopted it. But without a comprehensive and coherent political program, that choice is limited to what is "pragmatic and realistic." Washington-generated realism often has little to do with what the rest of the country is ready for. Politicians are afraid of risk. But now it is a question of leadership and, as a nation, we have a crisis in leadership.

That leadership can come from the peace movement, which will indeed move from protest to policy when it models itself after the vision it has for society as a whole.

NOTES

CHAPTER 1: SECURITY PAST AND PRESENT

1. Robert Karl Manhoff, Proceedings of symposium, "The New Cold War and the Assault by the Right" (Cambridge, Mass.: Institute for Peace and International Security, January 31–February 2, 1987).
2. Everett Mendelsohn in discussing disarmament strategies with author, September 1987.
3. E. P. Thompson, letter to the author, January 1986.
4. Professor Philip Morrison states that 100,000–110,000 are at work today in the direct production and manipulation of nuclear weapons compared to 40–50 in 1945. Planning at the federal level—in agencies such as the Departments of Defense and Energy—is focused almost entirely on worst-case scenarios. The National Security Council releases each year the "stockpile paper." This paper assumes an escalating threat from the Soviets and is the blueprint for warheads and special nuclear materials required to build up the nuclear weapons anticipated for five-year periods.
5. Mary Kaldor, Proceedings of symposium, "Demilitarized Regions and the Future of the Alliances" (Cambridge, Mass.: Institute for Peace and International Security, January 31–February 2, 1987).
6. Quoted in Roger Chickering, *Imperial Germany and a World Without War* (Princeton, N.J.: Princeton University Press, 1975), pp. 98–99. Throughout the late nineteenth and early twentieth centuries, the "peace societies" focused peace movement efforts on developing international mechanisms to control conflict and war, such as the International Court of Arbitration.

Political support led to the establishment of the court, the League of Nations, and later, the United Nations. "The secular, humanitarian, and liberal doctrines of the [peace societies in Europe] had begun to predominate over the religious antiwar thinking of most of the Anglo-American groups. And in an era enchanted with science, this liberal opposition to war took on the accents of positivism: the development of a community of nations, linked by economic, cultural and ultimately by political ties, was now characterized as the natural product of social evolution. Although there remained severe philosophical tensions, which surfaced whenever the problem of defensive war was raised, all elements in the peace movement continued to agree on the need for arbitration, and, particularly with the acceleration of the arms race at the turn of the century, on some kind of comprehensive arms agreement" (Chickering, *Imperial Germany*).

7. Ibid.

8. Ruth Sivard, *World Military and Social Expenditures 1986* (Washington, D.C.: World Priorities, 1986), p. 26. *Merchants of Death* (H. C. Engelbrecht and F. C. Hanighen, New York: Dodd and Mead, 1934) exposed the emerging arms industry. The economic and industrial base of the arms race was beginning to be established, alongside the growing technological imperative.

9. Lawrence Wittner, *Rebels Against War* (Philadelphia: Temple University Press, 1984). Wittner argues that the "peace movement appealed perhaps most strongly to women. In the decades following the granting of women's suffrage, politicians kept a wary eye on the peace issue, convinced that it exercised a strong influence over the feminine ballot. A visit by Mrs. Carrie Chapman Catt, who represented the eleven largest women's organizations in the country, occasioned considerable attention and respect from uneasy legislators" (Wittner, *Rebels Against War*, p. 6). The American Friends Service Committee, the Fellowship of Reconciliation, the War Resisters League, and the Women's International League for Peace and Freedom were all founded in this period.

10. Ibid., p. 17.

11. Ibid., p. 16.

12. Peter Goodchild, *J. Robert Oppenheimer: Shatterer of Worlds* (Boston: Houghton Mifflin, 1981), p. 44.

13. Ibid., p. 17. In *The Abandonment of the Jews* (New York: Pantheon, 1984), David S. Wyman writes: "The pervasiveness of anti-Semitism in the United States during the late 1930s and the war years was confirmed by national public-opinion polls. . . . The results indicated that over half the American population perceived Jews as greedy and dishonest and that about one-third considered them overly aggressive . . . Jews were consistently seen as more of a threat than such other groups in the United States as Negroes, Catholics, Germans, or Japanese (except during 1942, when

Japanese and Germans were rated more dangerous). . . . An alarming set of polls taken between 1938 and 1945 revealed that roughly 15 percent of those surveyed would have supported an anti-Jewish campaign. Another 20 to 25 percent indicated that they would have actively opposed it. In sum, then, as much as 35 to 40 percent of the population was prepared to approve an anti-Jewish campaign, some 30 percent would have stood up against it, and the rest would have remained indifferent" (p. 15).

14. E. Berkeley Thompkins, *Anti-Imperialism in the United States: The Great Debate 1890-1920* (Philadelphia: University of Pennsylvania Press, 1972) is a history of early anti-interventionist and antiexpansionist movements and their sources and arguments. This important period in American history and the central political debates of those years illustrate the conflicting principles and views about the U.S. global role from early on. "The anti-imperialists contended not only that the problems of administering a colonial empire were myriad, complicated and often highly distasteful, but also that imperialism, per se, represented a flagrant violation of the fundamental principles upon which the government of the United States was based. They emphasized that the United States had stood as the champion of liberty, democracy, equality and self-government throughout the world and that imperialism, by its very nature, was a denial of the universal validity of these tenets" (p. 2). Anti-imperialist leaders also argued against annexation of Hawaii, the Philippines, and other countries, despite claims of the strategic necessity to the United States. Some in the anti-imperialist movement, however, built racist arguments: either an annexed territory would have to be fully integrated into the political system of the United States—giving those occupied the right to vote—or that very denial of participation would violate basic tenets of American democracy. Knowing that integration into the political system was essential, this anti-imperialist argument appealed to racist sentiments by reminding the public that such integration would give people of color the right to vote.

15. Daniel Yergin, *A Shattered Peace: Origins of the Cold War and the National Security State* (Boston: Houghton Mifflin, 1977), p. 5.

16. Martin J. Sherwin, *A World Destroyed: The Atomic Bomb and the Grand Alliance* (New York: Vintage Books, 1977), pp. 186–192.

17. Adam B. Ulam, *The Rivals: America and Russia Since World War II* (New York: Viking Press, 1971), p. 63.

18. Harry Truman, quoted in David Holloway, *The Soviet Union and the Arms Race* (New Haven, Conn.: Yale University Press, 1983), p. 15.

19. Ibid., pp. 15–28.

20. Yergin, *Shattered Peace*, p. 5.

21. Ibid., p. 10.

22. National Security Council, *Report to the President Pursuant to the President's Directive of January 31, 1950* (Document 68, 7 April 1950. The

declassified version of NSC-68 is available at local libraries in the government documents section.

23. John Lewis Gaddis, *Strategies of Containment: A Critical Appraisal of Postwar American National Security Policy* (London: Oxford University Press, 1982), p. 90.

24. Richard Rubenstein, *The Cunning of History: The Holocaust and the American Future* (New York: Harper/Colophon, 1975), p. x of the Introduction by William Styron.

25. The MIT faculty has recently initiated an exploration of the military's influence on faculty and students and on the long-term implications for the university.

26. Mary Kaldor and Robert Karl Manhoff elaborate on these ideas in "Demilitarized Regions and the Future of the Alliances" and "The New Cold War and Assault by the Right," respectively (Cambridge, Mass.: Institute for Peace and International Security, Spring 1987).

27. NSC-68, pp. 44–48.

28. Paul Walker, "Seizing the Initiative: Independent Reciprocal Initiatives," (American Friends Service Committee and the Fellowship of Reconciliation, 1982).

29. Analyses of NSC-68 can be found in Gaddis, *Strategy of Containment*, and Jerry W. Sanders, *Peddlars of Crisis* (Boston: South End Press, 1983).

30. Luciana Castellini, Italian member of European Parliament, in an address to the END Convention, Evry, France, June 1986.

31. Thomas Merton, *Gandhi on Non-violence* (New York: New Directions, 1964), pp. 7–8.

32. Mary B. Anderson elaborates on human vulnerability and development.

33. Tom Graham, Fellow at the Center for Science and International Affairs at Harvard's Kennedy School of Government, estimates the national security elite to be 10,000 people, with high-level security clearance as the primary indicator. Many in academia who had top secret clearances and were advisors to previous presidents had their clearances cancelled upon Reagan's election.

34. James Skelly, "Power/Knowledge: The Problems of Peace Research and the Peace Movement" (Paper for International Peace Research Association biannual meeting, Sussex, England, April 13–18, 1986), pp. 28–30.

35. A phrase coined by one of the right wing's political architects, Irving Kristol.

CHAPTER 2: NAMING THE PROBLEM

1. Seymour Melman, *The War Economy in the United States* (New York: St. Martin's Press, 1971).

2. Labs Conversion Project workers Steve Ladd, Martha Henderson, Wendy Batson, and others in the Bay Area went on to start the Northern California Freeze Campaign. Steve Ladd served on the national and executive committees and was national cochair of the Freeze from July 1984 to September 1986.

3. The demonstration at Rocky Flats was proposed by the Colorado AFSC and supported by the disarmament program of FOR. FOR's Michael Jendrejczyk had two years earlier spotted the national potential of the Rocky Flats campaign and had asked me to consider when we would call for a national demonstration there. Together, in May of 1977, we proposed to our two organizations and to MOBE that Rocky Flats be the site of a national demonstration.

4. NWFTF was affiliated with MOBE during MOBE's first year. When the groups sponsoring MOBE pulled out of the coalition after the United Nations Special Session (for which it was formed), MOBE became yet another organization. NWFTF remained as a network supported by AFSC and FOR, working with a wide range of groups from the peace and environmental movements, including MOBE as a separate organization. Its ad hoc nature also allowed it to remain free of the constraints likely to come from affiliation with any single organization.

5. Sam Day, ed., *Makers of the Nuclear Holocaust* (AFSC/FOR Nuclear Weapons Project, 1980).

6. See note 4 above.

7. This is one of the reasons that the merger between SANE and the Freeze is both historically interesting and a promising sign. Peace opinion has always been small in the United States, able to influence the debate far beyond its numbers. It has done so when it focuses its resources and emphasizes personal and organizational cooperation and collaboration. The merger between these two groups could signal a forthcoming burst of political activity.

8. Estimates of the number of atomic veterans range from 250,000 to 400,000.

9. U.S., Congress, *Joint Hearing before the Subcommittee on Oversight and Investigation of the Committee on Interstate and Foreign Commerce, House of Representatives, and the Health and Scientific Research Subcommittee of the Labor and Human Resources Committee and the Committee on the Judiciary, U.S. Senate*, 96th Cong., 1st sess., 1979, p. 151.

10. The Environmental Policy Institute is one of the best informed resources on the status of radiation victims. For further information, contact them at 218 D Street, S.E., Washington, D.C. 20003, 202-544-2600. Local groups got support not only from the Environmental Policy Institute but also from AFSC, FOR, the Natural Resources Defense Council, the Envi-

ronmental Defense Fund, and the Union of Concerned Scientists. UCS was at that time primarily focused on nuclear power.

11. PSR was originally founded in 1961 to educate physicians and the public about the medical consequences of nuclear weapons and nuclear war.

12. Organizing within AAAS was initiated by NWFTF, working jointly with Harvard and MIT faculty members, including Jonathan King, Everett Mendelsohn, Bernard Feld, Philip Morrison, Joseph Weizenbaum, and the AAAS president, Kenneth Boulding of the University of Colorado.

13. A shareholder resolution requesting that Monsanto withdraw its contracts with the Department of Energy was filed in 1985. On 6 November 1986, Monsanto announced that it would not renew its contract with the DOE for the production of non-nuclear electrical parts for nuclear weapons. This contract will expire on 30 September 1988. For further information on initiatives involving corporate divestment from the production of weapons, contact Valerie Heinonon at the Interfaith Center on Corporate Responsibility, 475 Riverside Drive, Room 566, New York, NY 10115, 212-870-2293. Also involved in efforts to stop nuclear weapons production is INFACT, 256 Hanover Street, Boston, MA 02113, 617-742-4583.

14. Thomas L. Perry and Dr. James G. Foulks, ed., *End the Arms Race: Fund Human Needs*, Proceedings of the 1986 Vancouver Centennial Peace and Disarmament Symposium (Seattle: University of Washington Press, 1986).

15. The early committee involved Harvard's president, James B. Conant; the academic-military relationship was already in place in the early cold war years. The fifties' committee supported NSC-68: the United States needed to continue a military buildup to maintain its position of world dominance.

16. Max M. Kampelman, *Alerting America: The Papers of the Committee on the Present Danger* (Washington, D.C.: Pergamon-Brassey's 1984), p. xv.

17. Memo from Freeze National Clearinghouse to referendum campaign coordinators, 20 October 1982. ASC had been formed in Chicago in 1955. While it was originally founded as "a personnel security and investigation consulting firm," it soon "sought to become a broad-based political lobby for defense-oriented corporations." (*Interchange*, Anti-Freeze File Report No. 2, 20 January 1983.) In 1964 the American Conservative Union (ACU) was founded. By 1982 it was one of the largest conservative political lobbies, claiming "more than 325,000 supporters and contributions totalling [in 1979] $3.1 million." Before tackling the Freeze movement, ACU had "led the fight against ratification of the Panama Canal treaty and the SALT agreements." (*Interchange*, ACU Profile, 9 December 1982.)

18. For more on the acknowledgment of these limits, particularly in the Trilateral Commission, see Holly Sklar, ed., *Trilateralism* (Boston: South End Press, 1980).

19. Paul Walker, *MX: A Threat to American Security* (Cambridge, Mass.: Union of Concerned Scientists, 1980) and Gordon Thompson, *The Deadly Footprint* (Cambridge, Mass.: Union of Concerned Scientists, 1980).

20. For more details, see Ward Sinclair, "Church Perceived as Apostate Fearful of Election Disaster," *Washington Post*, 12 October 1979.

21. Jane Sharp analyzes the permutations in Allied positions on the U.S. negotiating posture and the relationship with the Soviet Union. She concludes that the Allies fear being abandoned when the United States moves too far in the direction of détente; then they press for evidence of the U.S. security guarantee. When the United States becomes more hostile and bellicose in relation to the Soviets, the Allies fear confrontation and press the United States to renew ties and commit to negotiations. And the cycle continues. Jane Sharp, "Belief Systems and Arms Control Possibilities," Australia National University Peace Research Center, Working Paper No. 12, September 1986.

22. For instance, FOR opposed SALT II for doing too little on arms control. AFSC, on the other hand, supported SALT II and urged that ratification be followed by other steps toward disarmament.

23. Robert Leavitt, "Freezing the Arms Race: The Genesis of a Mass Movement" (Kennedy School of Government Case Program, C14-83-557, 1983), p. 10.

24. Barnet reiterated the proposal in "A Way to End the Arms Race," *Washington Post*, 9 September 1979. The freeze idea was first proposed by Gerard Smith, U.S. negotiator in the Johnson administration, in the early 1970s.

25. The Boston Study Group went on to publish *The Price of Defense: A New Strategy for Military Spending* (New York: Times Books, 1979).

26. Leavitt, "Freezing the Arms Race," p. 18.

27. Groups represented at that first meeting were AFSC, CALC, FOR, IDDS, the Institute for Policy Studies (IPS), and Sojourners.

28. FOR, memo to Nyack, New York consultation participants, 20 February 1980.

29. Jerome Grossman, quoted in Leavitt, "Freezing the Arms Race," p. 18.

30. Leavitt, "Freezing the Arms Race," p. 17.

31. Elizabeth Drew, "A Reporter in Washington, D.C.," *New Yorker* 3 May 1982.

CHAPTER 3: TO THE VILLAGE SQUARE

1. Paulo Freire, *Pedagogy of the Oppressed*, trans. Myra Bergman Ramos (New York: Seabury Press, 1970).

2. George Sommaripa and Randall Forsberg, "Strategy for a Concerted National Effort to Halt the Nuclear Arms Race," first draft, 25 August 1980, p. 2.

3. Ibid., pp. 8–9.

4. Ibid., pp. 6–7.

5. "Strategy for a Concerted National Effort to Halt the Nuclear Arms Race," internal Freeze document.

6. Members of the strategy committee were Terry Provance, Patsy Leake, Marta Daniels, and Frances Crowe from AFSC; Pam Solo, Mike Jendrzejczyk from AFSC/FOR; George Sommaripa of the Boston Study Group; Carol Jensen from CALC; Mark Shanahan from the Coalition for a New Foreign and Military Policy; Randy Forsberg from IDDS; Bob Moore from MOBE; Marty Bartlett from Peacemakers Fellowship; Randy Kehler from the Traprock Peace Center; and Jonathan Fine.

7. Bruce Cronin, quoted in Leavitt, "Freezing the Arms Race," p. 26.

8. Randy Kehler, interview with author, Amherst, Mass., 23 September 1984.

9. To ensure that there would be representation from various parts of the country, regional caucuses were formed; each designated an interim representative to the national committee.

10. The initial task forces were International, Media, Fund-raising, Nominations, Government Relations, Resources, National Events, and Minority. Barbara Roche and Pam McIntyre (St. Louis staff for the Freeze campaign), interview with Deborah Mapes, 17 December 1985.

11. As ESR has grown, so has its organizational goals. It now promotes the teaching of controversial issues in the classroom and, in particular, places a heavy emphasis on U.S.-Soviet relations.

12. For information about peace studies programs at colleges and universities, consult Deborah Mapes, Peter Steven, Elizabeth Bernstein, et al., eds., *Peace Resource Book: A Comprehensive Guide to Issues, Groups, and Literature 1986* (Cambridge, Mass.: Ballinger, 1986) or Barbara Wein, ed., *Peace & World Order Studies: A Curriculum Guide* (New York: World Policy Institute, 1984).

13. Robert Scheer, "Pentagon Plan Aims at Winning Nuclear War," *Los Angeles Times*, 15 August 1982.

14. Carlucci and Lehman made these remarks before the Senate Armed Services Committee on 13 January 1981 and 5 February 1981, respectively. Wade was speaking before the House Appropriations Subcommittee on 15 September 1981, and Weinberger's comment was elicited at a 27 July 1981 press conference. The Center for Defense Information compiled a 21 March 1982 report, from which these quotations are taken, entitled "Recent Reagan Administration References To Nuclear Warfighting and Winning."

15. T. K. Jones, quoted in Robert Scheer, "Civil Defense Program to Be Revived," *Los Angeles Times*, 15 January 1982.

16. Douglas Waller, *Congress and the Nuclear Freeze: An Inside Look at the Politics of a Mass Movement* (Amherst, Mass.: University of Massachusetts Press, 1987), p. 47.

17. Peter Franchot, quoted in Ibid., p. 47.

18. Ibid., p. 49.

19. Ibid., pp. 52–54.

20. Bob Sherman, quoted in Ibid., p. 48.

21. David Doerge, quoted in Ibid., p. 51.

22. Randy Kehler, interview with author, Amherst, Mass., 23 September 1986.

23. Ibid.

24. Randall Forsberg, interview with author, Brookline, Mass., 30 September 1986.

25. James Reston, "Reagan's Forgotten Issue," *New York Times*, 23 March 1982.

26. Secretary of State Alexander Haig, Jr., told a Senate appropriations subcommittee, "This is not only bad defense policy, but it is a bad arms control policy as well."

27. Judith Miller, "58 Senators Back Alternative Plan on Nuclear Arms," *New York Times*, 31 March 1982.

28. "Several authorities in the field, including former undersecretary of State George Ball and Herbert Scoville, former top level official with the CIA and the US ACDA, rejected [administration criticisms of the freeze] in testimony on the Hill. . . . Scoville said the 'window of vulnerability' that Reagan wants to close, primarily with the MX, was a 'figment of some imaginative minds.' Ball added that 'each side already possesses such a massive amount of overkill that a numerical parity in warheads or throw weight or even qualitative advantage loses much of its relevance.'" Benjamin Taylor," Nuclear Arms-Freeze Push Gains Support in Congress," *Boston Globe*, 28 March 1982.

29. Elizabeth Drew, "A Reporter in Washington, D.C.," *New Yorker*, May 1982, p. 138.

30. By late April, several other arms control measures had been introduced in the Senate. Senators John Glenn of Ohio and Joseph Biden of Delaware introduced resolutions aimed at reviving SALT II; others used the threat of SALT II Treaty ratification as a means of pushing Reagan to the negotiating table. Senator Gary Hart circulated a "Dear Colleague" letter "urging ratification of the treaty unless the Administration began talks with Moscow by July 1."

31. Leslie Gelb, "U.S. Forging a New Concept for Curbing Strategic Arms," *New York Times*, 2 May 1982.

CHAPTER 4: SUSTAINING THE MOVEMENT

1. Robert Reinhold, "Scientists Urge More Effort to Cut Atom Risk," *New York Times*, 28 April 1982.
2. Randy Kehler, "The Real Mandate," a Freeze Campaign press statement, Fall 1982.
3. ABC News/Washington Post poll, taken 21–25 April 1982.
4. For a bibliography of publications on arms and disarmament, Bernstein, Elias, Forsberg, et al., eds., *Peace Resource Book*, "Guide to Peace-Related Literature."
5. Editorial, "Ferocious Mr. Reagan and the Freeze," *New York Times*, 16 March 1982.
6. Roger Molander, quoted in Judith Miller, "Effort to Freeze Nuclear Arsenals Spreads in U.S.," *New York Times*, 15 March 1982.
7. Eugene Rostow, "Memorandum for the Assistant to the President for National Security Affairs," *Washington Post*, 9 May 1982.
8. Sid Lens, memo to all projects and staff regarding Reagan's disarm-rearm proposal, 13 May 1982. NSC-68 reads as follows on the issue of negotiations: "The Soviet Union possesses several advantages over the free world in negotiations on any issue: It can and does enforce secrecy . . . allowing it to know more about the free world than the free world knows about its positions. . . . It does not have to be responsive to public opinion, it does not have to consult and get agreement from other countries, it can influence public opinion in other countries while insulating the peoples under its control."

    NSC-68 goes on to state that these advantages, combined with unfavorable trends in "our power position . . . militate against successful negotiation of a general settlement. . . . For although the U.S. probably now possesses . . . a force, principally in atomic weapons, adequate to deliver a powerful blow upon the Soviet Union and to open the road to victory in a long war, it is not sufficient by itself to advance the position of the United States in the cold war. . . . In short, it is impossible to hope that an effective plan for international control can be negotiated unless and until the Kremlin design has been frustrated to a point at which a genuine and drastic change in Soviet policies has taken place" (pp. 44–45).
9. The 12 June rally organizing committee in New York and in Boston was often bitterly divided. The committee included a fairly wide spectrum of groups: from those with left, sectarian politics to those representing the Freeze campaign, who in this context were viewed as the moderate or centrist part of the coalition. Heated disputes threatened to crack the coalition apart. Finally, the Reverend William Sloane Coffin and others were able to facilitate an agreement more or less acceptable to all forces.
10. *Interchange*, anti-Freeze file, report no. 2, 20 January 1983, and *Interchange*, memo on anti-Freeze initiatives, 9 December 1982.

11. Frank Donner, "The Campaign to Smear the Nuclear Freeze Movement," *Nation*, 6 November 1982, pp. 456–465.

12. John Barron, "The KGB's Magical War for 'Peace,'" *Reader's Digest* (October 1982). John Barron is also the author of the book on *KGB: The Secret Work of Soviet Secret Agents* (New York: Reader's Digest Press, 1983).

13. John Rees, "How the Left Is Manipulating the U.S. Nuclear 'Freeze Movement,'" *Human Events*, April 1982.

14. Donner, "Campaign to Smear," p. 458.

15. State Department, "World Peace Council: Instrument of Soviet Foreign Policy," Foreign Affairs Note, April 1982.

16. Vladimir Bukovsky, "The Peace Movement and the Soviet Union," *Commentary* (May 1982): 32, 36.

17. "Moscow and the Peace Offensive," Heritage Foundation "Backgrounder," May 1982.

18. Donner, "Campaign to Smear," p. 464.

19. Frank Chapple, "Masters of Manipulation," *Reader's Digest*, June 1982, p. 68.

20. Donner, "Campaign to Smear," p. 464.

21. Dorothy Rabinowitz, "The Building Blocks of the Freeze Movement," *Wall Street Journal*, 10 June 1982, p. 30, and Rael Jean and Erich Isaac, "The Counterfeit Peacemakers: Atomic Freeze," *American Spectator* 15, no. 6 (June 1982).

22. Donner, "Campaign to Smear," p. 460.

23. Rabinowitz, "The Building Blocks."

24. David McReynolds, quoted in Donner, "Campaign to Smear," p. 460.

25. State Department "Soviet Active Measures: An Update," Special Report No. 101, July 1982.

26. Donner, "Campaign to Smear," p. 465.

27. Jeremiah Denton, the Senator from Alabama, was then the head of the Security and Terrorism Subcommittee of the Senate Judiciary Committee.

28. Donner, "Campaign to Smear."

29. Barron, "KGB's Magical War," p. 211.

30. Editorial, "Hot Words for the Freeze," *Washington Post*, 6 October 1982.

31. Editorial, "Indecent Debate," *New York Times*, 6 October 1982. The CIA would later admit "in a statement filed in connection with the settlement of a Freedom of Information Act lawsuit that it had been using journalists not only to gather information but also to promote and disseminate CIA-inspired or -produced stories in support of U.S. foreign policy" (Donner, "Campaign to Smear," p. 463).

32. Donner, "Campaign to Smear," p. 458.

33. Robert McCloskey, "The Editorials on the Peace Groups," *Washington Post*, 12 October 1982, p. A12. McCloskey's article comments on the editorial, "The Peace Groups," from the *Washington Post*, 9 October 1982, p. A18.

34. Jon Sawyer, "Reagan Moves to Blunt Nuclear Freeze Drive," *St. Louis Post-Dispatch*, 17 October 1982, pp. 1, 5.

35. Ibid., p. 5.

36. Cited in Sawyer, "Reagan Moves to Blunt Drive," p. 5.

37. Ibid.

38. Rael Jean Issac, "Do You Know Where Your Church Offerings Go?" *Reader's Digest*, January 1983.

39. "Communism, the Churches and the Peace Movement: A Response by the Fellowship of Reconciliation," Fellowship of Reconciliation, February 1983.

40. Judith Miller, "Effort to Freeze Nuclear Arsenals Spreads in U.S.," *New York Times*, 15 March 1982.

41. Randy Forsberg, interview with author, Brookline, Mass., 30 September 1986.

42. Randy Kehler, interview with author, Peace Development Fund, Amherst, Mass., 23 September 1986.

43. Steve Waldman, "The Hiroshima Hustle," *Washington Monthly* (October 1986): 35.

44. Ibid., pp. 35–36.

45. Ibid., p. 38.

46. Patrick H. Caddell, quoted in David B. Richardson, "What's Next for the Nuclear Freeze Movement?" *U.S. News and World Report*, 21 June 1982, p. 24.

47. Adam Clymer, "Democrats Cheer Call for Freeze on Nuclear Arms," *New York Times*, 25 June 1982.

48. Matt Reese, quoted in Adam Clymer, "The Nuclear Freeze: Politicians Unsure of Its Influence," *New York Times*, 6 July 1982.

49. Peter Hart, quoted in Clymer, "Politicians Unsure."

50. Ibid.

51. Ibid.

52. An attempt to counter this trivialization was made in Jeremy Stone and Herbert F. York's editorial, "The Freeze is Not a Joke" (*Washington Post*, 19 March 1982). "The freeze has been proposed every six years for two decades. In 1964, at Geneva, President Johnson proposed a verified freeze on the number and characteristics of strategic nuclear offensive and defensive vehicles. In 1970, the Senate passed a resolution, by a vote of 73 to 6, calling for 'an immediate suspension . . . of the further deployment of all offensive and defensive nuclear strategic weapons' at a time when, we now know the director of the Arms Control Agency, Gerard C. Smith, was urging President Nixon to consider the same proposal to 'stop where we are.' In 1976, candidate Jimmy Carter made this proposal."

CHAPTER 5: EXTERNAL AND INTERNAL CONFRONTATION

1. By mid-December 1982, Soviet SS-20s numbered 245 in Europe and 100 in Asia.

2. There had been a shake-up in the U.S. negotiating team when Reagan fired Eugene Rostow as head of the Arms Control and Disarmament Agency in early January 1983. He was replaced by Kenneth Adelman. Paul Nitze was chief negotiator for the INF talks.

3. For example, meetings would be convened by KADEA—one of the large Greek peace movements—in Athens, for the purpose of dialogue with Communist bloc and Soviet peace committees.

4. Provance and the task force coordinated the 1982–83 work at the U.N. Their efforts resulted in the U.N. votes for a freeze. On 23 November 1982, the First Committee of the U.N. General Assembly voted for both a U.S.-Soviet freeze on testing, production, and deployment of nuclear weapons and a similar freeze by all countries with nuclear weapons. Three weeks later, the General Assembly voted 122–16 in favor of a freeze.

5. Grass-roots organizers, however, instinctively moved on the issue of U.S.-Soviet relations. For example, trips to the Soviet Union by churches local groups, "twinning" with Soviet cities, and coordinated youth programs were numerous during this same period.

6. "Bilateral accords are widely viewed as the hard-headed practical means to end the arms spiral. In fact, bilateralism is naive, ignorant, or cynical about the institutional momentum behind the nuclear build-up. Unilateral initiatives are dismissed as either naive or treasonous: in fact they are a realistic way to counter the inertia of destruction. They may be our only hope. If the movement can impart this truth, it will have served a profound historic mission." (Bob Borosage, "The Bilateral Box," *Working Papers* [May/June 1983] : 40).

7. Some of the European peace movement representatives were Ulrich Albrecht, Mary Kaldor, Mient Jan Faber, Wim Bartels, Andreas Zumach, Johann Galtung, Meg Beresford.

8. Waller, *Congress and the Freeze*, pp. 166–167.

9. Haynes Johnson, "A Preacher for 'Peace Through Strength' or, Maybe, the Bomb," *Washington Post*, 3 April 1983.

10. As quoted in Leslie Maitland, "FBI Rules Out Russian Control of Freeze Drive," *New York Times*, 26 March 1983.

11. George C. Wilson, "Reagan Reportedly Ready to Accuse Soviets," *Washington Post*, 16 April 1983.

12. Lou Cannon and Walter Pincus, "Reagan Rejects, for Now, Advice to Discuss Soviet Arms Breaches," *Washington Post*, 22 April 1983.

13. In its typical fashion, the Connecticut Freeze campaign soon produced an in-depth publication on Soviet treaty compliance. Throughout the life of the Freeze, the Connecticut campaign frequently provided well-researched and substantive information for the movement.

14. Elizabeth Drew, "A Political Journal," *New Yorker*, 20 June 1983, pp. 48–49.

15. In January 1983, the bipartisan Scowcroft Commission replaced the Townes Commission, which had been charged in May 1982 to study the idea of a closely spaced basing system for the MX, known as "densepack."

16. Drew, "Political Journal," p. 46.

17. Paul A. Walker and John A. Wentworth, "Midgetman: Missile in Search of a Mission," *Bulletin of Atomic Scientists* vol. 42, no. 42 (November 1986): 20–26.

18. Les Aspin, as quoted in Drew, "Political Journal," p. 55.

19. Ibid., p. 56.

20. Ibid., p. 69.

21. Christopher Lasch, *The Minimal Self: Psychic Survival in Troubled Times* (New York: W.W. Norton, 1984), p. 78.

22. "In 1960, Herman Kahn was one of the first to maintain that the United States could make preparations that would insure not merely the physical survival of the population—or a significant fraction of it—but the material and cultural resources necessary to rebuild the American way of life. Today this kind of thinking—which goes beyond deterrence and seeks to assure victory in a nuclear exchange—appears to have become official U.S. policy. In this view, the survivors will envy the dead only if Americans persist in the "misguided" belief that a nuclear war is unthinkable and that their efforts should therefore be directed toward preventing war instead of surviving it." Herman Kahn is author of *Thinking the Unthinkable* and has been a well-known nuclear weapons strategist since the beginning of the post-World War II era. Lasch, *The Minimal Self*, p. 80.

23. Carol Nadelson, M.D., in an unpublished paper. Dr. Nadelson is the former president of the American Psychiatric Association; she is now professor and the vicechairman of the Department of Psychiatry at Tufts University.

24. Robert Coles, "Freezeniks Are Elitists," *Washington Post*, 11 November 1984.

25. Ibid., p. D4.

26. Ibid., p. D4.

27. Ibid., p. D4. Coles borrows the phrase "mathematical certainty" from Caldicott, who said in a 1981 speech to a Harvard Phi Beta Kappa gathering, "If Ronald Reagan is reelected, accidental nuclear war becomes a mathematical certainty."

28. Randy Kehler, interview with author, held at Peace Development Fund, Amherst, Mass., on 25 November, 1986.

29. Randy Kehler, quoted in summary of the Freeze movement's meeting at Blue Mountain Center, New York, 13–16 May 1982, p. 7.

30. The Freeze launched a campaign to raise expectations for Reagan's performance at the 19 November 1985 Geneva summit meeting. One million signatures were gathered and delivered by SANE leaders to Mikhail Gorbachev. Reagan ignored the campaign.

31. Collaborative Change Associates, "Reflections on the Freeze Campaign Organization," October 1983.

CHAPTER 6: 1984

1. Editorial, "Evil Empire . . . Come in, Evil Empire," *New York Times*, 17 January 1984.

 2. Project '84 Task Force, "Targeting Work Group Report," presented to Freeze National Committee June 1983.

 3. Project '84 Task Force, "Draft Plan for Project '84," presented to Freeze National Committee June 1983.

 4. Randall Forsberg, President, Freeze Voter '84, letter to all Democratic candidates, 2 March 1984.

 5. Jim Matlack, AFSC Washington, D.C. office, memo to Asia Bennett, Joe Volk, et al. re meeting with Walter Mondale, 23 January 1984.

 6. Friends of Gary Hart, Advertisement, *New York Times*, 18 March 1984.

 7. Walter Mondale, speech to the Chicago Council on Foreign Relations, 14 March 1984.

 8. Fox Butterfield, "Mondale and Hart Trade Sharpest Words Yet, Over Arms Control," *New York Times*, 5 March 1984.

 9. "Draft Plank for Democratic Party Platform on Nuclear Arms Control," submitted to the Democratic party's platform committee and to the delegates to the 1984 Democratic National Convention, prepared at the request of Senator Alan Cranston by a special drafting committee chaired by Jerome Wiesner, MIT President Emeritus.

10. Karen Mulhauser, quoted in Betsy Taylor, "'If We Can't Change the Politicians' Mind . . . Let's Change the Politicians!': An Analysis of Six Peace PACs and Their Political Impact in 1984," unpublished report prepared by Taylor while a student at the John F. Kennedy School of Government, August 1985, p. 11.

11. Polling statistics and budget information as cited by Representative Patricia Schroeder, "The Fate of Women's Issues Under the Reagan Administration," speech before the Women's Health Services Tenth Anniversary Dinner, 22 April 1983.

12. *New York Times* poll conducted 11–20 November 1983, published 27 November 1983. Excluding Alaska and Hawaii, 1309 adults around the country asked, "Do you think Ronald Reagan has performed his job as Presi-

dent well enough to deserve re-election, or do you think it's time to give a new person a chance to do better?"

13. Project '84 Task Force, "Targeting Work Group Report."

14. Ibid.

15. Robert Karl Manhoff, speech before the Institute for Peace and International Security Conference on Generating the New Security Debate, 1 February 1987.

16. "Reagan Goes on the Attack," *Newsweek*, 16 April 1984.

17. Jay Wink, "Defense Policy for Democrats," *New York Times*, 20 June 1984, p. 27.

18. David Rosenbaum, "Poll Shows Many Choose Reagan Even if They Disagree with Him," *New York Times*, 19 September 1984.

19. Russell Watson et al., "Arms Control at the Crossroads," *Newsweek*, 1 October 1984.

20. Adam Clymer, "Americans in Poll View Government More Confidently," *New York Times*, 19 November 1984.

21. Actual figure: $1,490,549, based on FEC reports for 1983 and 1984.

22. Based on FEC reports for 1983 and 1984, as cited in Taylor, "'If We Can't Change the Politicians' Mind . . . ,'" p. 3.

CHAPTER 7: THE HOPE IS IN THE ACTION

1. The Campaign for Mutual Security was a program proposed by the Detroit Freeze. It drew on themes from Common Security but emphasized bilateral security concerns, for which it was criticized.

2. See Melinda Fine, Jennifer Leaning, Everett Mendelsohn, and Pam Solo, "The Future in Our Hands: A Call to Common Security," in *The Deadly Connection: Nuclear War and U.S. Intervention*, ed. Joseph Gerson (Philadelphia: New Society Publishers, 1985).

3. The work around the comprehensive test ban was led primarily by the grass-roots organizers who formed the American Peace Test (APT). APT worked congenially with the Freeze campaign even though the Freeze had formally rejected civil disobedience as a tactic. When the time had come to escalate demands, these organizers had simply formed a new organization with the flexibility to act. APT was invaluable in keeping the grass-roots network energized and focused during 1985–86. Once again, however, no consistent voice and political representative emerged to whom the press could immediately turn for response as news developed.

4. Published as *Common Security: A Program for Disarmament*, Report of the International Commission on Disarmament and Security Issues, Olaf Palme, Chair (London: Pan Books, 1982). See also Joseph Gerson, ed., *The Deadly Connection: Nuclear War and U.S. Intervention* (Philadelphia,

New Society Publishers, 1985), and Fine, Leaning, Mendelsohn, and Solo, "The Future in Our Hands."

5. I am grateful to Professor Naomi Chazan for her help in articulating this strain in peace movement cultures, which, judging from our discussions and from my experience with movements around the world, may not be peculiar to only the United States but may be a problem for Peace Now in Israel and for European peace movements as well.

INDEX

ABOUT THE AUTHOR

Pam Solo is co-director of the Institute for Peace and International Security in Cambridge, Massachusetts. As a political organizer and movement strategist, she is the former national coordinator for disarmament programs for the American Friends Service Committee; a founder and organizer of the Rocky Flats campaign in Colorado; and coordinator of the Nuclear Weapons Facilities Task Force, a nationwide network of campaigns focused on nuclear weapons production, testing, and deployment sites.

She helped found the Nuclear Weapons Freeze campaign, served as chair of the Strategy Committee, and coordinated the Freeze's development of Freeze Voter, and served on its founding board. In addition to local and national organizing, Solo has organized and coordinated international efforts for the Freeze, particularly in Europe. In 1985 she organized the Women Parliamentarians for Peace, working with Ambassador Maj Britt Theorin and Congresswoman Pat Schroeder.

Pam Solo was the 1985–86 Peace Fellow at the Mary Ingraham Bunting Institute, Radcliffe College; an adjunct research fellow at the Center for Science and International Affairs, Kennedy School of Government in 1985–87; and a visiting scholar at Radcliffe College in 1986–88.